MACROMOLECULES AND BEHAVIOUR

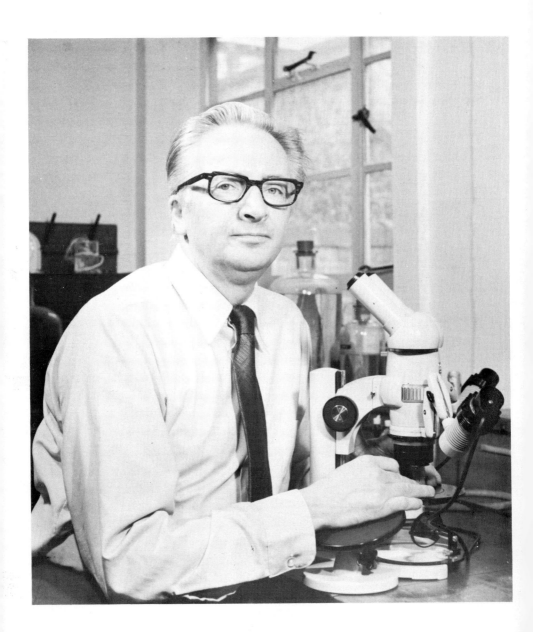

Professor Holger Hydèn

MACROMOLECULES AND BEHAVIOR

Lectures and Proceedings of the International Symposium held at the University of Birmingham Medical School in March 1971 to mark the visit of its first Arthur Thomson Visiting Professor, Professor Holger Hydén of the University of Göteborg.

Edited by G. B. Ansell and P. B. Bradley
University of Birmingham Medical School

UNIVERSITY PARK PRESS
Baltimore · London · Tokyo

© 1, 2 and 3. H. Hydén
© 4. E. Glassman and J. E. Wilson
© 5. S. P. R. Rose, P. P. G. Bateson and G. Horn
© 6. D. A. Booth
© 7. G. W. O. Oliver
© 8. J. T. Rick
© 9. W. Agranoff
© 10. G. Ungar
© 11. P. Mandel, R. Di Carlo, S. Simler and H. Randrianarisoa
© 12. G. Raisman
© 13. T. V. P. Bliss, A. R. Gardner-Medwin and T. Lømo
© 14. G. Adam
© 15. M. Berry, T. Hollingworth, R. Flinn and E. M. Anderson
© 16. G. A. Kerkut, P. Emson and R. J. Walker

All rights reserved. No part of this book may be reproduced or transmitted, in any form or by any means, without permission.

First published 1973 by
THE MACMILLAN PRESS LTD
London and Basingstoke
Associated companies in New York Toronto
Dublin Melbourne Johannesburg and Madras

SBN 333 13471 0

Published in North America by
UNIVERSITY PARK PRESS
1973
Printed in Great Britain

Library of Congress Cataloging in Publication Data

Main entry under title:

Macromolecules and behavior

1. Brain chemistry—Congresses. 2. Psychology, Physiological—Congresses. I. Ansell, Gordon Brian, ed. II. Bradley, P. B., ed. III. Birmingham, Eng. University. Faculty of Medicine.
QP376.M19   591.1'88   73-388
ISBN 0-8391-1022-7

Preface

This book is an attempt to place on permanent record some of the activities which took place in the Birmingham University Medical School during March 1971, on the occasion of the visit of the First Arthur Thomson Visiting Professor. How the Visiting Professorship came into existence is described by the Dean in his Introduction. The Visiting Professor had been nominated by the Faculty and when Professor Hydén accepted the invitation an Organising Committee was set up with representatives from each of the interested departments in the Faculty. This Committee was given the task of arranging the scientific programme for the visit, as well as the social programme, publicity, etc. and responsibility for the budget.

It was decided that the Visiting Professor should be asked to give three formal lectures in which to review his field of work, and which would be open to all. These are the 'Arthur Thomson Lectures' which form the three chapters in Part I of the book. The chapter headings correspond to the Lecture titles and the illustrations are largely taken from the slides used by the Lecturer. Each Lecture was followed the next day by an Advanced Seminar on the same topic before a smaller group of people and where questions were asked and a more active discussion took place. Unfortunately, it was not possible to record these seminars or the discussions for the purpose of publication. The fact that these seminars attracted visitors from a considerable distance and usually exceeded their allotted time was an indication of the interest which they, and the Lectures, aroused. There were also two live demonstrations. At the first of these Professor Hydén dissected out single neurones and their surrounding glia from the Deiters' nucleus of fresh rabbit brain, then removed the glia and cut open the neuronal perikaryon, no mean feat in a lecture theatre. The second demonstration was a beautifully presented photographic display of the methods used in his laboratory for the analysis of tritium-labelled proteins separated from a single cell.

The remainder of the time was occupied with visits to various departments in the Medical School and University where our Visiting Professor had the opportunity to talk to smaller groups and see something of their work. That some at least of this interchange was two-way is evidenced by the fact that we understand that Professor Hydén is now using a behavioural test on his animals which was developed in Birmingham and which he first learned about during his visit.

The original plan for the Arthur Thomson Visiting Professorship envisaged an International Symposium on a topic related to his field of interest. It seemed appropriate therefore for this Symposium, which took place during the last two days of the visit, to be entitled 'Macromolecules and Behaviour' and this was also chosen as the title for this book. The Symposium was attended by participants from the United States, France and Hungary as well as the United Kingdom. The papers presented, together with some of the discussion which ensued, form Part II of the book.

A number of those participating in the Symposium would consider biochemistry to be their primary discipline, and this reflects the growing interest of biochemists in the relationship between chemical processes and function in the nervous system. Conversely, it is apparent that more behavioural scientists are turning to other disciplines such as brain chemistry and neurophysiology in attempts to explain their observations. The increasing sophistication in biochemical techniques and meaningful co-operation with behavioural scientists has led to findings of considerable interest, some of which are described in this book. It is nevertheless apparent that the enthusiasm of a decade ago, when some investigators were hopeful of finding molecules which behaved like tapes in the world's largest tape recorder, have now been tempered. The neurochemical equivalent of the Holy Grail will not be found easily and those entering the field might recall the words of Alexander Pope*:

> "In vain the Sage with retrospective eye
> Would from th'apparent What conclude the Why"

An event which occurred in the weeks immediately preceding the visit by Professor Hydén, and which caused considerable problems for the Organising Committee, was the postal strike in the United Kingdom. As the telephone was the only means of communication, many of the participants in the Symposium arrived without any warning that it was to be published. We are grateful to these authors for producing manuscripts at short notice, and to Professor Hydén in particular for producing the text of his lectures from a recorded transcript. Thanks are also due to the publishers for their forbearance over the amount of editorial correction needed at various stages owing to lack of uniformity in the manuscripts. Our thanks are due to our colleagues on the Organising Committee, Drs M. Berry, J. B. Finean, J. T. Rick, Mr E. Turner and Professor J. H. Wolstencroft for all their hard work and for the confidence they placed in us in asking us

* *First Moral Essay*, lines 99–100 (1732).

to edit this book. We are especially grateful to Miss G. Bovill who provided a high level of secretarial help and put many of the decisions of the Organising Committee into effect; to Mr R. W. Blunn who recorded Professor Hydén's lectures and Miss J. Knight and Miss S. J. Clements for assistance with the editing. There must be many more, we think, who by their efforts helped to make the First Arthur Thomson Visiting Professorship the success it proved to be.

G. B. A.
P. B. B.

August 1972

List of participants

Dr G. Ádám, Department of Comparative Physiology, Eötvös Loránd University, Budapest, Hungary.

Dr B. W. Agranoff, Mental Health Research Institute, University of Michigan, Ann Arbor, Michigan 48104, USA.

Dr M. Berry, Department of Anatomy, Medical School, Birmingham B15 2TJ, England.

Dr T. V. P. Bliss, National Institute for Medical Research, Mill Hill, London NW7 1AA, England.

Dr D. A. Booth, School of Biological Sciences, University of Sussex, Brighton BN1 SQY, England.

Dr E. Glassman, Department of Biochemistry and the Neurobiology Program, University of North Carolina School of Medicine, Chapel Hill, North Carolina 27514, USA.

Dr G. Horn, Department of Anatomy, Cambridge, England.

Professor H. Hydén, Institute of Neurobiology, University of Göteborg, Fack S-400 33, Göteborg, Sweden.

Professor G. A. Kerkut, Department of Physiology and Biochemistry, University of Southampton, Southampton SO9 5NH, England.

Professor D. M. MacKay, Department of Communications, University of Keele, Keele, Staffs, England.

Professor P. Mandel, Centre de Neurochimie du CNRS, 11 rue Humann, 67-Strasbourg, France.

Dr G. W. O. Oliver, Department of Pharmacy and Pharmacology, Portsmouth Polytechnic, Portsmouth PO1 2DZ, England.

Dr G. Raisman, Department of Human Anatomy, University of Oxford, Oxford OX1 3QX, England.

Dr J. T. Rick, Department of Psychology, University of Birmingham, Birmingham B15 2TT, England.

Professor S. P. R. Rose, Department of Biology, The Open University, Walton, Bletchley, Bucks., England.

Mr E. A. Turner, Department of Neurosurgery, Queen Elizabeth Hospital, Birmingham B15 2TD, England.

Professor G. Ungar, Department of Anesthesiology, Baylor College of Medicine, Houston, Texas 77025, USA.

Professor P. D. Wall, Department of Anatomy, University College London, Gower Street, London WC1E 6BT, England.

Contents

Preface   v–vii
List of participants   ix–x
Introduction   xiii–xiv

PART I—Arthur Thomson Lectures

1. Changes in brain protein during learning   H. HYDÉN   3–26
2. Nerve cells and their glia: relationships and differences   H. HYDÉN   27–50
3. RNA changes in brain cells during changes in behaviour and function   H. HYDÉN   51–75

PART II—Symposium

Neurochemical correlates of behaviour with particular reference to learning
Chairman: P. B. BRADLEY

4. RNA and brain function   E. GLASSMAN and J. E. WILSON   81–92
5. Biochemistry and behaviour in the chick   S. P. R. ROSE, P. P. G. BATESON and G. HORN   93–104
6. Behavioural effects of protein synthesis inhibitors: consolidation blockade or negative reinforcement?   D. A. BOOTH and C. W. T. PILCHER   105–112
7. Neurochemical aspects of shock-avoidance learning in cockroaches   G. W. O. OLIVER   113–131
8. Neurochemical correlates of behavioural change: a problem in dynamics   J. T. RICK   133–139

Modifications of brain chemistry in relation to behaviour
Chairman: S. V. PERRY

9. Biochemical approaches to learning and memory   B. W. AGRANOFF   143–149

10	Molecular mechanisms in central nervous system coding G. UNGAR	151–162
11	Specific and nonspecific RNA synthesis in relation to behavioural changes P. MANDEL, R. DI CARLO, S. SIMLER and H. RANDRIANARISOA	163–179

Neuronal interactions, learning and memory
Chairman: J. T. EAYRS

12	Anatomical evidence for plasticity in the central nervous system in the adult rat G. RAISMAN	183–191
13	Synaptic plasticity in the hippocampal formation T. V. P. BLISS, A. R. GARDNER-MEDWIN and T. LØMO	193–203
14	Conditioned evoked potential: an electrical sign of memory G. ÁDÁM	205–215
15	Morphological correlates of functional activity in the nervous system M. BERRY, T. HOLLINGWORTH, R. FLINN and E. M. ANDERSON	217–240
16	Learning in the lower animals G. A. KERKUT, P. EMSON and R. J. WALKER	241–257

Round table discussion: neurobiological models of learning

Chairman: S. M. HILTON	261–283
General summing up G. A. KERKUT	285–286
Concluding remarks H. HYDÉN	287
Author index	289
Subject index	291

Introduction

Ladies and gentlemen, it must be well over two years, I suppose, since Professor Hugh McLaren suggested that it would be an excellent idea if we were able to invite to this Medical School a distinguished visiting lecturer and surround him with a Symposium. He went, as one does on these occasions, to Sir Arthur Thomson, who is our benefactor, and suggested the idea to him. As a result we are going to hear this evening the first of the Arthur Thomson Lectures by the first Arthur Thomson Lecturer, a very distinguished visitor from abroad, and as originally planned he is being surrounded by a Symposium. This is a very important occasion for the School and we are very glad to welcome you, Sir, as our first Arthur Thomson Visiting Professor.

Professor Hydén is at present Director of the Institute of Neurobiology at the University of Göteborg, but before this has been many things. Talking to him over a cup of tea this evening, I discovered he has been a Professor of the Karolinska Institute and a Research Fellow of the Nobel Institute for Cell Research. He is the Head of the Department of Histology at the University of Göteborg, and he has been both Vice-President and President of the University of Göteborg. When I asked him whether he was still President, he said no, he had resigned, and what is more, he had resigned from all his Committees as well, so he is a truly fortunate man as well as a distinguished one.

Professor Hydén originally worked on microspectrographic methods for the determination of nucleic acids in fixed nervous tissue but his major studies have been on the relationship between the neurones and glial cells. He has developed methods for the isolation of single neurones and associated glial cells, and the separation of neuronal surface membranes and cell nucleus. Because of the small amounts of material involved he has had to devise elegant micro-methods for the analysis of the constituents of these cells which include the isolation of RNA and DNA and determination of the base composition at the picogram level. Enzymic studies on neurones and glia have indicated changes with the diurnal rhythm which would be impossible by other methods. More recently he has been interested in changes in the RNA of neurones and glia during learning procedures. He has demonstrated changes in the base composition of nuclear RNA during learning and an increase in the synthesis of proteins in neurones during behavioural changes. One other possibly higher significant chemical finding was the demonstration of an aberrant RNA in the glia isolated from the globus pallidus of patients suffering from Parkinson's disease.

Neurobiology is certainly one of the most exciting scientific disciplines that confront us today. It interests many others who work in many different related fields: psychology, psychiatry, neurology, neurochemistry and so on, and it is a discipline which is fundamental to all these subjects. I think, therefore, it is highly appropriate that we should have to talk to us a scientist who is particularly distinguished in this field.

It gives me special pleasure, therefore, to introduce Professor Hydén as the First Arthur Thomson Visiting Professor.

W. H. TRETHOWAN,
The Medical School,
Birmingham.

PART I
Arthur Thomson Lectures

Changes in brain protein during learning
H. HYDÉN
Institute of Neurobiology, University of Göteborg
Fack S-400 33, Göteborg, Sweden

Arthur Thomson Visiting Professor

Professor Trethowan, Members of the Faculty, Ladies and Gentlemen. First, I should like to present my thanks for being chosen by the Faculty for the first Arthur Thomson Visiting Professorship which is a great honour to me. It is not only an honour, but an encouragement and great stimulus when you are in a field which is multidisciplinary, and where you sometimes feel as if you were at sea, in stormy weather—but without a boat. I would also like to pay homage to the benefactor of this University, Sir Arthur, whose many testimonials we can see all around us, and who made this Visiting Professorship possible. He is, as was said at his retirement, a fine physician, a philosopher, a wise leader of the medical profession, and he must also have been, as a friend said, a 'sturdy oak' indeed.

I would like to begin these discussions with an account of some observations on proteins and behavioural experiments. "What is matter? Never mind! What is mind? Never matter!" The problem hidden in this pun is a serious matter in neurobiology today but one which can now be tackled. When new information is presented to an organism, it is registered, encoded and stored, and is available for retrieval. Registration may take only a thousandth of a second, and the processing and storage, minutes to one hour or more. The first period is most vulnerable to interference of various kinds. Storage of information into long-term memory requires a high level of arousal; no learning is possible during sleep, for example, although information which we have stored while we are awake can be retrieved during sleep. Who has not heard of a mother awoken by a light sound from her child? That arousal is required, suggests that the old parts of the brain are important in learning, and we know that the so-called 'limbic system' is essential for memory formation. Within the limbic system, the hippocampus is the main integrating system (Figure 1.1). We should consider first some of the anatomical facts. The hippocampus is connected to the frontal lobes by the entorhinal cortex and the dentate gyrus. Subcortical regions are connected to the hippocampus by

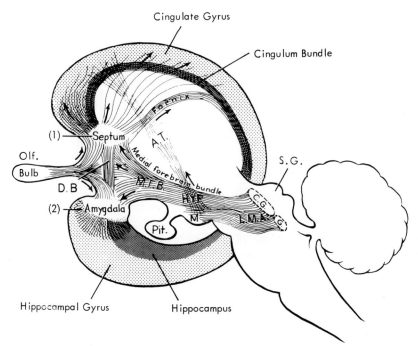

Figure 1.1. The limbic system comprises the limbic cortex and structures of the brain stem with which it has primary connections. AT, anterior thalamic nuclei; CG, central gray of midbrain; DB, diagonal band of Broca; G, ventral and dorsal tegmental nucleus of Gudden; HYP, hypothalamus; LMA, limbic midbrain area of Nauta; M, mammillary body; PIT, pituitary; SG, superior geniculate. (From MacLean, 1967.)

the septum and the fornix, the dentate gyrus with its granular cells; the hippocampus is further subdivided into different parts, called CA1 to CA4. The hippocampus constantly influences the hypothalamus and one knows that the hippocampus must be intact for formation of long-term memory, but no memories are stored within the hippocampus itself. It is worthwhile pointing out that in mammals there seems to be no strict localisation of memory and no memory cells in the strict sense exist, but certain parts are more important than others and we can assume that certain changes within the brain cells enable them to form pathways which encode information. Most of these data come from Lashley (1964) who worked for thirty years with rats, trying to trace the engram, or memory trace. Every organism has a set of complicated reflexes and behaviour ready, if not in overt activity, from birth. Simple triggers in the environment can activate them, and in some species, such as insects, the degree of freedom between genotype and behaviour is small. They work like small machines, exhibiting a strict genetically programmed activity.

In the higher phyla, it is harder to reveal a relationship between behaviour and genotype. As you all know, the brain is the most complicated structure in the body. Each nerve cell has 10–10 000 synapses on its surface, and approximately 250 000 fibres (Fox and Barnard, 1957) pass through the dendrites of one cerebellar nerve cell. There is therefore an enormous number of possible combinations. Only about 10 per cent of the nuclear genes are active in a nerve or glial cell. The rest are silent as in every other highly differentiated cell, although some can be activated by factors in the environment. Then we can ask, do 'instinct learning' and 'experience learning' involve the same mechanism, one superimposed upon the other? These phylogenetic remarks lead to the question of whether a molecular mechanism exists for storage of information that specifies all these possible combinations that are given by the phylogenetic pathways. When an animal learns, it reacts in a new or modified way as a result of experience. If one tries to define memory, and it can be defined in many ways depending upon the approach to this problem, it is the capacity to store information that can be retrieved with a high correlation to the function that was related to the new information.

Posing some problems

One important aspect of the learning and memory problem is the structure of the brain. The synaptic connections between the neurones, of which there are approximately 10^{10}, are beyond the possibility of computation, and the formation of synapses and sprouting continues during the first post-natal period. After 1920, the synapses became one of the central issues in the study of learning, and repeated synaptic use and impulse activity were believed to strengthen certain synaptic connections. The problem was considered—and is still by many—primarily as a problem of growth (see, for example, Eccles, 1970).

In my opinion, mere strengthening and outgrowth of excitatory and inhibitory synapses would not meet the requirement of simultaneous identification of a significant signal by a vast number of neurones. I should like to stress the idea that some of the requirements for the storage of new information in the brain are met by the connective possibilities of the complex brain structure with the synapses as crucial organs. Other requirements are met by a molecular mechanism for identification. When the molecules involved are considered, there seems to be agreement that small molecules can be excluded although biogenic amines have been suggested as reinforcing agents for consolidation of synapses during learning (Kety, 1970; Wada, Wrinch, Hill, McGeer and McGeer, 1963), but experimental evidence is lacking. Among macromolecules, proteins seem to me to be likely candidates as executive molecules in learning and memory mechanisms: they undergo conformational changes, they have sites for absolute recognition and they can be incorporated in the membranes of nerve cells, synapses and glia, thereby enabling recognition in a vast number of neurones simultaneously. In addition, because they can react rapidly and significantly to changes in the micro-environment caused by alterations in electric field, they may constitute the mechanism whereby electrical changes are transformed into molecular and cellular effects.

In this lecture, I will attempt to show that protein synthesis increases during the processing of new information in different brain areas according to a certain temporal sequence. The most pronounced response is found in the limbic system. One of the responsive proteins is the brain-specific protein S-100, and I shall present data to show that during the establishment of a new behaviour this protein responds specifically and that it undergoes a conformational change. I shall also examine the types of RNA changes that have been reported to occur in behavioural experiments.

From work in many laboratories during the last ten years, it is known that if the bulk of RNA and protein synthesis is inhibited in the brain by puromycin or cycloheximide, during or immediately after training, long-term memory will not be formed (Barondes, 1970; Agranoff, 1973). But there is no evidence that memory molecules exist which encode any information from experience within their own structure, like a tape-recording. As regards RNA—and I should like to return to this during the third lecture—one has to distinguish between large-scale changes in RNA, i.e. increase in amounts of 15–50 per cent in the nerve cells, and smaller changes (Hydén, 1967a). Large-scale RNA changes are induced by synaptic stimulation only (Peterson and Kernell, 1970) and occur during increased motor and sensory activity, stress or other chemical actions, and also during or after training. More specifically, there occurs during training a synthesis of small amounts of nuclear RNA with characteristic base ratios, with high adenine and usually low uridine values (Hydén, 1967b), which has not yet been found after stress or stimulation, whether chemical, motor or sensory.

Time-sequence protein changes in different brain areas during learning

During the last two years we have analysed proteins in different brain areas during training of animals. We have used two approaches. In the first, the unit approach, we used isolated nerve cells or clumps of glial cells and concentrated on brain-specific protein and conformational changes in uniform groups of nerve cells

(Hydén and Lange, 1970). There is also a need for system analysis in the brain, and in the second approach we applied time-sequence analysis of protein from the reticular formation to the limbic system and the cortex (Hydén and Lange, 1972). Here we sharpened up an old experiment in psychology from the early thirties involving reversal of handedness in rats (Peterson, 1934; Wentworth, 1942). To determine first whether the rats were left-handed, right-handed or ambidextrous, each was placed in a cage with a narrow glass tube into which it had to introduce a paw to grasp protein pills one by one. Then, using a right-handed rat, a wall was placed parallel and very close to the tube, making it difficult

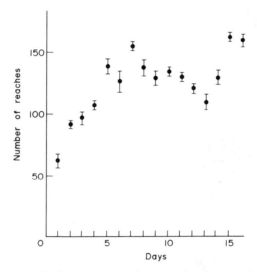

Figure 1.2. Performance curve of a group of twelve rats, given as the average number of reaches as a function of number of training sessions (2 × 25 minutes per day).

for the rat to use its right paw. As a result, it quickly learnt to use the left paw. The performance curve was linear up to the seventh or eighth day (Figure 1.2) and, once learned, this behaviour remained stable for more than 300 days. The animals were injected intraperitoneally with tritiated leucine, trained for one hour after the injection and then killed. We found that the specific radioactivity of 100 μg protein samples increased during the first forty minutes and then decreased slowly and that the specific activity values were the same from the left and the right hemispheres. The rats were trained for reversal of handedness in two 25-minute sessions each day for four days. Then after an intermission of fourteen days, during which they lived in the cages, they were trained for another two days, again with two 25-minute sessions per day. This was followed by another intermission and a final two days of training giving eight days of training in all. The establishment of the new behaviour proceeded quite rapidly and the performance was good after the first four days of the initial training. In the schematic drawings, the ratio of corrected specific activities of the trained animals to those of control animals is indicated by colours; blue indicates low values and red an increase, indicating an increase in protein synthesis (Figure 1.3). After the initial training, there was a high incorporation of leucine into the protein, indicating an increase in the amount of protein synthesis in the hippocampus, the dentate nucleus and the mammillary bodies, but at the same time, there were low values, i.e. a decrease in the cortex, the reticular formation, the entorhinal cortex and the septum. Given free choice at the finish of the first training period, some rats made errors and occasionally used their normally preferred paw.

Table 1.1

Ratios, $\left(\dfrac{I_p\,(\text{Tr})}{I_p\,(\text{C})}\right) \times 10^{-2}$, between corrected specific activities of total protein in different brain areas of trained animals and corresponding values of control animals. The values are given for three training periods of 4, 6, and 8 days. In each case, four trained and three control animals were used.

Brain area	$\left(\dfrac{I_p\,(\text{Tr})}{I_p\,(\text{C})}\right)_4$	$\left(\dfrac{I_p\,(\text{Tr})}{I_p\,(\text{C})}\right)_6$	$\left(\dfrac{I_p\,(\text{Tr})}{I_p\,(\text{C})}\right)_8$
Cortex	27	46	34
Formatio reticularis	34	40	29
Entorhinal cortex	28	40	24
Gyrus dentatus	46	20	33
Hippocampus	97	→28	→25
Thalamus, dorso-medial nucl.	23	32	51
Corpus mammillare	51	46	23
Septum	26	25	31

After the second training period, few errors were made and the specific activities of the protein were the inverse of those found after the first: there were low incorporation values in the hippocampus and dentate, but high ones in the cortex and reticular formation. The new establishment persisted for a long time. After the last intermission and the last two days of training, we found low values very close to the control values in all parts with one exception, the dorso-medial part of the thalamus. Thus, during a period which we could call the processing state of learning, there was a shift, as well as reversal in protein synthesis, from the limbic system to the cortical structures according to a certain time sequence (Table 1.1). The ratios of the corrected specific activities are given in Table 1.1. They demonstrate another main result of the study. The incorporation values into protein of [^{3}H]leucine are on average lower in the trained animals than in the controls.

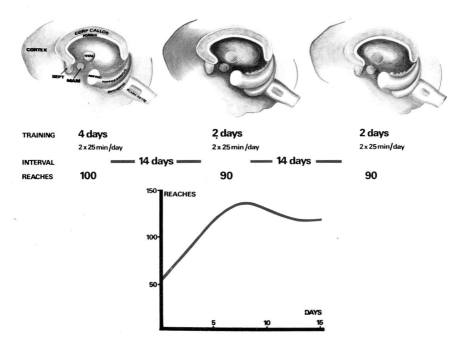

Figure 1.3. Sequential changes in the incorporation of [^{3}H]-leucine into total soluble protein. Light blue denotes medium quotient values corrected specific activity trained/corrected specific activity control. Darker blue denotes a decrease in this quotient. Light orange denotes slight increase in the quotient corrected specific activity trained/corrected specific activity control. Dark orange denotes a marked increase in this quotient. Abbreviations: amygd, amygdala; corp callos, corpus callosum; entorhin, cortex entorhinalis; form retic, formatio reticularis; mam, corpus mammillare; sept, septum; thal, thalamus.

This is the case even if no correction for ^{3}H-activity of the supernatant was made. Such a correction only slightly sharpened the significant difference. This is an unexpected finding and is corroborated by autoradiography. The figures in Table 1.1 further demonstrate the high values occurring initially in the hippocampus which then decrease considerably. The cortex goes the other way, from low values to high values. This was the first attempt we made to determine, according to a time sequence, the changes that occur in the total proteins, i.e. nonseparated proteins, in various parts of the brain, using very small samples.

Effect of training on protein synthesis of the hippocampus

I will now discuss the response of specific protein in defined groups of nerve cells determined by micro-analyses of 0·5 μg of protein extracted from dissected nerve cells. Recently attention has been focused on brain-specific proteins chiefly for two reasons: they occur only in the nervous tissue, and one of them, the so-called S-100 protein, cross-reacts with antiserum from man to fish (Moore, 1965). It has a molecular weight of 21 000, three subunits and a high content of glutamic and aspartic acids, and it binds calcium selectively (Kessler, Levine and Fasman, 1968; Calissano, Moore and Friesen, 1969). It is mainly a glial protein, being localised in the glial bodies (Hydén and McEwen, 1966; Mihailovic and Hydén, 1969). This has been shown by specific fluorescence after Coons' reaction with antiserum against the S-100 (Coons, 1957), as well as by precipitation reactions, in this case in the brain stem. We can see that the protein is localised in the bodies of the glia and in the nuclei of the neurones but that the localisation varies in different parts of the brain. In the hippocampus the S-100 protein is confined to the nuclei of nerve cells. If S-100 is isolated from the brain and separated by gel electrophoresis, several fractions are obtained. Each reacts with antiserum against S-100 protein and has a different turnover rate, two of them being rather high.

Calcium produces a conformational change in S-100. The protein specifically binds two calcium ions which produce a partial unfolding of the molecule at the tryptophan residues and probably allow oxidation of two sulphydryl groups. Calcium also stabilises the ordered native form and antigenicity of the molecule against thermal denaturation (Kessler *et al.*, 1968). In the hippocampus, the main integrating part of the limbic system, there is an excellent opportunity to observe this specific brain protein in isolated pyramidal nerve cells. This is known as unit cell analysis, a prerequisite being pure material from a defined group of uniform cells or glia; these have therefore to be separated from each other, for even in a few micrograms of tissue, nerve cells and glia will be present in equal amounts. Nerve cells and glia often respond biochemically in an inverse way, so that the net biochemical change in the glia/nerve cell ratio is zero and unobservable. These reverse changes reflect a two-cell collaboration, but I will return to this in the next

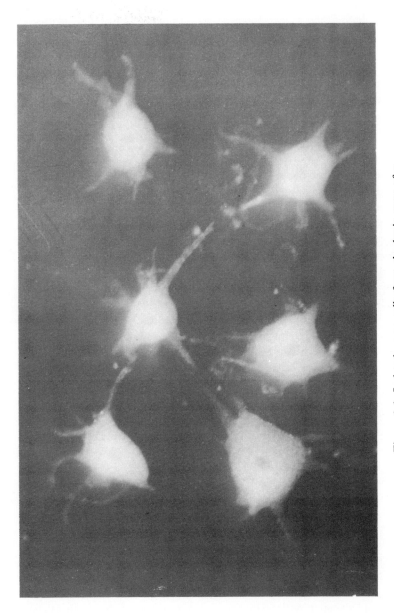

Figure 1.4. Isolated nerve cells from the brain stem of a rabbit microdissected free-hand from the fresh tissue and photographed with incident light in Ringer's solution. Magnification ×325.

lecture. Neuronal bodies and glia can be separated either by bulk separation (Blomstrand, 1971) which I will discuss later on, or by a micro-approach, in which a group of nerve cells (Figure 1.4, photographed in incident light) is first freed from glia by free-hand dissection and then further separated by microsurgery using small knives made from Swedish stainless steel. The isolated nerve cells phosphorylate, they have good oxygen consumption, and they have a membrane potential which indicates that they have closed the wounds afflicted by cutting off the dendrites. We therefore think that they are good material for biochemical studies. Staining with methylene blue or by silver impregnation after isolation demonstrates that the synaptic knobs still adhere to the isolated nerve cell perikarya and dendrites and, in small numbers, to the first part of the axon (Figure 1.5).

Table 1.2

Anti-Deiters' glia Antiserum, dilution 1:512

AG: N. D. homogenate
AG dilution $8 \cdot 0 \rightarrow 0 \cdot 01$ $\mu g/\mu l$
Ppt from $0 \cdot 85 \rightarrow 0 \cdot 1$ μg protein$/\mu l$

Anti-Deiters' glia Antiserum, dilution 1:512

AG: D glia homogenate
AG dilution $0 \cdot 67 \rightarrow 0 \cdot 02$ $\mu g/\mu l$
Ppt from $0 \cdot 67 \rightarrow 0 \cdot 16$ μg protein$/\mu l$

AG: antigen.

My collaborators, Drs Hamberger, Hansson and Sjöstrand (1970) have demonstrated the synaptic knobs on the cell surface by scanning electron microscopy (Figure 1.6). They have also demonstrated that a change occurs during retrograde reaction which temporarily causes the synaptic knobs to detach from the cell surface on removal of the glia.

It is quite clear that there are differences in protein composition between neurones and glia. Dr Mihailovic and I (1969) prepared antiserum against nerve cells and glial cells of Deiters' nucleus in the lateral vestibular area, and found that they differ in antigenicity. Using the glial antiserum we found good precipitation when we used as an antigen protein of a whole homogenate from the area (Table 1.2) containing both nerve cells and glia. When we used the same glial antiserum and only glial homogenate, we found the same type of precipitation within the same range. Only glial protein gave precipitation, not neuronal material (Table 1.3), but if the antiserum was absorbed with glia or with spleen, the glial reaction was removed when glial protein was used as antigen, suggesting the presence of specific antigens in the neurone (Table 1.4), localised close to the nerve

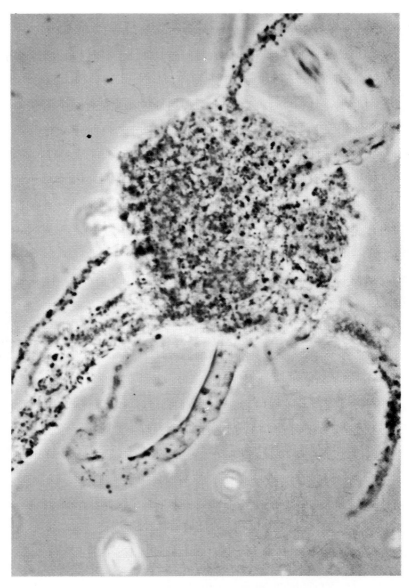

Figure 1.5. Isolated nerve cell with synapses.

cell membrane. The antigens of the glial protein differed from those of the neurones, but were not glia-specific.

To isolate the S-100 protein and the 14-3-2 protein, which is another brain-specific protein, we used discontinuous electrophoresis on polyacrylamide gel in capillaries (Figure 1.7, Hydén, Bjurstam and McEwen, 1966; Hydén and Lange,

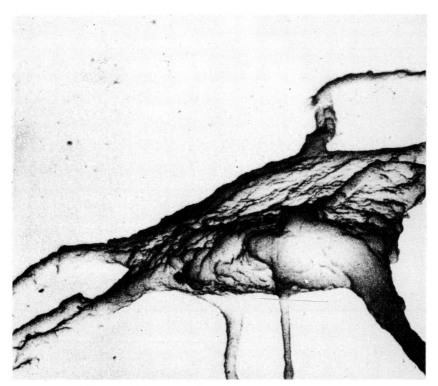

Figure 1.6. Hypoglossal neurone 14 days after nerve crush. The perikaryal surface is free from spherical particles. No regular surface impressions are visible. Scanning electron micrograph. ×1300. (From Hamberger, Hansson and Sjöstrand, 1970.)

1968a). Figure 1.8 shows a protein sample from nerve cells, separated on such gels in capillaries 300 to 400 μm in diameter, and stained with brilliant blue; 0·5 μg of protein was applied on each gel. Very briefly, the experiments involved injecting tritiated leucine into the lateral ventricles of the rats and dissecting the cells in the CA3 hippocampal region, which is the main integrating centre of the hippocampus. After micro-electrophoresis of the gels, we used a Leitz interference microscopic system to determine the protein mass of the fractions we were

Table 1.3

Results of testing anti-Deiters' glial antiserum with extracts of a varying number of nerve cells and a corresponding amount of surrounding glia.

Deiters' neurones			Deiters' glia		
Number of cells	Calculated protein in 10^{-6} g	Precipitation	Glia corresponding to amount of cells	Calculated protein in 10^{-6} g	Precipitation
300	3·6	—	300	1·8	+2 bands
150	1·8	—	150	0·9	+2 bands
70	0·9	—	70	0·45	+2 sharp clear bands
60	0·72	—	60	0·36	+1 band thin and faint
30	0·36	—	30	0·18	+1 band
15	0·18	—	15	0·09	negative
6	0·09	—	6	0·045	—
3	0·045	—	3	0·022	—

Values of $12\,000 \times 10^{-12}$ g protein/nerve cell and 6000×10^{-12} g protein/glia corresponding to that of nerve cell were obtained by X-ray spectrography and used as basis for calculation. Antiserum was diluted 1:512.

Table 1.4

Results of testing anti-whole Deiters' nucleus antibody with extracts of nerve cells and glia before and after its absorption with Deiters' glia.

		Antigen	
Serum	Dilution	70 Deiters' nerve cells (0.9×10^{-6} g protein/3 μl)	Deiters' glia (0.45×10^{-6} g protein/3 μl)
Anti-whole Deiters' nucleus antiserum unabsorbed	1:2	+(2 bands)	+(2 bands)
	1:4	+(4 bands)	+(2 bands)
	1:8	Not clear	
	1:16	+	+
Anti-whole Deiters' nucleus antiserum absorbed with Deiters' glia	1:2	+	—
	1:4	+	—
	1:8	+	—
	1:16	+	—
Normal serum taken prior to immunisation	1:2	—	—
	1:4	—	—
	1:8	—	—
	1:16	—	—

interested in. These were then sectioned under a microscope and placed in a capillary and combusted for one hour at 650°C together with zinc particles to transform the tritium into gas form. In order to compare different parts of one brain, or one part of the brains from different animals, we determined the activity of the free leucine in the same area to obtain a correction factor. In these extremely small

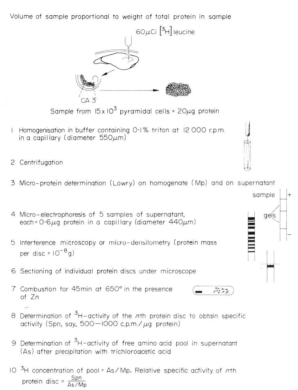

Figure 1.7. Outline of the microdisc electrophoresis procedure for separation of 10^{-7} to 10^{-9} g of protein and evaluation of incorporation of radioactive amino acid into the individual fractions. Volume of sample is proportional to weight of total protein in sample.

samples, it is chiefly the intracellular pool which is determined. This is an advantage in correcting for the pool. The radiometry is determined in a special tube. The basis for this computation is our finding that there is a linear relationship between the amount of leucine injected and the uncorrected specific activity. The localisation of the S-100 and the 14-3-2 protein in the electrophoretic pattern is indicated in Figure 1.8. My collaborator, S. Larsson (unpublished observations), has developed and perfected the apparatus for determination of very small activities of tritium (Figure 1.9). The sample is enclosed in a 0·5 mm diameter capillary, together with zinc particles, and combusted for one hour at 650°C. The capillary is placed inside the plastic tubing of the measuring system which contains helium and isobutane, and crushed in order to release the gas inside the capillary. The unit provides a very low background of about 1 c.p.s. The activity is measured by an anticoincidence unit.

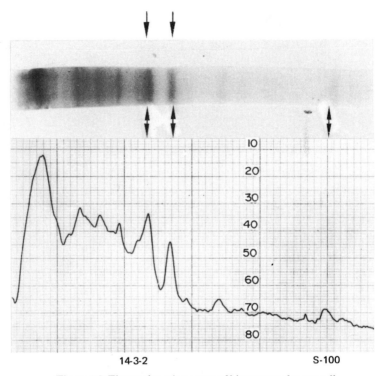

Figure 1.8. Electrophoretic pattern of hippocampal nerve cell soluble protein with densitometric recording below. Arrows indicate the localisation of the S-100 and 14-3-2 proteins.

When we looked at the S-100 protein fraction of the hippocampal material of the trained animals, we found two S-100 fractions in the electrophoretic pattern as opposed to one in the material of the controls. Figure 1.10 gives two examples of densitometric tracings from this material, and Table 1.5 gives the frequency of occurrence of the two S-100 fractions in seventy-one determinations from thirty-four rats. Training produced an increase in the amount of the S-100, because the sum of the integrated curves of the trained material of these two S-100 fractions was always greater than that of the same value from the control material of the

Changes in brain protein during learning

S-100 fraction. Since it is known that calcium causes conformational changes in S-100, Haljamäe and Lange (1972) at our laboratory studied the calcium content of hippocampal nerve cells from the CA3 region from trained and control rats by microflame photometry. They found a larger amount of calcium in material from the CA3 region of the trained animals than in material from the control animals

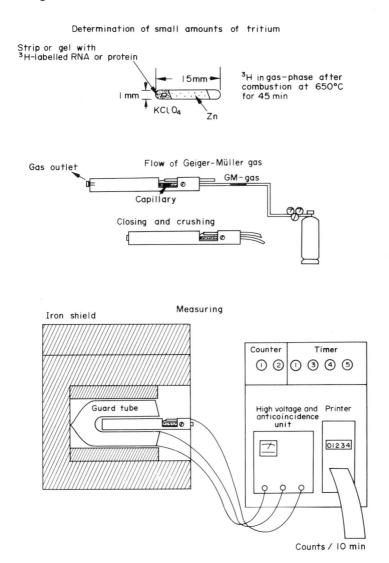

Figure 1.9. Apparatus for determination of very low tritium activity. (From Larsson, unpublished.)

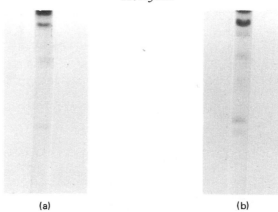

Figure 1.10. Photographs of nerve cell protein of the hippocampus, CA3 regions, separated on polyacrylamide gels 400 μm in diameter and stained by amido black. (a), From control rat; (b), from rat on day 5 of training with the non-preferred paw. The acidic proteins migrate toward the bottom of the gel.

(Table 1.6). They also found that the faster migrating band contained more calcium than the slower migrating band. Interference from magnesium and phosphate was controlled and sodium and potassium were not increased. According to our reasoning this excludes the possibility that the increased calcium content was due to an increased vascular bed. Thus, training produced an increase in the amount of S-100 in the hippocampal nerve cells. The split in the S-100 complex, the increased calcium content and the larger amount of calcium in the faster migrating band suggest that part of the S-100 produced during training has a different conformation from that of the S-100 from controls. One explanation may be that an increase in intracellular calcium occurs during the increased activity in the hippocampus, and causes an irreversible conformational change in S-100. Another

Table 1.5

Frequency of single- and double-frontal anodal proteins in the electrophoretic pattern of 75 polyacrylamide gels from 23 rats (7 controls, 4 resumed training on the 14th day, 12 resumed training on the 14th day and on the 30th day).

Controls		Resumed training on day 14		Resumed training on day 30	
1 fraction	2 fractions	1 fraction	2 fractions	1 fraction	2 fractions
20	0	5	10	20	20

explanation is, of course, that S-100 of a different conformation is formed during training. One may ask, why does not S-100 from control animals show these characteristics, since they have obviously learned quite a lot during their life? We have found that when the consolidation stage is completed, and the novelty of the task is over, the hippocampus does not give this analytical result. We therefore assume that the protein which has been produced during early training becomes incorporated into membranes and then exists in a tightly bound form, and we are studying this at the present time.

Table 1.6

Water, potassium, sodium and calcium content of brain samples from the CA3 region in the hippocampus of control rats and trained rats. Electrolyte values obtained both on wet weight and dry weight basis.

	%H_2O	Potassium, mEq/100 g		Sodium, mEq/100 g		Calcium, mg/100 g	
		dry weight	wet weight	dry weight	wet weight	dry weight	wet weight
Control ($n = 18$)	81·1	51·20	10·17	20·43	3·87	37·0	7·36
S.E.M. ±	0·4	1·60	0·38	0·35	0·07	1·9	0·27
Trained ($n = 20$)	81·0	50·42	9·99	20·04	4·04	44·0*	8·04†
S.E.M. ±	0·5	1·50	0·34	0·43	0·10	1·8	0·19

* $P < 0·001$.
† $P < 0·05$.
(From Haljamäe and Lange, 1972.)

To determine whether this response of the S-100 protein is specifically related to learning processes in the hippocampus, or whether it is completely unspecific, we attempted to block S-100 in the cells of the limbic system with antiserum against S-100. For a meaningful experiment, suitable controls are essential. Training involves a number of variables, such as motor and sensory activity, increased motivation, orientation reflexes, a certain amount of stress and learning processes *per se*, and all these factors must be identical in the experimental and control animals, except learning, which can be controlled behaviourally. We therefore trained a group of rats in an identical way for the first three days (Figure 1.11) and injected some intraventricularly with antiserum against S-100 on the fourth day between the two training periods. The performance curve was clearly deflected by further training (Figure 1.11). We then used antiserum against S-100 absorbed

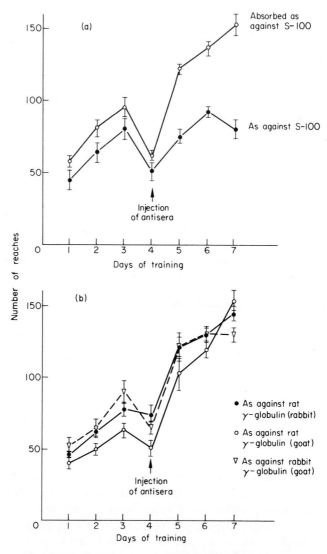

Figure 1.11. Performance curves of rats injected intraventricularly on day 4 with 2×30 μg of antiserum: (a), against S-100 protein and eight rats injected with 2×30 μg of antiserum against S-100 absorbed with S-100 protein; (b), against rat gamma globulin from rabbit (four rats), and from goat (four rats), and rabbit gamma globulin from goat (four rats).

with S-100 as a control and obtained a performance curve equivalent to an extrapolation of the curve before the injection. We also used various types of rat gamma globulins and rabbit gamma globulins as other controls, but with no visible result. In none of these experiments did the animals show any signs of motor disability. The globulins are big molecules, and the pertinent question is, therefore, whether they can penetrate the ependymal cells and reach the structures inside the cells of the hippocampus. To subject the question to an experimental test we used

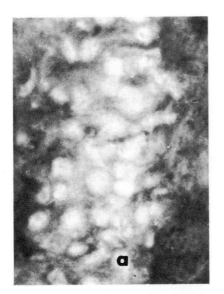 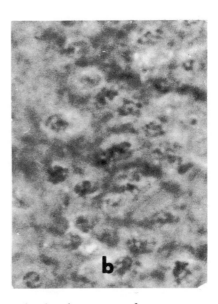

Figure 1.12. Specific fluorescence showing the presence of antibodies against the S-100 protein localised to the nerve cell nucleus in the CA3 region of the hippocampus (a). There is no specific fluorescence to be seen in the corresponding structures of rats injected with antiserum against S-100 protein absorbed with S-100 protein (b).

Coons' indirect method for specific fluorescence in two steps. That is, we injected the antiserum intraventricularly in the live animals and applied the fluorescein-conjugated gamma globulin to cryostat sections. In the pyramidal nerve cells of the hippocampus we found a specific fluorescence, indicating that the antiserum had reached the cells (Figure 1.12). The same results were obtained in the case of the dentate nucleus. We concluded that the S-100 protein seems to be correlated with specific processes occurring during the training of animals, in the training test which we used, and that therefore the S-100 protein may mediate neuronal connections and functions.

Response of the 14-3-2 protein in the hippocampus during training

The other brain-specific protein that we have studied is the 14-3-2 protein, again an acidic protein, having a molecular weight of 38 000 and appearing as multiple bands in gel electrophoresis experiments which probably correspond to different aggregation states of a single protein (Moore and Perez, 1968). This may explain why it is localised in two fractions in the electrophoretic pattern. We recently performed an amino acid analysis of the 14-3-2 protein and found it to be rich (13–14 per cent) in aspartic and glutamic acids (Hydén and Lange, unpublished observations). Like the S-100 protein, it increased in amount during embryogenesis and early post-natally, and although it was also found both in glia and in

Table 1.7

Corrected specific activities of hippocampal CA3 nerve cell proteins, both unseparated and fractions 4 and 5. Corrected specific activity refers to counts per minute/μg $\pm$ S.E.M.

	Fractions 4 and 5			Unseparated protein	
	No. of rats	No. of gels	Corrected specific activity	No. of samples	Corrected specific activity
Group I (training 5 days)	5	10	3.3 $\pm$ 0.40	10	14.20 $\pm$ 1.90
Group II (resumed training day 14)	5	10	3.9 $\pm$ 0.48	10	15.50 $\pm$ 1.90
Group IIA (half training time)	2	5	13.0 $\pm$ 0.60		
Group III (resumed training day 30)	14	35	1.8 $\pm$ 0.17	28	5.10 $\pm$ 0.58
Control	10	24	1.5 $\pm$ 0.16	20	6.00 $\pm$ 0.92

nerve cells, it is chiefly a neuronal protein and not a glial protein like S-100. We performed the same type of reversal of handedness experiments and showed that the incorporation of [^{3}H]leucine into the 4 and 5 protein fractions—which contain the 14-3-2 protein—increased significantly as a function of training (Hydén and Lange, 1968b). Yet when we examined the data after repeated training, or resumed training after thirty days, there was no response at all over that of the control material (Table 1.7). If the increased protein synthesis had been an expression of increased neural function in general, the protein response should also have occurred when training was resumed one month after the initial training.

To summarise, at this point, when an animal is faced with a new situation which requires learning within the capacity of the species, there is a time-sequence response of protein which involves first the hippocampus and then gradually the reticular formation and the neocortex, with a concomitant decline in the limbic reaction. Among all the nerve cell proteins, there is the quantitative response of the two brain-specific proteins with an additional conformational change in the S-100 protein.

Side-lights on a protein identification mechanism in the brain

Finally, let me briefly discuss these results. The brain is a hierarchically organised system, and the time sequence of protein response reflects the integrative function of different brain areas when new information is processed. The fact that nerve cells within the limbic system increase their protein synthesis at the beginning of training agrees in time with the electrical changes which have been found in the hippocampus during early training, for example by Adey, Kado, Didio and Schindler (1963). Since it is well known that bilateral lesions to the hippocampus prohibit long-term storage of information (Meissner, 1966; Ojemann, 1966), the protein response in the limbic cells seems to be a chemical correlate of function in this part of the brain. New protein synthesis was inhibited in the neocortex when it was stimulated in the hippocampus, and this temporary inhibition may well be another correlate to learning processes. If absolute incorporation values are considered, it is clear that these values of trained animals are lower than the values of the control animals. It is important to keep this in mind when we consider the extensive incorporation of precursors into specific brain proteins during early training. The S-100 and 14-3-2 proteins constitute only 0·3 per cent of the nerve cell 'soluble' protein. Even if the overall protein synthesis is inhibited in the neocortex during processing of information, this does not exclude an increase of, for example, S-100 protein. This does not mean that S-100 is specific for the ability 'reversal of handedness'. Nor is there reason to believe, as I stressed before, that the molecule could register a specific memory within its structure, but it is reasonable to assume that the enormous number of combinations that are possible between neurones, plus a molecular identification mechanism using conformation of specific protein, enables pathways to store information.

How could such a mechanism function? Let us start from the early post-natal period. The brain-specific proteins studied here are produced pre-natally and are present in neurones as well as in glia at birth. The fact that such proteins respond quantitatively and qualitatively in brain cells as a function of experience, implies a protein differentiation which occurs in vast numbers of brain cells but differently in different groups of cells.

If we assume that proteins of the S-100 type can be part of synaptic, nerve cell body or glial membranes, the selective uptake of calcium in nerve cells which we found during the behavioural test could have a dual effect: it could induce a conformational change in the S-100 protein and it could increase the impulse activity (Rasmussen, 1970); it would therefore induce protein synthesis (Rasmussen and Nagata, 1970) and even regulate the release of transmitters (Banks, 1970). The selective ion-effect and the conformational change of protein could be the mechanism of translating electrical activity into remaining macromolecular patterns and could constitute the identification mechanism.

Millions of neurones sharing the protein pattern of their synaptic membranes would respond to the same signals, whether they came from the environment or from the cell interior. The experience of an activity of the identification mechanisms in their three-dimensional shape would be an actualisation of stored information. Seen in this light, the engram is a process, not a trace.

References

ADEY, W. R., KADO, R. T., DIDIO, J. and SCHINDLER, W. J. (1963). Impedance changes in cerebral tissue accompanying a learned discriminative performance in the cat. *Expl Neurol.*, **7**, 259–81.

AGRANOFF, B. W. (1973). Biochemical approaches to learning and memory. In: *Macromolecules and Behaviour* (ANSELL, G. B. and BRADLEY, P. B., Eds.), pp. 143–149. Macmillan, London.

BANKS, P. (1970). Involvement of calcium in the secretion of catecholamines. In: *A Symposium on Calcium and Cellular Function* (CUTHBERT, A. W., Ed.), pp. 148–62. Macmillan, London.

BARONDES, S. H. (1970). Multiple steps in the biology of memory. In: *The Neurosciences Second Study Program* (SCHMITT, F. O., Ed.), pp. 272–8. The Rockefeller University Press, New York.

BLOMSTRAND, C. (1971). *Studies on Protein Metabolism in Neuronal and Glial Cell-Enriched Fractions from Brain Tissue*. Thesis. Göteborg.

CALISSANO, P., MOORE, B. W. and FRIESEN, A. (1969). Effect of a calcium ion on S-100, a protein of the nervous system. *Biochemistry*, **8**, 4318–26.

COONS, A. H. (1957). The application of fluorescent antibodies to the study of naturally occurring antibodies. *Ann. N.Y. Acad. Sci.*, **69**, 548–662.

ECCLES, J. C. (1970). *Facing Reality*. Springer-Verlag, New York.

FOX, C. A. and BARNARD, J. W. (1957). A quantitative study of the Purkinje cell dendritic branches and their relationship to afferent fibres. *J. Anat.*, **91**, 299–313.

HALJAMÄE, H. and LANGE, P. W. (1972). Calcium content and conformation changes of S-100 protein in the hippocampus during training. *Brain Res.*, **38**, 131–142.

HAMBERGER, A., HANSSON, H.-A. and SJÖSTRAND, J. (1970). Surface structure of isolated neurons. Detachment of nerve terminals during axon regeneration. *J. cell. Biol.*, **47**, 319–31.

HYDÉN, H. (1967a). Biochemical changes accompanying learning. In: *The Neurosciences* (QUARTON, G. C., MELNECHUK, T. and SCHMITT, F. O., Eds.), pp. 765–71. The Rockefeller University Press, New York.

HYDÉN, H. (1967b). Behavior, neural function and RNA. In: *Progress in Nucleic Acid Research and Molecular Biology*, Vol. 6, p. 187. Academic Press, New York.

HYDÉN, H., BJURSTAM, K. and MCEWEN, B. (1966). Protein separation at the cellular level by microdisc electrophoresis. *Analyt. Biochem.*, **17**, 1–15.

HYDÉN, H. and LANGE, P. W. (1968a). Micro-electrophoretic determination of protein and protein synthesis in the 10^{-9} to 10^{-7} gram range. *J. Chromat.*, **35**, 336–51.

HYDÉN, H. and LANGE, P. W. (1968b). Protein synthesis in the hippocampal pyramidal cells of rats during a behavioural test. *Science, N.Y.*, **159**, 1370–3.

HYDÉN, H. and LANGE, P. W. (1970). S-100 brain protein: correlation with behaviour. *Proc. natn. Acad. Sci., U.S.A.*, **67**, 1959–66.

HYDÉN, H. and MCEWEN, B. (1966). A glial protein specific for the nervous system. *Proc. natn. Acad. Sci., U.S.A.*, **55**, 354–8.

KESSLER, D., LEVINE, L. and FASMAN, G. (1968). Some conformational and immunological properties of a bovine brain acidic protein (S-100). *Biochemistry*, **7**, 758–64.

KETY, S. S. (1970). The biogenic amines in the central nervous system: their possible roles in arousal, emotion and learning. In: *The Neurosciences Second Study Program* (SCHMITT, F. O., Ed.), pp. 324–36. The Rockefeller University Press, New York.

LASHLEY, K. S. (1964). *Brain Mechanisms and Intelligence*. Hafner Publishing Company, New York.

MACLEAN, P. D. (1967). In: Brain organization. In: *The Neurosciences* (QUARTON, G. C., MELNECHUK, T. and SCHMITT, F. O., Eds.), p. 506. The Rockefeller University Press, New York.

MEISSNER, W. W. (1966). Hippocampal functions in learning. *J. Psychiat. Res.*, **4**, 235–304.

MIHAILOVIC, L. and HYDÉN, H. (1969). On antigenic differences between nerve cells and glia. *Brain Res.*, **16**, 243–56.

MOORE, B. W. (1965). A soluble protein characteristic of the nervous system. *Biochem. biophys. Res. Commun.*, **19**, 739–44.

MOORE, B. W. and PEREZ, V. J. (1968). Specific acidic proteins of the nervous system. In: *Physiological and Biochemical Aspects of Nervous Integration* (CARLSON, F. D., Ed.), pp. 343–59. Englewood Cliffs, New Jersey.

OJEMANN, R. G. (1966). Correlation between specific human brain lesions and memory changes. *Neurosci. Res. Progr. Bull.*, **4**, 1–70.

PETERSON, G. M. (1934). Mechanisms of handedness in the rat. *Comp. Psychol. Monogr.*, **9**, 1–67.

PETERSON, R. P. and KERNELL, D. (1970). The effects of nerve stimulation on the metabolism of ribonucleic acid in a molluscan giant neurone. *J. Neurochem.*, **17**, 1075–87.

RASMUSSEN, H. (1970). Cell communication, calcium ion, and cyclic AMP. *Science, N.Y.*, **170**, 404–11.

RASMUSSEN, H. and NAGATA, N. (1970). Renal gluconeogenesis. Effects on parathyroid hormone and dibutyryl 3′,5′-AMP. *Biochim. biophys. Acta*, **215**, 17–28.

WADA, J. A., WRINCH, J., HILL, D., McGEER, P. L. and McGEER, E. G. (1963). Central aromatic amine levels and behaviour. *Archs Neurol., Paris*, **9**, 69–80.

WENTWORTH, K. L. (1942). Some factors determining handedness in the rat. *Genet. Psychol. Monogr.*, **26**, 55–117.

Nerve cells and their glia: relationships and differences

H. HYDÉN (GÖTEBORG)

In this lecture I should like to discuss nerve cells and their glia, particularly the glia around the nerve cells. Sir Hans Krebs was among the first to recommend that the regulatory mechanisms of the metabolism of both isolated and complete cells should be studied, and he suggested that in this way the relationship between live cells could be clarified. There are difficulties, however, in the interpretation of data because of the heterogeneity of cells and because of our lack of understanding of signals between the cells. In neurones and glia, there are indications of the presence of intercellular regulatory and feedback systems, particularly of macromolecules, RNA and proteins.

Although both glia and nerve cells develop from the same stem cells, the interest in nerve cells has always been dominant; the description of the development of neuroblasts by His (1890) is appealing to say the least, but until now the glia have not been discussed very much. It may be appropriate, however, to review briefly some early papers. Although there was a general interest in glia, it was chiefly Weigert (1895) and Ramón y Cajal (1910) who initially defined the different types morphologically and Glees (1955) who sharpened the criteria. It was recognised early in comparative studies that the appearance of glia varied widely through the phyla. In invertebrates they are often large cells which harbour several nerve cells, whereas in mammals there is the intricate relationship between the processes of many glial cells and a single neurone. The higher up in the phyla, the greater is the ratio of glial cells to neurones. Virchow (1846) was the first to describe the glia cell as a special type of brain cell, and it is not surprising, therefore, that his many followers in pathology have kept an observant eye on glial changes. Spielmayer (1922) reviewed a number of interesting phenomena which indicated their participation in pathological changes and in the formation of the so-called Büngner bands during, for example, retrograde reaction. The intimate relationship between the nerve cell and glia was described in detail by Holmgren in a series of papers between 1899 and 1910 and his pictures show how the glial cells may form invaginations into ganglion cells. Figure 2.1 demonstrates a spinal ganglion cell

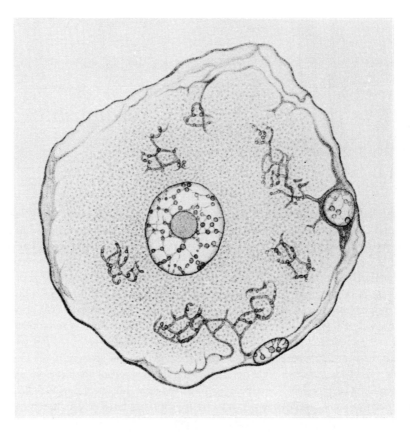

Figure 2.1. Section through spinal ganglion cell of calf exposed to osmic acid fumes. Rays of granules from the satellite cells are invading the perikaryon-like channels. (From Holmgren, 1902.)

which Holmgren had treated with osmium. He depicts how the satellite cells form channels which invaginate the cell cytoplasm and proposed that the glia transfer substances of some kind from their own bodies into the cytoplasm of the nerve cells and that they act as food suppliers to the nerve cells.

Among the observers of glia in the past was the Arctic explorer Nansen (1886), but none was more original than Carl Ludwig Schleich. In 1916 he wrote a book called *Vom Schaltwerk der Gedanken* in which he maintained that the glia pulsate and massage the neurones, either stimulating the neurones or breaking their connections. He regarded them as 'muscles of the brain' which could be trained for better performance, like a runner, and which beat the time. But he was a rather pathetic person, and some of what he wrote was based on a misunderstanding of information he received in a letter from the anatomist Benda, at that time in Berlin. A generation later, Pomerat in his elegant experiments during the 1950s, recorded genuine glial pulsations in cultures. At present there is good evidence that astrocytes with their capillary feet serve as ion exchangers, that oligodendroglia capture and release potassium, and that they both generally mediate transport. And if we look at the results of Adey, Kado, Didio and Schindler (1963), we may or may not agree with their conclusion that glia form diffuse pathways for extrasynaptic and extraneuronal currents.

The isolation of glia

I shall now discuss biochemical differences between nerve cells and glia, which can be studied both by microchemical and macrochemical methods, and then ask whether we are still at the describing stage, collecting stamps, or whether we can draw some conclusions about function. In our laboratory, we have used both micro- and macro-procedures to obtain nerve cell and glial samples. The microsamples consist partly of nerve cells and partly of collections of those glial cells which surround the perikarya (Figure 2.2). We used scanning X-ray microspectrography at 0·8 to 1·2 nm (Brattgård and Hydén, 1952, 1954; Rosengren, 1959) to determine the dry weight of the isolated nerve cells and found that, per volume unit, the glial and the nerve cell material had the same weight. The technique consisted, therefore, of isolating a volume of glia matching that of a particular nerve cell. Great care was taken to ensure that the glial material taken was that surrounding the nerve cell body. The glial and nerve cell data could then be compared since the samples have the same weight (Hydén and Larsson, 1956). Such a collection of glia contained four or five nuclei. Capillaries and dendritic fragments, if visible, were removed during the dissection from the glial sample. The weight of such a glial sample from the big vestibular nerve cells was around 10^{-8} g. Figure 2.3 shows an example of bulk separation of nerve cell bodies by Rose's (1967) method modified by my collaborators, Blomstrand and Hamberger (1969). Many processes have been broken off close to the cell body, but otherwise the sample is quite pure and is also the cleanest of the bulk-separated fractions. Figure 2.4 shows a less pure sample of glia collected in the same way; astrocytes, microglia and oligodendrocytes are clearly visible.

There are a number of advantages in using the micro-procedure. It takes five to ten minutes to obtain a sufficient number of microsamples from the newly-killed animal, and they can be obtained from a defined small area (Hydén, 1959), namely, as I have stressed, that surrounding the nerve cells which are also sampled. The microsamples are more pure, less damaged and free from blood, vessels and capillaries. The samples can be frozen rapidly and in some cases—but only in some—the loss of material by diffusion into the solvents is smaller than that which occurs in the macrofractions. These are some of the advantages. On the other hand, there is only a limited number of analytical methods available

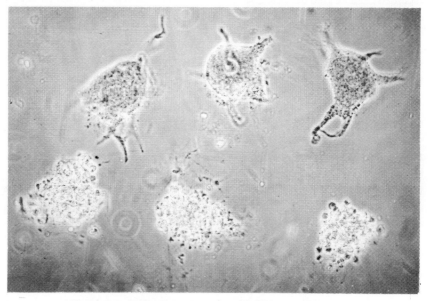

Figure 2.2. Three isolated nerve cells. Below each cell is a collection of neuronal glia of the same volume as that of the nerve cell, i.e. around 90 000 μm^3, and with the same weight, 20 000 pg.

at the 10^{-8} to 10^{-10} g level and subfractionation of glia into astrocytes, oligodendrocytes and microglia can be done by microseparation in only a few situations and then only with a low degree of accuracy.

The macro-procedure has, however, greater disadvantages. It takes hours, not minutes, to prepare bulk preparations and soluble substances are easily lost. Furthermore, such fractions cannot be obtained from small defined areas, but only from whole brain areas such as the cortex. Contamination with dendritic debris is greater, especially in the case of the glial fractions. The numerous so-called synaptic globules seem to be glial membrane debris posing as synaptic globules. One obvious advantage of the macrofractions is that almost any biochemical method of analysis can be applied.

Nerve cells and their glia: relationships and differences 31

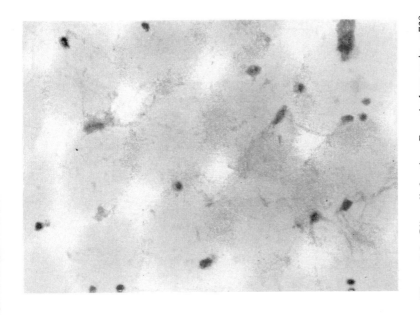

Figure 2.4. Glia cell fraction. Papanicolaou stain. ×720. (From Blomstrand and Hamberger, 1969.)

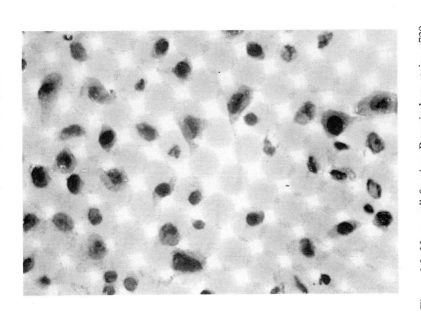

Figure 2.3. Nerve cell fraction. Papanicolaou stain. ×720. (From Blomstrand and Hamberger, 1969.)

In the preparation of the bulk separation (Figure 2.5), the cortices are sliced in 0·4 mm sections and incubated in a Krebs Ringer solution at 37°C for half an hour. They are then passed through two nylon nets, the first with a 1 mm mesh, the

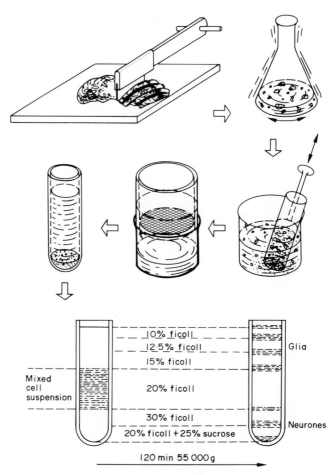

Figure 2.5. Outline of the neurone–glia preparative procedure. (From Blomstrand, 1971.)

second with a 50 μm mesh. This produces a primary suspension of mixed cells and small particles free from larger cell aggregates. The suspension is centrifuged at low speed to sediment the cells, the cell debris remaining largely in the supernatant. An important feature of this procedure is the use of Ficoll in a discontinuous 10–30 per cent gradient for centrifugation. The glial fraction remains at the 12 per cent Ficoll concentration, and the nerve cells can be sampled at the 30 per cent Ficoll level.

Biochemical differences between nerve cells and glia

Next let us consider some of the differences between nerve cells and glia. The oxygen consumption is five to ten times higher in neurones than in the glia (Figure 2.6). The glia also have a greater capacity for anaerobic glycolysis, and there is a pronounced glucose shunt metabolism. It seems, therefore, that the respiratory rate of the oligodendrocytes is higher than that of the astrocytes. The histochemical observations of Friede (1963) revealed an inverse relationship between

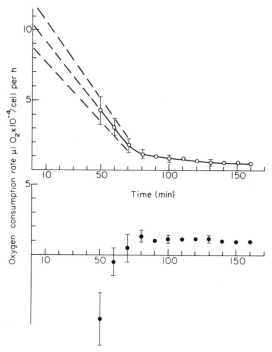

Figure 2.6. The oxygen consumption rate of nerve cells and glia expressed as $\mu l \; O_2 \times 10^{-4}$/sample, as a function of time after removal of the cells from the living animal. The standard deviation of the means (standard error) is given for the first four sets of values used for the extrapolation and for two further sets of values measured at the decreased oxygen consumption rate. The averages of the first four sets of values for the nerve cells (○) are significantly different from the zero (blank) level with a high degree of significance, contrary to those of the glial cells (●) which are not significantly different from zero.

the oxidative enzyme activities of axons and the Schwann cells, which suggests a symbiotic relationship between the two. Our study of the oxygen consumption was made with a micro-manometric method involving the Cartesian microdiver (Hydén and Pigon, 1960). Table 2.1 gives some data on the differential way in which substrates are oxidised by nerve cells and the glial cells immediately surrounding them and by the glia which surround capillaries. This differentiation of the glia is based on their location and not on a histological characterisation. The cytochrome oxidase activity in both types of glia is almost three times as high as that of the nerve cells and the rate of succinate oxidation is higher in the glia and highest in the capillary glia. Oxidation of α-ketoglutarate is also highest in the capillary glia, but surprisingly, it is of the same value in the nerve cell and

Table 2.1

Enzyme activity in nerve cells, neuronal and capillary glia of Deiters' nucleus: Enzyme activity expressed as 10^{-4} μl O_2/hour. Mean values ±S.E.M.

	Nerve cell	n	Neuronal glia	n	Capillary glia	n
Cytochrome oxidase	4·2 ± 0·6*	16	11·5 ± 0·8*	17	11·6 ± 1·1	10
Succinate oxidation	2·2 ± 0·3*	17	4·2 ± 0·5	9	6·9 ± 0·7	9
α-Ketoglutarate oxidation	2·2 ± 0·4	9	2·1 ± 0·2	12	4·0 ± 0·7	13
Glutamate oxidation	2·2 ± 0·3†	21	1·1 ± 0·2	9	1·6 ± 0·4	10

* From Hydén & Pigon (1960).
† From Hamberger (1961).

the neuronal glia. In the presence of glutamate, the oxygen uptake was higher in the nerve cell than in the adjacent glia.

It is relevant to consider adenosine triphosphatase (ATPase) activity. From the results of his experiments with leech glial cells Kuffler (1967) showed that they possessed a mechanism which allowed potassium to enter during the rising phase of the slow potential; presumably this is a reflection of membrane capacitance. In 1962 Dr Cummins and I made a study of some compartments in Deiters' nucleus with respect to the ATPase activity. We determined hydrolysis of radioactive ATP by isolated nerve cells, isolated cell membranes and neuronal and capillary glia. The data we obtained furnished another aspect of a regulatory function of the glia as a potassium regulator and as a safety mechanism for the nerve cell.

Figure 2.7 demonstrates the microsurgical preparation technique. The isolated nerve cell bodies are cut open by hand with a knife and the contents of the cell including the nucleus are removed by micropipette and careful dissection. The remaining outer part of the cell is folded back against the glass surface and more

Nerve cells and their glia: relationships and differences   35

material is removed from the interior surface. The remaining thin membranous structure has a thickness of about 0·2 μm measured interferometrically.

The glia samples had a high ATPase activity (Table 2.2), whether intact or homogenised, whereas whole nerve cells showed no ATPase activity except when homogenised, when they too had high activity. The nerve cell membranes had a definite

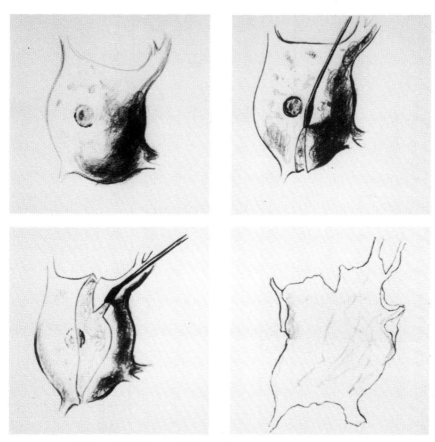

Figure 2.7. Microsurgical procedure to obtain isolated nerve cell membrane. Whole nerve cell, initial cut, cut along dendrite and prepared membrane.

activity. We concluded that there is no ATPase activity on the surface of nerve cells freed from their glia, but that the interior of the nerve cell close to the cell membrane has a considerable capacity to hydrolyse ATP. We then studied some of the requirements of this ATPase activity and found that with sodium, magnesium and buffer, the activity was 0·14 pmol. This value was doubled in the

Table 2.2

ATPase activity in Deiters' nerve cells, nerve cell membranes and oligodendroglia.

Medium	A		B		C	
	NaCl 128 mM–Tris 25·0 mM MgSO$_4$ 0·7 mM KCl 5·0 mM CaCl$_2$ 0·9 mM (pH 7·4)		NaCl 100 mM–Tris 25·0 mM MgSO$_4$ 5 mM (pH 7·4)		Sucrose 200 mM–Tris 25·0 mM MgSO$_4$ 5 mM (pH 7·4)	
	Nerve cells	Glia	Nerve cells	Glia	Nerve cells	Glia
Whole cells	0 to 0·3	2·0 ± 0·4 (6)	0	2·4 ± 1·1 (6)	0	1·7 ± 0·3 (4)
Homogenised	0·7 ± 0·5 (4)	1·3 ± 0·7 (3)	0·9 ± 0·47 (6)	1·0 ± 0·5 (7)	0·76 ± 0·11 (3)	1·0 ± 0·6 (4)
Isolated nerve cell membranes	0·27 ± 0·07 (7)	—	0·24 ± 0·02 (7)	—	0·23 ± 0·06 (4)	—

Values expressed in pmol of ATP hydrolysed per sample/hour (mean ± s.D.). Number of rabbits: 41. Number of analyses: given in parenthesis, each consisting of 8–15 cells or equal volume of glia.

nerve cell membranes by adding potassium, suggesting that this type of ATPase activity is highly potassium dependent; it is also dependent upon sodium, and it is obliterated by ouabain. What part of the total nerve cell ATPase activity is contributed by the cell membrane? In a cell weighing about 20 000 pg, the cell membrane constitutes about 2000 pg and has a quarter of the ATPase activity of the whole cell. There is therefore a high specific activity in this structure. From these studies we conclude that the glia can capture and release potassium.

Neurones and glia also differ in the amount and base ratios of their RNA. Per unit dry weight, glia contain only one tenth as much RNA as the big nerve cells. This difference is due to the large amount of ribosomal RNA in the nerve cell. The amount of DNA-dependent RNA-polymerase is correspondingly higher in nerve cells. The high values of adenine and uracil in the glial RNA in the

Table 2.3

RNA base composition of hypoglossal nerve cells and glia from rabbits.

Base	Nerve cells	Glia	P
Adenine	21·1 ± 0·63	28·1 ± 1·30	<0·001
Guanine	24·8 ± 0·60	23·5 ± 1·47	
Cytosine	31·9 ± 0·53	21·8 ± 1·15	<0·01
Uracil	22·2 ± 0·53	26·6 ± 1·83	<0·05

RNA base composition is expressed as mean values of molar percentages of the sum ±S.E.M. (From Daneholt and Brattgård, 1966.)

hypoglossal cells (Table 2.3) (Daneholt and Brattgård, 1966) probably arise because the nuclear RNA is dominant in the glial samples. Taking the big nerve cells of Deiters' nucleus and their glia as examples (Table 2.4), it can be seen that the proportion between the guanine and cytosine values varies inversely. The quantity and composition of RNA differ in different types of neurones and their glia, and a statement about values should be accompanied by an accurate description of cell type and locus. This is usually overlooked. The results of our incorporation studies indicated that the rate of the synthesis of glial RNA is twice that of the nerve cell.

I should like to remind you of the localisation of one of the brain-specific proteins I spoke of in the last lecture. The S-100 protein is localised in the bodies of the glia and in the nucleus of the nerve cell. Differences in the lipid composition of glia and nerve cells have been reported by Derry and Wolfe (1967). They used isolated cells and found a ganglioside content which was several times higher in nerve cells than in glia. On the other hand, Norton and Poduslo (1969), using enriched bulk fractions, found that the glia were twice as rich in gangliosides as the nerve cells. In our

Table 2.4

The composition of the RNA in control Deiters' nerve cells and their oligodendroglial cells in rabbits. Micro-electrophoretic analysis of the RNA.

	Nerve cell		Glia mean		
	Mean	v	Mean	v	P
Adenine	19.7 ± 0.37	4.2	20.8 ± 0.28	3.0	
Guanine	33.5 ± 0.39	2.6	28.8 ± 0.64	5.0	0.001
Cytosine	28.8 ± 0.36	2.8	31.8 ± 0.27	2.0	0.001
Uracil	18.0 ± 0.18	2.3	18.6 ± 0.55	6.7	0.001

v = the coefficient of variation, $\dfrac{S \times 100}{\text{Mean}} \times$ P = probability after t test.

Nerve cell: 1500 pg of RNA per cell. Average dry weight: 20 000 pg.
Glia: 125 pg of RNA per sample. Average dry weight: 20 000 pg.
Purine and pyrimidine bases as molar proportions in percentages of the sum.
Number of animals: 5.
Number of analyses: 49.

own laboratory, Hamberger and Svennerholm (1971) also used enriched fractions and obtained the same result as Norton. They separated gangliosides by thin-layer chromatography and found that the concentration of gangliosides and sulphatides in the nerve cell was 50 per cent of that in the glia. The fatty acid composition of the

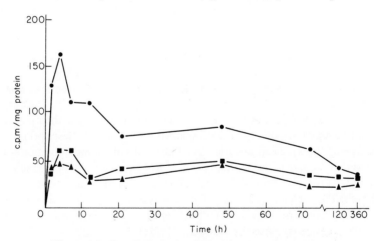

Figure 2.8. Protein-bound radioactivity in fractions from cerebral cortex against time after injection of [³H]leucine. (●), Nerve cell fraction; (■), glial cell fraction; (▲), myelin fraction. (From Blomstrand and Hamberger, 1969.)

Nerve cells and their glia: relationships and differences

phosphoglycerides was similar in the two types of cells. Figure 2.8 shows the difference between the incorporation of tritiated leucine into glial protein and nerve cell protein. It is two to three times higher in the nerve cell fraction and has a half-life of approximately fifteen hours (Blomstrand and Hamberger, 1969).

The *in vitro* experiments which Blomstrand and Hamberger (1970) recently performed at different oxygen concentrations gave interesting results (Figure 2.9). They showed that if slices of the cortex are incubated for thirty minutes with tritiated leucine in an oxygen-saturated atmosphere with succinate as oxidisable substrate, the incorporation of leucine in the nerve cell protein is about five times larger than that in the glia. But a decrease in the oxygen tension affects the nerve cells

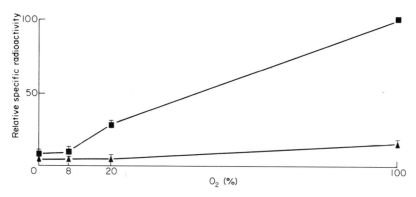

Figure 2.9. [^{3}H]leucine incorporation into the trichloroacetic acid-precipitable residue of the neuronal (■——■) and glial (▲——▲) fractions in relation to rate of oxygenation during the incubation of cortical slices. Glucose was used as oxidisable substrate. Incubation time thirty minutes. Each point shows the mean ± S.E.M. of five experiments. (From Blomstrand and Hamberger, 1970.)

more than the glia, reflecting the fact that the glia have a greater capacity for anaerobic glycolysis than the nerve cells. Figures 2.10–2.12 compare the neuronal and glial incorporation of [^{3}H]leucine into subcellular fractions (Hamberger, Blomstrand and Yanagihara, 1971) of bulk isolated nerve cells and glia (Figure 2.10), cortex slices (Figure 2.11) and cell-enriched fractions after incubation with [^{3}H]leucine (Figure 2.12). It can be seen that the unfractionated neuronal material had a higher level of protein-bound [^{3}H]leucine than the glial material. It is interesting to note from the subcellular fractions that there was a marked neuronal-glia difference in microsomes and soluble proteins.

A more striking difference between nerve cells and glia was observed by Hamberger (1971). Amino-isobutyric acid is not metabolised or incorporated by

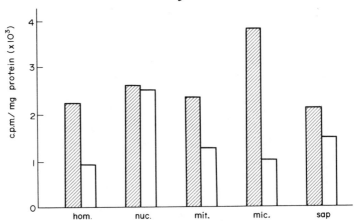

Figure 2.10. Protein-bound radioactivity in homogenate (hom.), nuclei (nuc.), mitochondria (mit.), microsomes (mic.) and sap from neuronal (▨) and glial (□) fractions of cerebral cortex after two injections of [^{3}H]leucine 120 and 180 minutes before sacrifice (100 µCi/kg body weight each time). Mean values of two experiments. (From Blomstrand, 1971.)

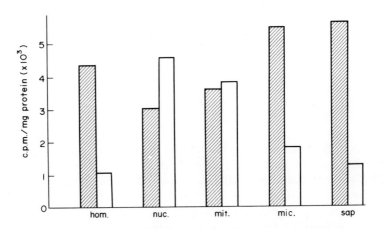

Figure 2.11. Protein-bound radioactivity in homogenate (hom.), nuclei (nuc.), mitochondria (mit.), microsomes (mic.) and sap from neuronal (▨) and glial (□) fractions prepared after incubation of cortex slices for 30 minutes with [^{3}H]leucine (10 mCi/mmol). Mean values of two experiments. (From Blomstrand, 1971.)

cells, and therefore it is suitable for transport studies. The glial fraction concentrated amino-isobutyric acid five to six times more than the nerve cells. The potassium concentration strikingly affected the leucine uptake in the glia (Figure 2.13). With no potassium, the leucine concentration in both glia and neurones was low, but with 5 mM potassium, there was a big peak in the glia but not in the

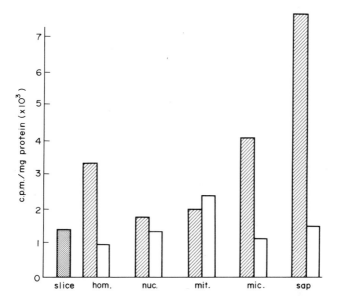

Figure 2.12. Protein-bound radioactivity in homogenate (hom.), nuclei (nuc.), mitochondria (mit.), microsomes (mic.), and sap from neuronal (▨) and glial (□) fractions after incubation of each cell-enriched fraction with [^{3}H]leucine (10 μCi/ml, 100 mCi/mmol) for thirty minutes. Left (▨) column represents the radioactivity in unfractionated cortex slices. Mean values of two experiments. (From Blomstrand, 1971.)

neurones. Thus it could be concluded that there is a higher rate of transport of amino acids into glia than into nerve cells, but not that there is a higher rate of incorporation of amino acids into protein in nerve cells than in the glia. The possibility that the higher uptake of amino acids in the glia is due to damage of the membrane can be ruled out since the ratio of incorporation of amino acid into nerve cells and glia is not lower in isolated fractions than in slices. Whether or not these results reflect a transport mechanism for amino acids or proteins from glia to nerve cells where the main part of the protein synthesis occurs is a question I shall return to

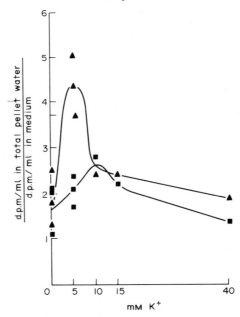

Figure 2.13. Effect of K^+ levels in the medium on amino acid (leucine, 0.1 mM) uptake into neuronal (■) and glial (▲) cell suspensions. d.p.m.: Disintegrations per minute. (From Hamberger, 1971.)

after discussion of some metabolic changes which indicate a close collaboration between nerve cells and their glia.

Inverse neurone–glia changes as a function of stimulation

Vestibular stimulation back and forth was produced by oscillating the animal's head through an arc of 120°. After such stimulation and inhibition for twenty-five minutes a day for seven days, we found an increase in the RNA and protein content of the nerve cells in the lateral vestibular nucleus and a slight but significant decrease of these substances in the glia and inverse changes with respect to the cytochrome oxidase activity in both types of cells (Figure 2.14) (Hydén and Pigon, 1960). When the cytochrome oxidase activity in the glia decreased, the anaerobic glycolysis increased by 70 per cent, but decreased in the nerve cells by 23 per cent. This suggests that there is a close collaboration between these two types of cells with a possible exchange of RNA and proteins. As a function of such a stimulation we found in a further experiment (using succinate as the oxidisable substrate) that the rate of activity increased in the nerve cells as a function of stimulation, three to five times, but that the glia was not greatly affected (Hamberger and Hydén, 1963).

In kinetic studies, the effects of both stimulation and hypoxia indicated that the neurone has energy priority over the glia during a change of functional equilibrium. There is an oscillation which indicates a metabolic coupling between two levels of enzyme activities. Using brains from sleeping rabbits, we obtained results we had not expected, and which showed the advantage of micro-techniques. In nuclei throughout the brain stem, we found the greatest change in the nucleus reticularis

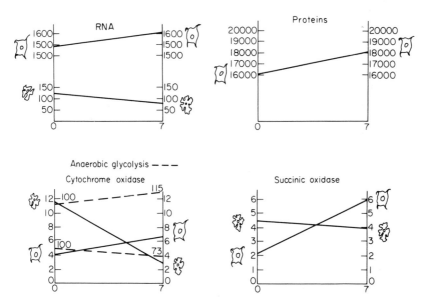

Figure 2.14. Survey picture of quantitative macromolecular changes in vestibular nerve cells after stimulation.

giganto-cellularis in the caudal part of the reticular formation during the transition from wakefulness to sleep (Hydén and Lange, 1965). The rabbits were trained to sleep for three hours per session and to kill them, because we could not shoot them or use poison or gas, we constructed according to old principles an automatic guillotine which killed the rabbits on the twelfth day when the recordings showed sleep activity from the cortex. We rapidly dissected out nerve cells and glia from various parts of the brain in the cold, and found, using succinate as a substrate, that during wakefulness the enzyme activity was highest in the glia, and that during sleep it was highest in the nerve cells (Table 2.5). In the oralis part of this reticular nucleus, we found only slight changes in the nerve cells, reflecting such an oscillation and no changes in the glia. For controls we used nerve cells and glia from the mesencephalic nucleus and the hypoglossal nuclei where we did not find similar changes.

I would like to stress that the nuclei we studied were not separated by more than 0·5 to 2 mm from each other. Such rhythmic inverse changes during sleep may reflect the biological clock behind the sleep rhythm, although it may not be the ultimate factor in the physiological sleep mechanism. On the other hand there were

Table 2.5

Succinoxidase activity of neurones and glia isolated from rabbits. The results are expressed as 10^{-4} μl O_2/sample per hour. Group 1, sleep; group 2, wakefulness; group 3, cage controls.

Group	Nerve cells		Glia	
	Activity (10^{-4} μl O_2)	No. of analyses	Activity (10^{-4} μl O_2)	No. of analyses
Nucleus reticularis giganto-cellularis				
1	3·41 ± 0·51	29	2·34 ± 0·18	25
2	1·30 ± 0·25	24	3·06 ± 0·24	28
3	2·74 ± 0·21	39	2·16 ± 0·18	33
Nucleus reticularis pontis oralis				
1	6·38 ± 0·58	35	3·50 ± 0·30	19
2	4·01 ± 0·52	15	2·94 ± 0·21	17
3	5·41 ± 0·39	32	3·72 ± 0·58	12
Nucleus trigeminus mesencephalicus				
1	2·68 ± 0·29	9	1·46 ± 0·23	8
2	3·08 ± 0·83	5	1·11 ± 0·12	5
3	3·21 ± 1·16	5	1·15 ± 0·15	13
Nucleus hypoglossus				
1	1·03 ± 0·17	13		
2	0·83 ± 0·08	13		
3	0·68 ± 0·13	3		

When wakefulness was compared to sleep, the difference between the enzyme values in nucleus reticularis giganto-cellularis proved to be significant both for nerve cells ($P < 0.001$) and glia ($P < 0.02$). Values for group 1 compared to those for group 3 were not significant. The difference between the values for the nerve cells in the nucleus reticularis pontis oralis of groups 1 and 2 was significant ($P < 0.01$).

no inverse enzyme changes in nerve cells and glia during barbiturate sleep when all values were low in comparison with the controls.

Rabbits can withstand a decrease in oxygen tension without apparent pathological changes. In our experiment we used 8 per cent oxygen and 92 per cent nitrogen for fifteen hours and found that in the nerve cells the RNA content and respiratory enzyme activity increased significantly (Hamberger and Hydén, 1963), the latter by more than three times. The anaerobic glycolysis of the nerve cells also increased by 57 per cent. In contrast, the glia did not respond in any of these cases, a result which tallies with the old experience that glia can withstand a considerable lack of oxygen. The response of the nerve cells we interpreted as a defence reaction. All these changes were reversible.

Neurone–glia interaction in two neuropathological conditions

In collaboration with Professor G. Gomirato of the University of Pisa, we had the unique opportunity to observe the quantitative and base ratio changes in RNA from cases of Parkinson's disease and Huntington's chorea (Gomirato and Hydén, 1963; Hydén, 1966). The biopsies were taken in connection with therapeutic operations

Table 2.6

RNA base ratios of nerve cells in globus pallidus in Huntington's chorea and Parkinson's disease, expressed as molar per cent of total base.

	Chorea (7 cases)	Parkinson (8 cases)	Controls (4 cases)
Adenine	21.5 ± 0.38	20.7 ± 0.65	18.3 ± 0.42
Guanine	23.7 ± 0.42	28.8 ± 0.25	30.5 ± 0.44
Cytosine	35.3 ± 0.68	34.4 ± 0.79	35.3 ± 0.60
Uracil	19.4 ± 0.29	16.1 ± 0.38	15.9 ± 0.36
$\frac{G + C}{A + U}$	1.41	1.71	1.93

Number of nerve cells analysed per case: 100.

and from the globus pallidus. We found surprisingly large changes in the glia in these carefully chosen cases and in both the Parkinson and the Huntington material, the amount of RNA in both the nerve cell and the glial samples was greater than the controls by 25–30 per cent. In Table 2.6 it can be seen that the nerve cell RNA composition differed significantly with respect to the adenine and guanine values only in Parkinsonism. In the glial samples, surprisingly large RNA changes had taken place (Table 2.7), the trend being similar in both types of material, although there were some differences. In two cases it was interesting to find that these RNA changes, which clearly reflected a primary biochemical error, began in the glia and were later observed in the nerve cells apparently simultaneously with the onset of clinical symptoms. When only glial RNA changed, very few clinical symptoms could be found. These biochemical findings demonstrate a differentiation in response of the glia and the neurones they surround with a dependence of the neurones on the glia.

Table 2.7

RNA base ratios of glia samples in globus pallidus in Huntington's chorea and Parkinson's disease, expressed as molar per cent of total base.

	Chorea (7 cases)	Parkinson (8 cases)	Controls (4 cases)
Adenine	30·7 ± 0·61	30·8 ± 0·70	19·0 ± 0·78
Guanine	22·1 ± 0·47	20·3 ± 0·90	29·1 ± 0·15
Cytosine	28·3 ± 0·52	33·2 ± 1·70	33·7 ± 0·72
Uracil	19·0 ± 0·37	15·7 ± 0·60	18·2 ± 0·36
$\dfrac{G+C}{A+U}$	1·04	1·74	1·68

Number of samples analysed per case: 90.

Neurone: increase 550 pg RNA

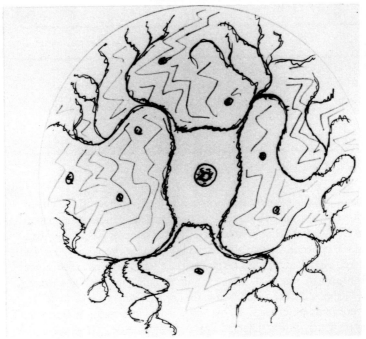

Adenine 22·5 ± 1·61
Guanine 37·7 ± 1·66
Cytosine 21·0 ± 2·0
Uracil   18·8 ± 0·91

Adenine 21·6 ± 1·10
Guanine 37·8 ± 3·0
Cytosine 23·0 ± 3·33
Uracil   17·6 ± 1·50

Glia: decrease 500 pg RNA

Figure 2.15. Schematic representation of concomitant changes in the glial and neuronal compartment with induced RNA changes, indicating transfer of RNA from glia to neurone.

To return to a more general question, because amino acids are transported faster into the glia than into the nerve cells whereas they are incorporated into protein at a faster rate in the nerve cells, it is likely that there is a mechanism for transporting amino acids from the glia to the neurone. Other studies with RNA also provided evidence for such a glia–neurone relationship. Thus, tricyanoaminopropene induced an increase in the RNA of the nerve cells in many parts of the brain and a decrease in the surrounding glia (Egyhazi and Hydén, 1961). This substance also caused certain base ratio changes, indicating that the RNA—mostly ribosomal RNA—formed during the first hour after the injection was different to the original. One hour after the injection of 20 mg into a rabbit, the amount of RNA in the big nerve cells of the lateral vestibular nucleus increased from 1500 pg to 2070 pg; that in the glial sample decreased by 55 pg. Then using the volume values for the cell and dendritic territories of such cells determined by Sholl (1960), Schadé, Backer and Colon (1964) and others, we calculated a loss of 500 pg of RNA from the nerve cells' immediate glial territory compared with the neuronal increase of 550 pg (Hydén and Lange, 1966). We also calculated the composition of the RNA lost in the glia and of the RNA fraction increased in the nerve cells. Figure 2.15 shows these values to be remarkably similar, and together with other results, they are a good indication that polymerised RNA is transferred from the glia to their neurone. The energy requirements for macromolecules to pass membrane structures in carrier systems did not seem to pose any difficulties (Eigen and Maeyer, 1971).

Some remarks on glial function

A summary of these observations suggests some glia functions. The response of the nerve cell and its surrounding glia, at changed functional equilibrium, indicates that they are linked metabolically. The rate of biosyntheses can swing between two levels and, from a cybernetic point of view, such a system is a stable one. The capture and release of potassium by the glia; the localisation of brain-specific protein to the glia and the differences with respect to the neurones; the finding of a high amino acid uptake capacity of the glia; a higher incorporation of amino acids into the nerve cell protein; and the indication of a transfer of RNA from glia to the neurone all suggest a programming of the neurone by the glia. And if these observations are linked to what is known about the rapid transport of protein and precursors in the axon and the possibility of local synthesis of protein in the axon, one gets a picture of the function of the glia, not only as a metabolic auxiliary system or stabiliser of the neurone, but also as a partner at almost all levels in a two-cell collaboration.

References

ADEY, W. R., KADO, R. T., DIDIO, J. and SCHINDLER, W. J. (1963). Impedance changes in cerebral tissue accompanying a learned discriminative performance in the cat. *Expl Neurol.*, **7**, 259–81.

BLOMSTRAND, C. (1971). *Studies on Protein Metabolism in Neuronal and Glial Cell-Enriched Fractions from Brain Tissue.* Thesis. Göteborg.

BLOMSTRAND, C. and HAMBERGER, A. (1969). Protein turnover in cell-enriched fractions from rabbit brain. *J. Neurochem.*, **16**, 1401–7.

BLOMSTRAND, C. and HAMBERGER, A. (1970). Amino acid incorporation *in vitro* into protein of neuronal and glial cell-enriched fractions. *J. Neurochem.*, **17**, 1187–95.

BRATTGÅRD, S.-O. and HYDÉN, H. (1952). Mass, lipids, pentose nucleoproteins and proteins determined in nerve cells by X-ray micro-radiography. *Acta radiol.*, **94**, Suppl. 15, 1–48.

BRATTGÅRD, S.-O. and HYDÉN, H. (1954). The composition of the nerve cell studied with new methods. *Int. Rev. Cytol.*, **3**, 455–76.

CUMMINS, J. and HYDÉN, H. (1962). Adenosine triphosphate levels and adenosine triphosphatases in neurons, glia and neuronal membranes of the vestibular nucleus. *Biochim. biophys. Acta*, **60**, 271–83.

DANEHOLT, B. and BRATTGÅRD, S.-O. (1966). A comparison between RNA metabolism of nerve cells and glia in the hypoglossal nucleus of the rabbit. *J. Neurochem.*, **13**, 913–21.

DERRY, D. M. and WOLFE, L. S. (1967). Gangliosides in isolated neurons and glial cells. *Science, N.Y.*, **158**, 1450–2.

EGYHAZI, E. and HYDÉN, H. (1961). Experimentally induced changes in the base composition of the ribonucleic acids of isolated nerve cells and their oligodendroglial cells. *J. biophys. biochem. Cytol.*, **10**, 403–10.

EIGEN, M. and MAEYER, L. DE (1971). Carriers and specificity in membranes. *Neurosci. Res. Progr. Bull.*, **9**, 299–437.

FRIEDE, R. L. (1963). The relationship of body size, nerve cell size, axon length, and glial density in the cerebellum. *Proc. natn. Acad. Sci., U.S.A.*, **49**, 187–93.

GLEES, P. (1955). *Neuroglia, Morphology and Function.* Blackwell, Oxford.

GOMIRATO, G. and HYDÉN, H. (1963). A biochemical glia error in the Parkinson disease. *Brain*, **86**, 773–80.

HAMBERGER, A. (1961). Oxidation of tricarboxylic acid cycle intermediates by nerve cell bodies and glial cells. *J. Neurochem.*, **8**, 31–5.

HAMBERGER, A. (1971). Amino acid uptake in neuronal and glial cell fractions from rabbit cerebral cortex. *Brain Res.*, **31**, 169–78.

HAMBERGER, A., BLOMSTRAND, C. and YANAGIHARA, T. (1971). Subcellular distribution of radioactivity in neuronal and glial-enriched fractions after incorporation of ^{3}H-leucine *in vivo* and *in vitro*. *J. Neurochem.*, **18**, 1469–78.

HAMBERGER, A. and HYDÉN, H. (1963). Inverse enzymatic changes in neurons and glia during increased function and hypoxia. *J. cell. Biol.*, **16**, 521–5.

HAMBERGER, A. and SVENNERHOLM, L. (1971). Composition of gangliosides and phospholipids of neuronal and glial cell enriched fractions. *J. Neurochem.*, **18**, 1821.

HIS, W. (1890). Histogenese und Zusammenhang der Nervenelemente. *Arch. Anat. Physiol.* suppl. **25**, 95–117.

HOLMGREN, E. (1902). Beiträge zur Morphologie der Zelle. I. Nervenzellen. *Anat. Hefte*, **18**, 267–325.

HYDÉN, H. (1959). Quantitative assay of compounds in isolated fresh nerve cells from control and stimulated animals. *Nature, Lond.*, **184**, 433–5.

HYDÉN, H. (1966). Production of RNA in neurons and glia in Parkinson's disease indicating genic stimulation. In: *Biochemistry and Pharmacology of the Basal Ganglia* (COSTA, E., CÔTÉ, L. J. and YAHR, M. D., Eds.), pp. 195–204. Raven Press, New York.

HYDÉN, H. and LANGE, P. W. (1965). Rhythmic enzyme changes in neurons and glia during sleep. *Science, N.Y.*, **149**, 654–6.

HYDÉN, H. and LANGE, P. W. (1966). A genic stimulation with production of adenine-uracil rich RNA in neurons and glia in learning. *Naturwiss.*, **53**, 64–70.

HYDÉN, H. and LARSSON, S. (1956). The application of a scanning and computing cell analyser to neurocytological problems. *J. Neurochem.*, **1**, 134–44.

HYDÉN, H. and PIGON, A. (1960). A cytophysiological study of the functional relationship between oligodendroglial cells and nerve cells of Deiters' nucleus. *J. Neurochem.*, **6**, 57–72.

KUFFLER, S. W. (1967). Neuroglial cells: physiological properties and a potassium mediated effect of neuronal activity on the glial membrane potential. *Proc. R. Soc.*, B., **168**, 1–21.

NANSEN, F. (1886). *The Structure and Combination of the Histological Elements of the Central Nervous System.* Bergens Museum Aarbs, Bergen.

NORTON, W. T. and PODUSLO, S. E. (1969). Isolation and some properties of whole neuroglia and neuronal perikaya from rat brain. *Abstr. Int. Soc. Neurochem.* 2nd Meet. (PAOLETTI, R., FUMAGALLI, R. and GALLI, C., Eds.), pp. 44–5. Tamburini, Milan.

RAMÓN Y CAJAL, S. (1910). *Histologie du système nerveux de l'homme et des vertébrés.* Maloine, Paris.

ROSE, S. P. R. (1967). Preparation of enriched fractions from cerebral cortex containing isolated metabolically active neuronal and glial cells. *Biochem. J.*, **102**, 33–43.

Rosengren, B. H. O. (1959). Determination of cell mass by direct X-ray absorption. *Acta radiol.* suppl., **178**, 1–62.

Schadé, J. P., Backer, H. van and Colon, E. (1964). Quantitative analysis of neuronal parameters in the maturing cerebral cortex. *Prog. Brain Res.*, **4**, 150–75.

Schleich, C. L. (1916). *Vom Schaltwerk der Gedanken.* Fischer, Berlin.

Sholl, D. A. (1960). Anatomical heterogeneity in the cerebral cortex. In: *2nd Int. Meet. Neurobiol.*, Amsterdam, 1959 (Tower, D. B. and Schadé, J. P., Eds.), pp. 21–7. Elsevier, Amsterdam.

Spielmayer, W. (1922). *Histopathologie des Nervensystems.* Berlin.

Virchow, R. (1846). Ueber das granulierte Ausschen der Windungen der Gehirnventrikel. *Allg. Z. Psychiat.*, **3**, 242–885.

Weigert, C. (1895). *Encyclopädie d. mikroskop. Technik.*

RNA changes in brain cells during changes in behaviour and function

H. HYDÉN (GÖTEBORG)

The relationship between brain RNA and the mechanism serving registration and storage of new information in the brain has certainly been the subject of much attention in the literature as well as in the mass media, and it is interesting or sad, depending on how you look at it, that every piece of news of that kind has contributed to an anatomy of confusion which would even make James Thurber reel. In the cross-talk between neurobiologists, chemists and psychologists, there have been misunderstandings in the interpretation of the data over the last ten years. There is also no clear agreement on a reproducible behavioural test which could be used by biochemists and psychologists alike. Progress in the field goes on as usual, however, with the slaughter of beautiful hypotheses by ugly facts, and some facts have emerged.

Posing some problems

In this lecture I should like to make two points. Firstly, large-scale changes and synthesis occur in the ribosomal type of RNA of brain cells which may have nothing to do with behaviour *per se*, but which are seen during changes in behaviour as well as under other functional conditions. Secondly, there is a more specific type of RNA change, a synthesis of small amounts of RNA with high adenine and uracil values which so far has been found only during change in behaviour. As with proteins I would like to stress that there is no evidence that RNA in brain cells can store experiential information within its own structure like a tape-recorder. That a tune by the Beatles, for example, could be stored in one molecule, and Tchaikovsky's B flat Concerto in another one, is not very likely.

One could argue that this would require too many bits even for the molecules of 10^{10} brain cells of the cortex. By analogy with evolution one could also say that knowledge of the structure and properties of DNA and RNA molecules is not likely to solve evolution, learning, or memory. Since the brain is a hierarchic system of highest complexity, I would postulate as does Bertalanffy (1970) that to analyse memory and learning mechanisms ultimately other tools will be needed and used in addition to molecular analysis and thermodynamics of hierarchically dynamic systems. Nevertheless, several molecular mechanisms have been suggested. For example, the question has been raised, whether part of the RNA in brain cells can undergo hysteresis, in the form of conformational changes of long duration. Katchalsky and his co-workers (1966, 1970, 1972) have shown in model experiments that macromolecules may undergo hysteresis as a function of pH change. They suggest that the hysteresis phenomena in RNA could well be involved in the storage of information in brain cells, because such changes are independent of time but dependent on previous experience. Through the hysteresis the molecules could become organised in some regions to hold a higher informational content. The molecule enters a metastable state which is not easily disturbed thermally. Such a procedure would require a small investment of free energy; for example, each adenine would require 1·5 kcal. Another hypothetical substrate for long-term storage of information is DNA, together with DNA changes induced by electrical field changes and mediated by RNA, and DNA-dependent DNA Polymerase.

Instead of expanding a hypothesis I should like to discuss some of the RNA changes that are known to occur in brain cells, both with respect to quantity and quality. One has to make this distinction between large-scale RNA changes which have also been found to accompany learning in whole brain samples and in cell samples, and the nuclear RNA changes that occur on a minute scale. I will give some examples of RNA changes in brain cells when there is an increased demand on the activity of nerve cells and glia with respect to sensory modalities, motor activity and the effect of chemicals and training. These large-scale changes could be contrasted with minute quantitative and qualitative changes which are seen in the training of animals.

The problem is therefore to determine whether at least two types of RNA changes occur during learning. First, our data suggest that a large-scale RNA increase occurs where the RNA produced is of the guanine-cytosine-rich type. This type of RNA response is seen as a prompt effect of many types of stimuli and seems unspecific in relation to the more specific processes related to learning. Second, during learning, small amounts of nuclear RNA are also produced in nerve cells which are predominantly of a type rich in adenine and uracil. Such an RNA fraction could imply an increase in the minute pre-existing RNA fraction, or it could imply the production of a new type of RNA which, as an assumption, is induced by the repression of the synthesis of specific proteins.

Age and neuronal RNA

Let us look next at some of the material we have used. An ultraviolet picture of a thin section through a nerve cell is an impressive sight (Figure 3.1). This photograph was taken at 260 nm, the absorption maximum of nucleic acids. The cells contain 1500 µg RNA which is mostly ribosomal. The cells were opened with a small knife by the technique described in Lecture I (Cummins and Hydén, 1962)

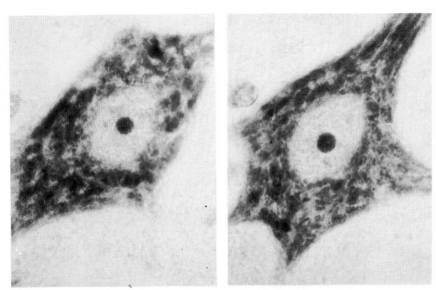

Figure 3.1. Micrograph taken at 260 nm of thin sections through nerve cells from the lateral vestibular nucleus of the rabbit.

and their contents were emptied in a small drop placed on the foil of an electron microscope grid. The polysomal RNA structures sediment and can then be studied in the electron microscope. They are delicate and easily destroyed, but by this technique they are not broken down by centrifugal forces and can be studied in a more native state. A frequency study showed that most polysomes in such nerve cells contain three to five ribosomes (Ekholm and Hydén, 1965) but several have many more. Using this microsurgical technique it was easy to show the presence of extensive polysomal structures in the nerve cell cytoplasm. The one in Figure 3.2 has more than twenty ribosomes attached to the messenger strand. There are also enormous polysomal structures containing more than a hundred ribosomes (Figure 3.3).

Some of the nerve cell samples we used for RNA analysis consisted of isolated nerve cell nuclei, thirty of which were used in each analysis. The nerve cells were

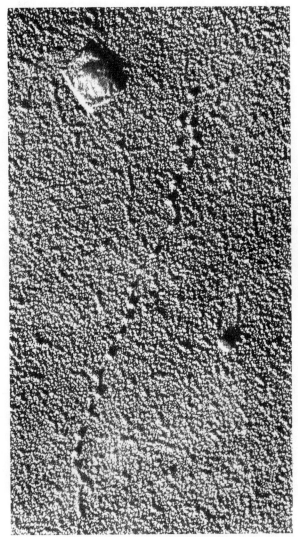

Figure 3.2. Shadowed preparation from normal Deiters' cells showing 10 nm particles in a linear formation. ×130 000.

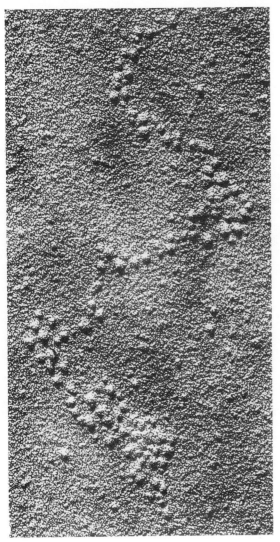

Figure 3.3. Shadowed preparation of normal Deiters' cells showing a huge cluster of ribosomes, possibly a giant polysome. ×120 000.

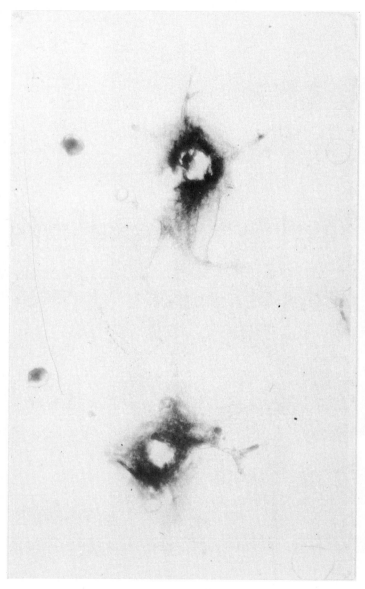

Figure 3.4. Two isolated Deiters' nerve cells cleaned from glia and treated with phenol–water. The nucleus from each cell has been taken out and the nuclei are seen situated above the nerve cells in the centre of which is seen the corresponding hole. Photographed at 257 nm. ×400.

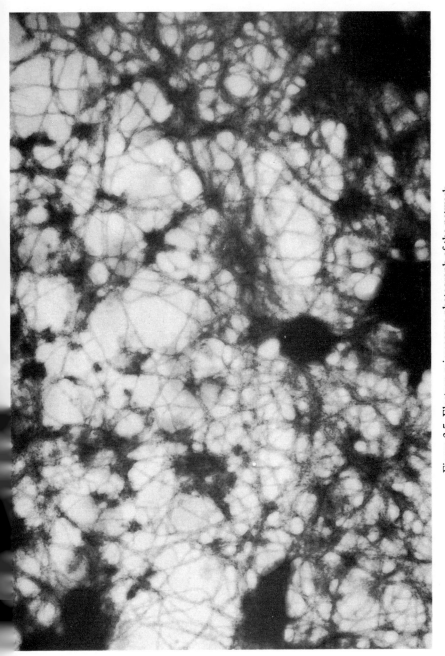

Figure 3.5. Electron microscope photograph of the network of 8 nm filaments close to the inner part of the nerve cell membrane. ×45 000, fixed with 1 per cent uranyl acetate.

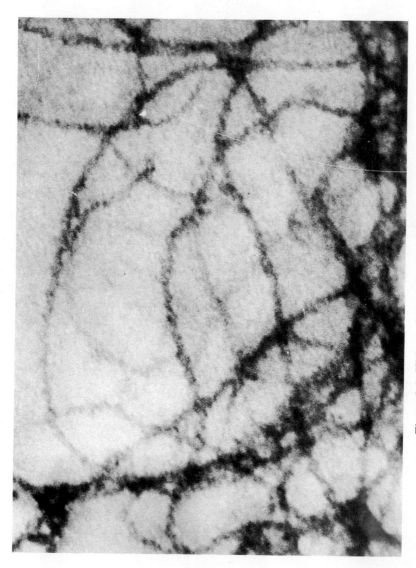

Figure 3.6. High resolution electron miscroscope photograph demonstrating that the filaments consist of intercoiled 2 nm unit-filaments. ×480 000.

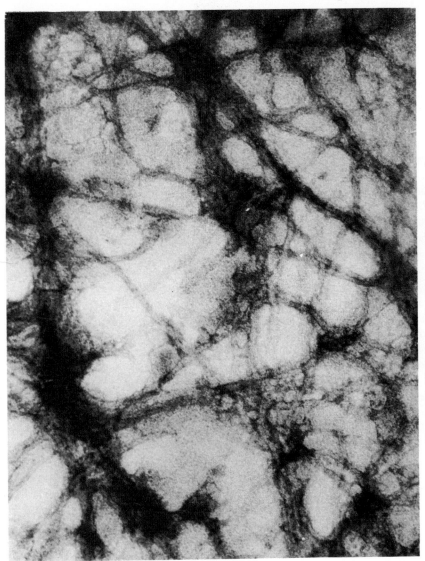

Figure 3.7. The effect of Ca^{++} is an uncoiling of the unit-filaments. ×480 000.

freed from glia and the nucleus of each cell was removed by microsurgery. Both the sampled nuclei and the nerve cell bodies, from which the nuclei had been removed, were used for RNA analysis (Figure 3.4).

In collaboration with Professor Metuzals, I have also demonstrated the existence of a structured protein close to the inner part of the nerve cell membrane (unpublished observations). Using the microsurgical technique, nerve cell membranes were prepared so that in parts they were only 20 nm in thickness. When these parts were photographed in the electron microscope, a reticulum of thin filaments was seen (Figure 3.5). At higher magnification the reticulum seemed to consist of two 2 nm filaments coiled around each other (Figure 3.6). No loose ends could be seen. The uncoiling in the presence of increased concentrations of Ca^{++} (Figure 3.7), its digestion by trypsin and its insolubility in water suggest highly structured protein. We have found that this continuous network consists of a protein with contractile properties. The filaments give arrow heads with heavy meromyosin. They do not contain RNA or DNA, but probably glycoproteins. They do not bind colchicine. This contractile network of continuous protein filaments could affect the tension of the membrane as a function of Ca^{++} and thus modulate its function (Hydén and Metuzals, unpublished observations).

The amount of RNA varies in nerve cells depending on the cell size and the ratio between the nuclear and the cytoplasmic volumes. Table 3.1 shows a variation from 70 pg to more than 1500 pg. Some of the cells in the cortex have a large nuclear to cytoplasm ratio. The base composition of the RNA also depends on some of these parameters. Table 3.2 gives some examples, but as yet the data are insufficient to make statements about RNA characteristics of nerve cells in phylogenetically different cell types. Table 3.3 demonstrates the difference in base ratios between vestibular nerve cells and the glia around the cells.

The rate of synthesis of RNA in the glia was found to be twice that in the nerve cells. Table 3.4 is from the study of the hypoglossal nerve cells and shows the *in vivo* incorporation of tritiated adenine and cytidine expressed as micromoles of labelled base per gram of RNA. The values for the glia were, with the exception of cytosine, twice the values for the nerve cells. When the incorporation is expressed as millimoles of labelled base per mole of base (Table 3.5), one sees that in glia each RNA base is labelled about twice as much as the corresponding base in nerve cells. Therefore, in these hypoglossal cells the labelled RNA of the nerve cells has a higher proportion of cytosine than that of the glia, and the synthesis of RNA is twice as rapid in glia as in nerve cells. This finding has been confirmed and extended by authors such as Volpe and Giuditta (1967a, b). Differential phenol extraction of the various RNA fractions of both nerve and glial cells revealed one small rapidly-labelled RNA fraction with a very high specific activity (Table 3.6).

Age also has an important bearing on the variation in the RNA content of nerve cells. Some years ago I made a study of the RNA content of neurones of the spinal

Table 3.1

RNA content in different types of nerve cells.

Type of nerve cell	RNA (pg/cell) mean values
Ganglion cells of the supraoptic nucleus, rabbit	70
Spinal ganglion cells, rabbit	1070
Hypoglossal cells, rabbit	200
Anterior horn cells, rabbit	530
Anterior horn cells, man 40–50 years	670
Anterior horn cells, man 60–70 years	540
Deiters' cells, rabbit	
Large type	1550
Small type	700

Table 3.2

Molar percentage of the bases in nerve cell RNA.

	N. Deiters' rabbit	N. Supraopt. rat	N. Deiters' rat	F. Reticul. rat	Glob. Pall. man
Adenine	19·7	18·9	20·7	19·5	17·1
Guanine	33·5	36·0	33·3	30·0	29·8
Cytosine	28·8	26·9	27·5	34·0	37·0
Uracil	18·0	18·2	18·5	16·5	16·1

Table 3.3

Composition of Deiters' nerve cell and glial RNA from control rats (base ratios expressed as molar proportions in per cent of the sum).

	Nerve Cells		Glia		P
	Mean	V	Mean	V	
Adenine	20·5 ± 0·54	5·5	25·3 ± 0·16	1·5	0·001
Guanine	33·7 ± 0·33	2·2	29·0 ± 0·24	1·9	0·001
Cytosine	27·4 ± 0·34	3·0	26·5 ± 0·43	3·7	
Uracil	18·4 ± 0·26	3·1	19·2 ± 0·27	3·1	
No. of animals	5		5		
No. of analyses	50		33		

V = variation coefficient, $(S \times 100)/\text{mean}$.

Table 3.4

In vivo incorporation of [³H]adenine and [³H]cytidine into RNA of hypoglossal nerve cells and glia from rabbits over 4 hours.

Base	Nerve cells	Glia
Adenine	2·6 ± 0·12	5·8 ± 0·66
Guanine	0·43 ± 0·05	1·0 ± 0·11
Cytosine	3·2 ± 0·16	2·8 ± 0·36
Uracil	0·90 ± 0·11	2·0 ± 0·30
A:G:C:U	2·9:0·48:3·6:1	2·9:0·50:1·4:1

The incorporation is expressed as μmol labelled base/g RNA (mean value ±S.E.M.). (From Daneholt and Brattgård, 1966.)

cord (C_5) of traffic accident cases from three to more than eighty years of age. Table 3.7 shows an increase in the RNA content per nerve cell from early age up to young adulthood, a plateau between forty and sixty, and a subsequent and significant decrease after the age of sixty. Similar findings in rats were reported by Ringborg (1966). The rate of RNA synthesis decreases post-natally, and the RNA polymerase activity in nuclei is higher in young than in adult brain cells. Up to 80 per cent of the ribonucleic acid precursors are incorporated into the nuclear fractions and in species of RNA larger than the 28S RNA. Presumably, fewer ribosomes are at the disposal of protein synthesis in old age than in the prime of life. The increase during the first period of life may reflect a continuous growth of the neurone, due

Table 3.5

In vivo incorporation of [³H]adenine and [³H]cytidine into RNA of hypoglossal nerve cells and glia from rabbits over 4 hours.

Base	Nerve cells	Glia
Adenine	4·1 ± 0·65	6·9 ± 0·62
Guanine	0·68 ± 0·09	1·3 ± 0·45
Cytosine	3·2 ± 0·19	5·6 ± 0·92
Uracil	1·4 ± 0·17	2·6 ± 0·34
A:G:C:U	2·9:0·49:2·3:1	2·7:0·50:2·2:1

The incorporation is expressed as mmol labelled base/mol base, (mean value ±S.E.M.). (From Daneholt and Brattgård, 1966.)

Table 3.6

Phenol–ribonuclease extraction of a highly-labelled RNA fraction from neurones and glia. Phenol extraction was performed at 3°. Ribonuclease was used as a 50 μg per ml aqueous solution and as 400 μg per ml of 0·2 N ammonium acetate, respectively.

		Ribonuclease 50 μg/ml			Ribonuclease 400 μg/ml		
	No. of expts.	% RNA released	% activity of RNA released	Specific activity c.p.m./μg	% RNA released	% activity of RNA released	Specific activity c.p.m./μg
Neurones	1 N	11·4	50	310	88·6	50	40
	2 N	4·8	35	285	95·2	65	27
	3 N	0·6	25	2500	99·4	75	46
	4 N	1·1	51	11,790	98·9	49	88
Glia	1 G	52·4	75	85	47·6	25	32
	2 G	5·5	9	932	94·5	91	540
	3 G	8·5	22	219	91·5	78	71
	4 G	0·7	2	4950	99·3	98	2270

Table 3.7

Total RNA content in human motor nerve cells (spinal cord, C_5, nucleus ventralis lateralis).

Age in years	RNA in pg/cell
0–20	402 ± 28
21–40	553 ± 38
41–60	640 ± 55
61–80	504 ± 31
over 80	420 ± 30

to usage and experience. From an experimental point of view, the changing amount of neuronal RNA during the life cycle stresses the necessity to have controls of the same age, preferably from the same litter.

Large-scale RNA changes induced by stimulation

By manipulating factors in the environment it is easy to induce RNA production in the nerve cells. For example, Jarlstedt (1963) studied the effect of increased sensory activity on the RNA content of Purkinje cells in the cerebellum by irrigating the outer ear with cold and warm water. It is interesting that in these experiments the effect can also be measured using physiological parameters. When the rabbit's left outer ear was irrigated with warm water for thirty minutes, there was a unilateral 30–60 per cent increase in the RNA of the Purkinje cells in the modulus as well as in those of the lobulus centralis. When he used cold water irrigation, on the other hand, he found that on the contralateral side the RNA

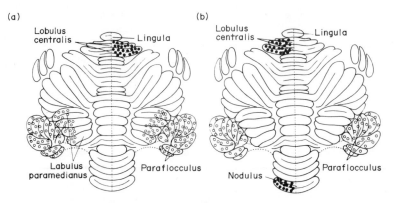

Figure 3.8. (a), Rabbit cerebellum unfolded in one plane. Surface view. (Redrawn after Brodal, 1940.) (•), Areas with *unilaterally higher* Purkinje cell RNA content after thirty minutes of *cold* water irrigation in the left outer ear. (○), Areas with *bilaterally similar* Purkinje cell RNA content after cold water irrigation in the left outer ear. In this figure and in (b), RNA is expressed as pg per nerve cell.

(b), Rabbit cerebellum unfolded in one plane. Surface view. (Redrawn after Brodal, 1940.) (•), Areas with *unilaterally higher* Purkinje cell RNA content after thirty minutes of *warm* water irrigation in the left outer ear or after right-sided vestibular neurotomy. (○), Areas with *bilaterally similar* Purkinje cell RNA content after warm water irrigation in the left outer ear or after right-sided vestibular neurotomy. (From Jarlstedt, 1963.)

of the Purkinje cells in the lobulus centralis of the cerebellum increased by 25–35 per cent (Figure 3.8, a and b).

In fish, I have found that motor activity can increase the level of the RNA in the motor nerve cells of the upper part of the spinal cord by 25 per cent. I used 60 cm Barracudas from the Caribbean which can exert quite a high degree of motor activity in swimming and attacking. Between attacks they hardly move but float quietly in waiting for the next victim and they are easily exhausted by twenty to thirty minutes of rapid swimming. Figure 3.9 shows the neuronal RNA changes over a period of five hours.

Brain RNA in relation to behaviour

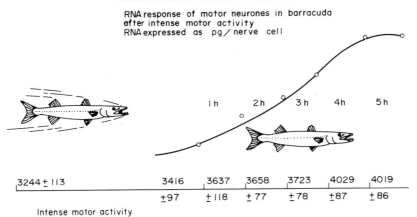

Figure 3.9. RNA response of motor neurones in barracuda after intense motor activity.

Table 3.8 summarises the effects of some other stimuli on nerve cell RNA. Intermittent rotation of animals results in an RNA increase within less than an hour. The experiment with vertical, direction changing rotation is a stress experiment, and was used as a control for stress in some of our behavioural tests to show

Table 3.8

RNA response of neurones to increased sensory stimulation.

Stimulus	Cell type	RNA increase in pg per cell	%	P
Intermittent horizontal rotation 25 min/day, 7 days	Deiters' neurones rabbit	1550 → 1750	10	0·01
Intermittent horizontal rotation 25 min/day, 7 days	Deiters' neurones rat	680 → 750	10	0·02
Intermittent vertical rotation 30 min	Deiters' neurones rat	680 → 850	25	0·001
Sodium chloride 1·5% 30 days	neurones of N. supraopticus rat	68 → 121	80	0·01
Thirst for 7 days	neurones of N. supraopticus rat	52 → 129		0·001

	Amount per kg	RNA changes		RNA base ratio changes		Protein changes	Cytochrome oxidase $\mu l\ O_2 \times 10^{-4}/h$	
		Nerve cell	Glia	Nerve cell	Glia	Nerve cell	Nerve cell	Glia
Controls		1545±45 pg	123 pg	A 19·7±0·37 G 33·5±0·39 C 28·8±0·36 U 18·0±0·18	A 20·8±0·28 G 28·8±0·64 C 31·8±0·27 U 18·6±0·055	16 000 pg	4·2±0·6	11·5±0·8
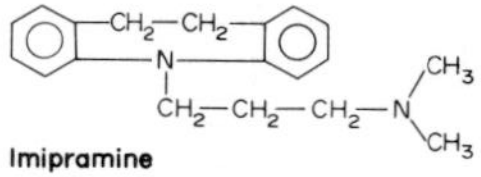 Imipramine	5 mg	0	−30%	0	A +25% C −20%	0	+400%	
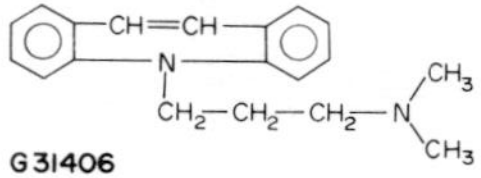 G 31406	4 mg	+18%	−45%	0	A +8% C −11%	+26%	+250%	
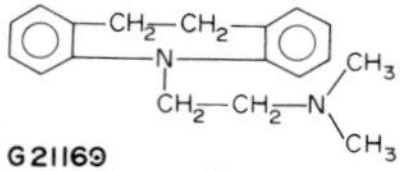 G 21169	5 mg	+26%	−45%	0	A +20% C −20%	+30%	+300%	
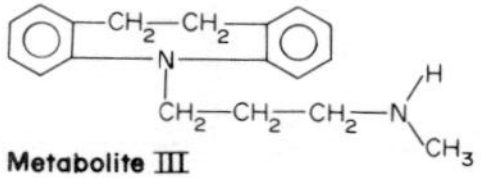 Metabolite III	5 mg	+12%		0	0			
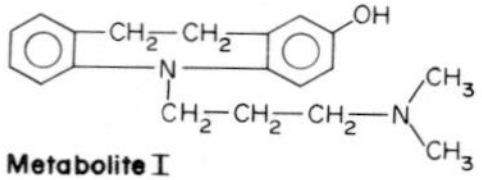 Metabolite I	5 mg	0					+100%	−13%
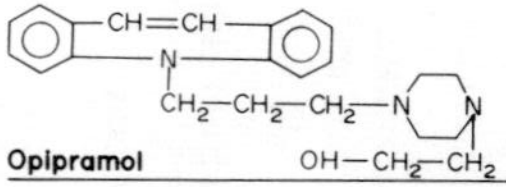 Opipramol	5 mg	0					+300%	−27%

Figure 3.10.

that stress induces production of G–C rich RNA in nerve cells, but that it does not increase production of nuclear RNA of the A–U type. Stimulation of supraoptic neurones with increased production of antidiuretic hormone resulted in a remarkable increase in the RNA content. I would like to state at this point that physiological stimulation, if strong enough, induces nerve cells to produce RNA which has the same base composition as the main part of the cell RNA, and which is of the ribosomal type.

Chemicals have also been found to affect the RNA of nerve cells. Psychotomimetics such as imipramine hydrochloride (Tofranil) and tranylcypromine (Parnate), had a reversible effect both on the amount and the content of RNA of many types of nerve cells in the brain, and also on their respiratory enzyme activities. The effect could remain for up to one week, but eventually it became reversible. Five mg/kg of imipramine hydrochloride, given intravenously to rabbits, produced an 18 per cent increase in the RNA content of the nerve cells studied and a decrease of 45 per cent in the glia outside the nerve cells, but it changed the base ratios only in the RNA of the glia. Derivatives of imipramine had a similar effect (Figure 3.10). The significant effect of the imipramine hydrochloride was on the glia in the part of the brain we studied, the vestibular nuclei. It is interesting to note how the glia, in some cases, responded with primary biochemical changes, whereas the neurones they surrounded did not. I would like to refer again to the biopsies from cases of Parkinson's disease (Hydén, 1964; Gomirato and Hydén, 1963; Hydén, 1966). The analysis showed that the glial RNA changes (increase of RNA, higher adenine and lower guanine values than the controls) were present before any nerve cell RNA changes could be noted. Such alterations surely represent long-lasting changes at the primary level in the cell organisation, and they reflect a biochemical error. The effect of 0·3 mg/kg of tranylcypromine was striking: not only did the RNA content of the nerve cells increase, but the guanine, cytosine and uracil values of the newly produced RNA were different from those of the controls (Tables 3.9, 3.10 and 3.11),

Table 3.9

The effect of 0·3 mg/kg of tranylcypromine on the amount of RNA per nerve cell and same weight of glia in rabbits killed one hour after injection or six days after daily injections of 0·3 mg/kg (values given in pg per cell).

	Nerve cells				Glial cells			
	Mean	P	N	n	Mean	P	N	n
Controls	1550 ± 62		24	187	123 ± 17·5		17	41
One hour	2012 ± 97	0·01	3	33	58 ± 6·4	0·01	3	17
Six days	1914 ± 87	0·01	3	30				

N = number of animals; P = probability level; n = number of analyses.

Table 3.10

Electrophoretic analyses of Deiters' nerve cells of rabbits injected with 0·3 mg/kg tranylcypromine and killed one hour later.

	Controls			Tranylcypromine		
	Mean	V		Mean	V	P
Adenine	19·7 ± 0·37	4·2		19·1 ± 0·25	3·2	
Guanine	33·5 ± 0·39	2·6		30·9 ± 0·44	3·5	0·001
Cytosine	28·8 ± 0·36	2·8		33·5 ± 0·45	3·3	0·001
Uracil	18·0 ± 0·18	2·3		16·5 ± 0·38	5·6	0·01
N	5			6		
n	40			60		

N = number of animals; P = probability level; n = number of analyses; V = variation coefficient.
The value for each base is expressed as a molar percentage of the total base present.

and the species were between 5S and 14S and thus rather small (Figure 3.11) and in the range of some species of messenger RNA.

These are examples of what can be called large-scale RNA changes in brain cells; they are reversible and usually amount to 15–30 per cent of the total (med-

Table 3.11

Electrophoretic analyses of glial cells surrounding Deiters' nerve cells of rabbits injected with 0·3 mg/kg tranylcypromine and killed one hour later.

	Controls			Tranylcypromine		
	Mean	V		Mean	V	P
Adenine	20·8 ± 0·28	3·0		19·6 ± 0·46	4·7	
Guanine	28·8 ± 0·64	5·0		22·3 ± 0·27	2·4	0·001
Cytosine	31·8 ± 0·27	2·0		38·7 ± 0·76	3·9	0·001
Uracil	18·6 ± 0·55	6·7		19·4 ± 0·52	5·4	
N	5			5		
n	50			40		

N = number of animals; P = probability level; n = number of analyses; V = variation coefficient.
The value for each base is expressed as a molar percentage of the total base present.

Brain RNA in relation to behaviour

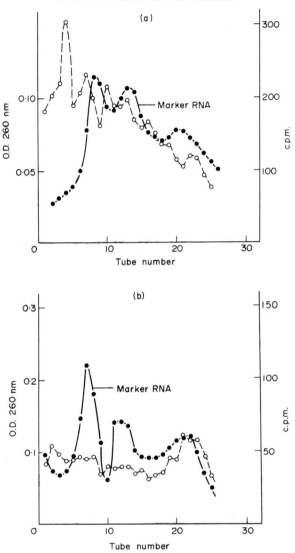

Figure 3.11. (a), Sucrose gradient profile of normal nuclear RNA of brain cells in the lateral vestibular nucleus. The [³H]orotic acid was administered intraventricularly one hour before the animals were killed. (●—●), Optical density at 260 nm. (○—○), Radioactivity.

(b), Sucrose gradient profile of nuclear RNA of the same area from tranylcypromine-treated rabbits (0.3 mg/kg), killed after one hour.

ium and large-size neurone) nerve cell body RNA, that is from 100 to 500 pg per cell. With an excessive stimulus such as motor exhaustion, a decrease in the RNA content or synthesis has been found. This is probably due to the lack of triphosphates of the four nucleotides. What this largely ribosomal RNA change, or what this ribosomal RNA species, is mediating, is not clear. A compilation of data and a discussion of their significance has been published by Pevzner (1966). A possible correlation of electrical phenomena and RNA changes in nerve cells is a much discussed possibility and a recent study has stressed the importance of synaptic stimulation for producing a macromolecular response in neurones. Using *Aplysia* neurones, Peterson and Kernell (1970) found that when the abdominal ganglion cells were electrically stimulated via the synapses, and the postsynaptic spikes were recorded, the synthesis of both ribosomal and nonribosomal RNA increased by some 30 per cent. Nonsynaptic stimulation produced no effect, and this result, I think, explains many of the negative results which add to the confusion in the literature. When the time sequence of the labelled RNA was followed, precursor species around 38S in the nucleus were found shortly after the labelling. A 14S fraction was also observed. I would suggest that this represents a type of RNA synthesis which antibiotics can inhibit by 90 per cent without preventing the formation of the so-called short-term memory. On the other hand, since this RNA synthesis is correlated with neural function in general, and there seems to be no doubt about that, this could be the reason why the 90 per cent inhibition prohibits long-term memory from being consolidated.

Neuronal RNA during learning

The large-scale RNA synthesis in nerve cells can be contrasted with the minute production of around 10 to 20 pg of nuclear RNA per nerve cell, which in a few experiments has been correlated with the establishment of a new behaviour, and not simply with neural function in general. We used the modified 'reversal of handedness in rats' experiment described in the first lecture (Hydén and Egyhazi, 1964), correcting for differences in performance by analysing material from animals which had been using the preferred paw for the same number of reaches and times.

In the part of the sensory motor cortex in front of the bregma which is of importance to the reversal of handedness, the cells within the fifth and sixth layer are especially sensitive to damage. In the nerve cells removed from these areas in rats trained to use the nonpreferred paw, we found a large nucleus and such cells were poor in cytoplasm. A large part of the total RNA, therefore, is nuclear RNA. After four days of training with two 25-minute training sessions per day, we found a significant increase of 10 pg of RNA per cell (Table 3.12). In control animals there was no difference between the RNA content of the right and left

Table 3.12

RNA content of cortical neurones in transfer of right- to left-handedness

	Controls (left side)	Learning (right side)	P
RNA pg	22 ± 2·3	31 ± 2·5	0·002

part of the cortex. Table 3.13 shows that there are significant changes in the base ratios of the cells from the trained rats. The ratio $\frac{G+C}{A+U}$ had changed from 1·72 to 1·51 in the trained rats. To control for performance we also analysed the nerve cell RNA of rats which had used the preferred paw for the same number of times, and found no such base ratio changes. The base ratio changes we found as a function of training cannot be attributed to an addition per cell of G–C rich RNA, and the ratio U to C increased in the material from trained rats.

In an earlier experiment rats were trained to balance on a wire 1 m long and 1 mm in diameter at an angle of 45° (Hydén and Egyhazi, 1962, 1963). We found a 10 per cent increase in the RNA content of the vestibular nerve cells, the so-called Deiters' cells which are clearly involved in this task. The nuclei of these cells were analysed separately, and the nuclear adenine to uracil ratio was higher than

Table 3.13

Changes in the RNA base composition of cortical neurones from the control (left) side and from the learning (right) side.

	Controls Mean	Learning Mean	% change	P
Adenine	18.4 ± 0.48	20.1 ± 0.11	+9.2	0.02
Guanine	26.5 ± 0.64	28.7 ± 0.90	+8.3	0.01
Cytosine	36.8 ± 0.97	31.5 ± 0.75	−14.4	0.01
Uracil	18.3 ± 0.48	19.6 ± 0.56	+7.1	0.05
$\frac{A+G}{C+U}$	0.81 ± 0.27	0.95 ± 0.035	+17.3	0.01
$\frac{G+C}{A+U}$	1.72 ± 0.054	1.51 ± 0.026	−12.2	0.02

that of the controls. The uracil to cytosine ratio of the trained rats had also increased. In control rats of the same age, subjected to vestibular stimulation by intermittent rotation or cage controls, neither vestibular nerve cells nor nerve cells from the reticular formation showed such a nuclear RNA change. The glial cells surrounding the nerve cells (same dry weight with both types of samples) also responded with a change of the base ratios, and had higher adenine and lower cytosine values than the controls.

These RNA changes during learning have recently been corroborated in another species and with another test. Shashoua (1968, 1970) used goldfish in a training and behavioural test and analysed the brain RNA with respect to base composition. When the animals established the new behaviour, Shashoua found that the newly synthesised RNA had a U to C ratio which was 20–80 per cent higher than the RNA which was formed under nonlearning conditions in his control experiments. These consisted of intense motor activity, convulsions and passive behaviour. The RNA formed during the proper training had a sedimentation constant of 14S.

Of the other studies of brain RNA during formation of long-term memory, I should like to comment briefly on two. Glassman and collaborators (1968, 1970) took great pains to eliminate the effect of nonspecific stimuli by using mice which were yoked to the trained mice. They also tried to divide the training situation in order to trap the 'behavioural trigger' which could elicit a specific response especially in the limbic system. Glassman demonstrated that an increased incorporation of uridine into polysomes occurred during a stage of the training which was characterised by adaptive responses.

In contrast to this increased incorporation of uridine, incorporation in cortical areas decreased, and moreover, in an overtrained mouse, there was no chemical response after further training. These results agree well with our findings of [^{3}H]leucine incorporation into protein during training. Glassman, who used sedimentation in sucrose gradients, could not find that the increased radioactivity was localised in a particular species of RNA, but my comment is that this technique is not sensitive enough to detect a small increase of, for example, 10 pg of RNA per cell.

Bowman and Kottler (1970) found a significant increase in the incorporation of cytidine into RNA of the hippocampus in rats in a spatial reversal test. They also found that the ratio of [^{3}H]RNA in the nucleus to that in the nucleus plus the cytoplasm was the same for both reversal and control rats. These findings strengthened the conclusion that the reversal learning had produced increased RNA synthesis in the hippocampus. Technically, they made the important point that only intravenous administration of the label gave correct results in these RNA studies. In the experiments of Glassman and Bowman, as well as in ours, it seems possible to exclude the idea that the RNA changes found were a result of differential stresses.

In addition to these data there is also the fact that the formation of long-term memory is prevented when RNA or protein synthesis is inhibited by antibiotics during and immediately after training (Flexner and Flexner, 1968; Agranoff, Davis, Casola and Lim, 1968; Barondes and Cohen, 1968).

Conclusion

Finally we must consider the question: what significance do these observations on brain RNA have in relation to mechanisms which underlie registration and storage of new information in brain? As I stressed in the first lecture, there is no evidence that macromolecules, such as RNA and protein, can encode and store experiential memory like a tape-recorder. There is no evidence that any brain cell RNA species go beyond their role as mediators between DNA and protein synthesis.

In this lecture I have presented some data of brain cell RNA in two groups: large-scale cytoplasmic RNA changes and small-scale, mainly nuclear RNA changes, in order to make two conclusions. Firstly, there occurs in neurones a production of RNA rich in guanine and cytosine which can be called a large-scale RNA production since it manifests itself as a 15–50 per cent increase in the total content of RNA, that is, it can amount to 500–600 pg of RNA in large nerve cells. This RNA increase is reversible and occurs as a response to motor, sensory, stress and chemical stimuli, and it also occurs during learning. Increase in total cell protein and defined proteins, such as the brain-specific protein S-100, and enzyme activities occur concomitantly with this RNA response. What detailed function this large-scale RNA production fulfils in brain cells is unknown, but it is clearly a biochemical substrate for neural function.

Secondly, in cortical neurones and in hippocampal nerve cells there occurs during change in behaviour a production of small amounts of RNA, mainly nuclear RNA, in addition to the large-scale cytoplasmic RNA increase. This nuclear type of RNA is characterised by adenine and uracil values which are higher than those of the guanine–cytosine rich RNA just discussed. This type of RNA may never leave the nucleus, but these species may also be messengers for cytoplasmic synthesis of brain-specific protein. The S-100 protein has a high content of aspartic and glutamic acids (Moore and McGregor, 1965), and the messenger which could be predicted would have adenine, guanine and uracil values similar to those we calculated for the nuclear RNA which was formed in the cortical neurones at the end of a training period of reversal of handedness.

Such calculations have also been made by Shashoua (unpublished observations) and Agranoff (1970). Based on this reasoning, my tentative conclusion would be that the neuronal RNA formed during learning in certain areas of the brain consists partly of a guanine–cytosine rich RNA, and partly of a formation of a messenger RNA specifically for synthesis of acidic protein. The base ratio change would reflect a quantitative increase of a species of RNA which already exists in these neurones. This RNA response would lead to a protein differentiation of neurones and their synapses (and glia) different for phylogenetically different areas of the brain to serve mechanisms for registration and storage of information in the hierarchically structured brain, as discussed in the first lecture.

References

ADAIR, L., WILSON, J. E., ZEMP, J. W. and GLASSMAN, E. (1968). Brain function and macromolecules, III. *Proc. natn. Acad. Sci., U.S.A.*, **61**, 606–13.

AGRANOFF, B. W. (1970). Current questions in brain and behaviour. In: *Biochemistry of Brain and Behaviour* (BOWMAN, R. E. and DATTA, S. P., Eds.), pp. 347–58. Plenum Press, New York.

AGRANOFF, B. W., DAVIS, R. E., CASOLA, L. and LIM, R. (1968). Actinomycin D blocks formation of memory of shock-avoidance in goldfish. *Science, N.Y.*, **158**, 1600–1.

BARONDES, S. H. and COHEN, H. D. (1968). Arousal and the conversion of 'short-term' to 'long-term' memory. *Proc. natn. Acad. Sci., U.S.A.*, **61**, 923–9.

BERTALANFFY, L. V. (1970). Chance or law. In: *Beyond Reductionism* (KOESTLER, A. and SMYTHIES, J. R., Eds.), pp. 56–84. Macmillan, New York.

BOWMAN, R. E. and KOTTLER, P. D. (1970). Regional brain RNA metabolism as a function of different experiences. In: *Biochemistry of Brain and Behaviour* (BOWMAN, R. E. and DATTA, S. P., Eds.), pp. 301–26. Plenum Press, New York.

CUMMINS, J. and HYDÉN, H. (1962). Adenosine triphosphate levels and adenosine triphosphatases in neurons, glia and neuronal membranes of the vestibular nucleus. *Biochim. biophys. Acta*, **60**, 271–83.

DANEHOLT, B. and BRATTGÅRD, S.-O. (1966). A comparison between RNA metabolism of nerve cells and glia in the hypoglossal nucleus of the rabbit. *J. Neurochem.*, **13**, 913–21.

EKHOLM, R. and HYDÉN, H. (1965). Polysomes from microdissected fresh neurones. *J. Ultrastruc. Res.*, **13**, 269–80.

FLEXNER, L. B. and FLEXNER, J. B. (1968). Intracerebral saline: effect on memory of trained mice treated with puromycin. *Science, N.Y.*, **159**, 330–1.

GLASSMAN, E. and WILSON, J. E. (1970). The effect of short experiences on macromolecules in the brain. In: *Biochemistry of Brain and Behaviour* (BOWMAN, R. E. and DATTA, S. P., Eds.), pp. 279–99. Plenum Press, New York.

GOMIRATO, G. and HYDÉN, H. (1963). A biochemical glia error in the Parkinson disease. *Brain*, **86**, 773–80.

HYDÉN, H. (1964). Biochemical and functional interplay between neuron and glia. In: *Recent Advances in Biological Psychiatry* (WORTIS, J., Ed.), Vol. VI, pp. 31–54. Plenum Press, New York.

HYDÉN, H. (1966). Production of RNA in neurons and glia in Parkinson's disease indicating genic stimulation. In: *Biochemistry and Pharmacology of the Basal Ganglia* (COSTA, E., CÔTÉ, L. J. and YAHR, M. D., Eds.), pp. 195–204. Raven Press, New York.

HYDÉN, H. and EGYHAZI, E. (1962). Nuclear RNA changes during a learning experiment in rats. *Proc. natn. Acad. Sci., U.S.A.*, **48**, 1366–73.

HYDÉN, H. and EGYHAZI, E. (1963). Glial RNA changes during learning experiment in rats. *Proc. natn. Acad. Sci., U.S.A.*, **49**, 618–24.

HYDÉN, H. and EGYHAZI, E. (1964). Changes in RNA content and base composition in cortical neurons of rats in a learning experiment involving transfer of handedness. *Proc. natn. Acad. Sci., U.S.A.*, **52**, 1030–5.

JARLSTEDT, J. (1963). Functional localization in the cerebellar cortex studied by quantitative determinations of Purkinje cell RNA. *Acta physiol. scand.*, **67**, 243–54.

KATCHALSKY, A. and OPLATKA, A. (1966). Hysteresis and macromolecular memory. *Neurosci. Res. Progr. Bull.*, **4**, 71–93.

KATCHALSKY, A. and NEUMANN, E. (1972). Hysteresis and molecular memory record. *Int. J. Neurosci.*, **3**, 175–82.

MOORE, B. W. and MCGREGOR, D. (1965). Chromatographic and electrophoretic fractionation of soluble proteins of brain and liver. *J. biol. Chem.*, **240**, 1647–53.

NEUMANN, E. and KATCHALSKY, A. (1970). Thermodynamische Untersuchung der Hysterese im System Polyriboadenyl-Polyribouridylsäure-Modell einer makromolekularen Gedächtnis-Aufzeichnung. Vorgetragen von E. NEUMANN anlässlich der 69. Hauptversammlung der Deutschen Bunsengesellschaft für Physikalische Chemie e. V. 9 p. Mai 1970 (Heidelberg).

PETERSON, R. P. and KERNELL, D. (1970). Effects of nerve stimulation on the metabolism of RNA in a molluscan giant neurone. *J. Neurochem.*, **17**, 1075–85.

PEVZNER, L. Z. (1966). Nucleic acid changes during behavioural events. In: *Macromolecules and Behaviour* (GAITO, J., Ed.), pp. 43–70. Appleton-Century-Crofts, New York.

RINGBORG, U. (1966). Composition and content of RNA in neurons of rat hippocampus at different ages. *Brain Res.*, **2**, 296–8.

SHASHOUA, V. E. (1968). RNA changes in goldfish brain during learning. *Nature, Lond.*, **217**, 238–40.

SHASHOUA, V. E. (1970). RNA metabolism in goldfish brain during acquisition of new behavioural patterns. *Proc. natn. Acad. Sci., U.S.A.*, **65**, 160–7.

VOLPE, P. and GIUDITTA, A. (1967a). Kinetics of RNA labelling in fractions enriched with neuroglia and neurones. *Nature, Lond.*, **216**, 154.

VOLPE, P. and GIUDITTA, A. (1967b). Biosynthesis of RNA in neuron- and glia-enriched fractions. *Brain Res.*, **6**, 228–40.

PART II
Symposium

Neurochemical correlates of behaviour with particular reference to learning

Chairman: P. B. Bradley
Department of Pharmacology, Medical School, Birmingham

RNA and brain function

E. GLASSMAN and J. E. WILSON

Department of Biochemistry and the Neurobiology Program, University of North Carolina School of Medicine, Chapel Hill, North Carolina 27514, USA

Few neurobiologists, if any, believe that experiential information is stored or coded in macromolecules. Instead, the prevailing, though not universally accepted view is that the associative processes that go on in the brain during learning involve the formation of functionally new pathways or networks, the nature of which encode the memory. It is not known how the pathways or networks are selected, or what the relationship of the pathway or network is to the encoded memory, and this particular topic is beyond the scope of this paper. Instead, we shall confine the discussion to the role that molecules might play in pathway or network formation, since it is difficult to conceive of the formation of new functional relationships between neurones without the occurrence of molecular changes within these neurones. Many hypotheses have been proposed. In general, all involve some chemical changes that affect the efficiency of synaptic transmission. This would happen, for example, if there were changes in the amount of transmitter released or a change in its rate of destruction, and the papers by Professor Kerkut and his associates in this volume are excellent examples of the type of data available concerning this idea. Changes in the efficiency of synaptic transmission or the connectivity between neurones would also occur if there were changes in the size of the synapse or in the number of receptor sites for the transmitter. In addition, any agent that changes the level of polarisation of the postsynaptic membrane would affect the connectivity between neurones. Thus, the possible number of theoretical models along these lines is very large.

The major problem is the generation of data that will have bearing on the molecular events associated with changes in neuronal connectivity. The present volume contains some extremely interesting and promising attempts at attacking this problem. Our own approach is based on the research that suggests that the storage or consolidation of memory involves successive stages, and that the processes responsible for memory storage during and shortly after a learning experience differ from the processes responsible for maintaining the same memory at a later time (John, 1967; McGaugh and Dawson, 1971; Agranoff, 1973). During and just after training, memory seems to be retrievable from a short-lived form, short-term memory. This is thought to decay within hours, but by that time memory is retrievable from a more permanent form, long-term memory. A number of approaches indicate the existence of at least these two phases.

Firstly, in a variety of mammals including humans, lesions in the area around and including the hippocampus are reported to cause rapid forgetting after a new task has been learned (Douglas, 1967). Memory for events learned before the production of the lesion seems unimpaired. Removal of the ventral lobe of the octupus brain has a similar effect (Young, 1965). It appears that these lesioned animals can form short-term, but not long-term memory.

Secondly, the formation of long-term memory can be influenced by agents that have little effect on short-term memory, or on long-term memory once it has been formed. The period of sensitivity has generally been estimated to be seconds or minutes after the learning experience, depending on a variety of factors too complex to be discussed here (John, 1967). After the sensitive period ends, memory is no longer affected by these agents, and is said to be consolidated into long-term memory. The use of this term is somewhat unfortunate since it implies a mechanism involving a process that fixes the memory to prevent its being lost. A plausible alternative is that the retrieval of the memory encoded in the chosen pathways or networks is made easier (Quartermain and McEwen, 1970).

There are many reports of a correlation between a change in RNA or protein and learning experience (see Glassman, 1969, for a review). The cause and significance of such changes are not known, but few, if any, of the changes can be ascribed merely to neurophysiological stimulation. Edström and Grampp (1965) have shown that no detectable changes in RNA or protein take place when the neurone to the stretch receptor muscle of the crayfish is stimulated for periods up to eight hours. Nor is neurophysiological activity or information storage dependent on RNA or protein synthesis. For example, Schwartz, Castellucci and Kandel (1971) have found that extensive neurophysiological activity and behavioural phenomena (short-term habituation) can take place in *Aplysia* even though protein synthesis is inhibited over 95 per cent. In addition, one can inhibit RNA or protein synthesis extensively in the brains of goldfish (Agranoff, 1968) or mice (Barondes and Cohen, 1967; Flexner and Flexner, 1968), and not interfere with the primary acquisition of tasks involving conditioned avoidance. One must conclude that if macromolecules are playing a role in changes in neuronal connectivity in these short-term experiments, the mechanism probably involves conformational changes in pre-existing molecules rather than synthesis, although the possibility of a requirement for very low levels of synthesis is not ruled out.

Because memory deficits are produced when protein or RNA synthesis is inhibited by antibiotics during and immediately after training (Flexner, Flexner and Roberts, 1967; Agranoff, Davis, Casola and Lim, 1968; Barondes and Cohen, 1967), it seems likely that the formation of long-term memory depends on the synthesis of these macromolecules. The sensitivity to these inhibitors is short-lived, however, and thus the perpetuation of long-term memory is not specifically dependent on high levels of the uninterrupted synthesis of RNA or protein. Some form of excitement (arousal) seems to be necessary for this process to take place, as shown by McGaugh (1968) and Barondes and Cohen (1968). Indeed it is possible that certain types of novel or intense sensory stimulation and experience can produce this level of excitement and the subsequent chemical events without the presence of short-term memory. This would account for many of the chemical changes caused by novel sensory stimulation (Glassman, 1969).

If short-term memory does not involve macromolecular synthesis, and if the formation of long-term memory does involve the synthesis of RNA and protein as the data using antibiotics suggests, then it seemed to us that it might be possible to detect this synthesis through the use of radioactive tracers during short training experiences. Most of our research has been carried out using the mouse. A behavioural task rapidly learned by a mouse was used in order to measure the incorporation of precursors into RNA, proteins, lipids and other substances while the mouse was learning. In this way it was hoped that the synthesis of macromolecules associated with the formation of long-term memory might be detected. The mouse was chosen because it has been used extensively in behavioural, biochemical and genetical studies, but recent studies with the rat have also produced comparable data (Coleman, 1969; Coleman, Pfingst, Wilson and Glassman, 1971). To minimise genetic variation, only six- to eight-week-old males of the C57B1/6J strain supplied by the Jackson Laboratories were used, but female mice show the same chemical changes when conditions are right (Coleman, 1969; Coleman et al., 1971). The methods and the data have been published in detail elsewhere (Adair, Wilson and Glassman, 1968a; Adair, Wilson, Zemp and Glassman, 1968b; Coleman et al., 1971; Coleman, Wilson and Glassman, 1971; Kahan, Krigman, Wilson and Glassman, 1970; Zemp, Wilson, Schlesinger, Boggan and Glassman, 1966; Zemp, Wilson and Glassman, 1967).

The training apparatus consisted of a box divided into two sections with a common electric grid floor (Zemp et al., 1966; Schlesinger and Wimer, 1967). One mouse was placed in each section. A light and a buzzer were attached to the outside of the box so that each mouse received equal stimulation. The sections were identical except that one side had an escape shelf. The light and buzzer were presented for three seconds after which an electric foot shock was applied. Initially, both mice jumped in response to the shock. The shock was terminated as soon as the animal that had the shelf used it as a haven. After fifteen seconds, the mouse was then removed from the shelf and placed on the grid floor and another trial commenced. The training lasted for fifteen minutes, and between twenty-five and thirty-five trials were carried out in this interval. The mouse that had the shelf would usually start to avoid the shock in response to light and buzzer by the fifth trial, and was performing to a criterion of nine out of ten by ten minutes. The untrained mouse also received equivalent handling at random during the training. Thus with respect to lights, buzzers, shocks, handling, and injection, the untrained mouse was yoked to the trained mouse.

It was planned to study the incorporation of radioactive precursors into RNA, protein, lipids, etc., but only RNA has been studied. The approach uses a double isotope-labelling method. One mouse of a pair was injected intracranially with [^{14}C]uridine, the other with [^{3}H]uridine. Thirty minutes later, one of the mice was trained for fifteen minutes in the jump-box while the other served as the yoked animal. After the training period, the brains of both mice were homogenised simultaneously in the same homogeniser, after which the homogenate was fractionated into nuclei, ribosomes, and supernatant fraction (Zemp et al., 1966). Uridine monophosphate (UMP) was isolated from the supernatant fraction and RNA was extracted from each of the subcellular components; the amount of ^{14}C and ^{3}H in each was determined (Zemp et al., 1966).

The purpose of using two labels in this way is to avoid the problem of differential losses of RNA that occur during the complicated manipulations we had to use to isolate the RNA. The amount of ^{14}C or ^{3}H in the RNA indicates the extent of incorporation of uridine into RNA of the mouse that was injected with ^{14}C or ^{3}H, respectively. The ratio of ^{3}H to ^{14}C in the UMP is a useful indication of the relative efficiency of the injection and of the relative amount of uridine that entered brain cells, and we have used it to correct the observed ratio ^{3}H to ^{14}C in the RNA. This double isotope-labelling method was used in all of these experiments to measure the incorporation of radioactive uridine into polysomes or into RNA extracted from nuclei or ribosomes.

Preliminary experiments indicated that more radioactive uridine was incorporated into the RNA extracted from brain nuclei or from brain ribosomes of the trained mouse, and coded blind experiments were carried out thereafter. Only after the biochemical analysis was completed and all the data were computed was it revealed which isotope (^{3}H or ^{14}C) the trained mouse had received. In twenty-five of such blind double labelling experiments, all trained mice incorporated more radioactivity into RNA than did the untrained mice (Zemp et al., 1966). It is of interest that if the mice were killed thirty minutes after training instead of immediately after, the differences were no longer observed. This, however, could be due to the fact that the total radioactivity in the RNA increases greatly during this time, and the differences due to the experience are obscured (Zemp et al., 1966). This is consistent with the finding that the differences between the amounts of uridine incorporated into polysomes of trained and untrained mice persist up to one hour after training (Adair *et al.*, 1968a; Coleman, 1969).

This difference between the incorporation into brain RNA of the trained and untrained mice cannot be unequivocally ascribed to increased synthesis of RNA in the trained animal. It could, for example, be due to decreased destruction of RNA, to increases in permeability of the cells or their nuclei to uridine, to a decrease in the synthesis of endogenous uridine, or to any one of a number of other alternatives. We have not been able to pursue this problem directly because of technical difficulties. Thus, we refer only to the change in incorporation and do not specify a mechanism. This is a crucial problem in the interpretation of these data. A similar uncertainty exists for most experiments involving the incorporation of a radioactive precursor into any molecule, whether it is in brain or in any other tissue. Usually, however, this problem is not taken into account.

To test whether there is an increased incorporation into brain RNA and polysomes in the trained mouse or a decreased incorporation in the yoked animal, the incorporation into brain RNA or polysomes in the yoked animal was compared with that in a 'quiet' mouse, that is, one that had been returned to its home cage after the injection of radioactive uridine. If the yoked animal was undergoing a decrease in incorporation due to its peculiar experience, the same decrease should have been observed when it was compared with the quiet animal. The data indicated that the yoked and the quiet animal had similar amounts of incorporation of radioactive uridine into brain RNA and polysomes (Adair *et al.*, 1968a; Zemp *et al.*, 1966).

Two conclusions can be drawn. Firstly, it seems clear that the increased amount of radioactivity in the RNA from the brain of the trained mouse is due, in fact, to an increased incorporation of uridine in the trained mouse, and not to a decreased incorporation in the yoked mouse. Secondly, since the yoked and quiet mice showed similar chemical responses, evidently the lights, buzzers, shocks and handling that the yoked mouse received are not sufficient to have any effect by themselves. To test this second idea further, the incorporation of radioactive uridine into RNA in the brains of quiet mice was compared with that in mice subjected to thirty electric shocks given at random over the fifteen-minute period. The radioactivity in the RNA and polysomes was similar in both mice, thus giving further support to the idea that mere stimuli and activity were not responsible for the effect we observed (Adair *et al.*, 1968a; Zemp *et al.*, 1966). It is possible, of course, that such stimuli can cause effects, but that the stress of the injection of solutions into the brain that all the mice undergo is large enough to mask the effects of other stimuli.

Trained and untrained animals showed no significant differences in the incorporation of radioactive uridine into liver and kidney RNA or polysomes, even though these same animals showed pronounced differences in the brain (Adair *et al.*, 1968a; Zemp *et al.*, 1966). It was concluded, therefore, that although tissues other than the liver and kidney might be responding, the effect is probably specific to brain.

The effect also seems to be limited to specific areas. Chemical analyses of brains after gross dissection have indicated that the changes in RNA occur primarily in the diencephalon and associated areas (Zemp *et al.*, 1967). Autoradiography has confirmed this (Kahan *et al.*, 1970). Most areas and cells of the brain seem to incorporate similar amounts of radioactivity in trained and untrained animals. This is an important point in autoradiography since there is no independent measure of the amount of radioactivity that gets into each brain, and it indicates that injections were equally effective and similarly distributed in both sets of animals. Neurones were the only cells to be consistently labelled, except for glial elements of the ependyma. The silver grains were concentrated over the neuronal nuclei.

There are, however, areas and cells in parts of the core-brain of trained mice that produce silver grains, while what appear to be the corresponding areas in the brains of untrained mice produce very few grains in the autoradiogram. Although our analysis has not proceeded to the point where we can catalogue all of the areas that show a difference between trained and untrained animals (especially where these differences are not so striking), there are nuclei throughout the olfactory and entorhinal cortices, hippocampus, amygdala, thalamus, hypothalamus and mammillary bodies in which there is incorporation in all trained mice with little incorporation into corresponding nuclei of their untrained yoked controls.

These data indicate the importance of knowing the extent of the involvement of the brain in chemical responses to behavioural stimuli. The significance of the changes in macromolecules associated with experience and behaviour will not be fully understood until the functional relationships between the cells in which the chemical changes take place are known. Autoradiography, and perhaps histochemistry, seem well suited for elucidating the cellular relationships (Beach, Emmens, Kimble and Lickey, 1969; Kerkut, Oliver, Rick and Walker, 1970). There are, however, two technical problems that must be solved before the results of autoradiographic studies can be interpreted definitively. Firstly, there is the problem of establishing that equal amounts of radioactive precursors are similarly distributed in the brains of the trained and the untrained mice. This is done by determining the radioactivity in UMP in biochemical experiments (Zemp *et al.*, 1966; and others), and appropriate modification of this technique might be applicable to autoradiographic studies. A second problem is the difficulty of reliably establishing that the same neurones of trained and untrained mice are being compared. Only careful attention to these possible sources of error will prevent investigators from drawing incorrect conclusions.

The behavioural or environmental agents that caused such chemical changes have not been elucidated. It may be that the learning *per se* or the special stresses and emotional and motivational effects of learning are responsible for triggering such chemical responses. It is also possible, however, that the changes in macromolecules are due to nonspecific stimuli or to the activity associated with the training experience. Visual (Appel, Davis and Scott, 1967; White and Sundeen, 1967; Talwar, Chopra, Goel and D'Monte, 1966), auditory (Hamberger and Hydén, 1945), rotary (Hamberger and Hydén, 1945, 1949a, b; Watson, 1965; Attardi, 1957; Jarlstedt, 1966a, b), olfactory (Rappoport and Daginawala, 1968) and stress stimulation (Bryan, Bliss and Beck, 1967; Altman and Das, 1966) have been reported to cause changes in RNA or polysomes in the nervous system, and it is not unexpected that such stimuli would be effective during training. Such stimuli have been eliminated in our research, but the exact mechanism has not been delineated. This does not necessarily mean that the encoding of the experience in the nervous system is the trigger for the chemical reactions. It may well be that the special stresses, levels of excitement, emotional responses, and other phenomena that may be related to the learning process are operating here. There are many differences between the trained mouse and the yoked mouse in addition to learning. For example, the trained mouse has a change in cue and his attention is now directed at a stimulus that the untrained mouse probably views as benign. Also, the stresses on the trained mouse are different, as are his responses to them. Finally, the trained mouse jumps more often than the yoked mouse, which does not get a shock if the trained mouse avoids. It is clear that the increased number of jumps is not responsible for the chemical change since a mouse given thirty shocks in fifteen minutes does not show any increase of radioactivity in RNA or polysomes (Adair et al., 1968a; Zemp et al., 1966). There is, however, a difference in the quality of the jump, in that the trained mouse quickly learns to organise his locomotion to reach the shelf, while the untrained mouse jumps with random purpose.

To study the nature of the RNA into which the increased incorporation took place, ^{14}C- and ^{3}H-labelled RNA mixtures from yoked and trained animals were sedimented in sucrose gradients to see if the increased radioactivity was located in a single species of RNA that might have a unique function (Zemp et al., 1966). In all cases, the increased radioactivity associated with the RNA of the trained mouse was quite heterogeneous with respect to sedimentation rate. The patterns of radioactivity were of the same general shape for RNA from the brain, liver or kidneys from both trained and untrained mice. Thus, the increased incorporation into brain RNA resembled that found after RNA synthesis had been stimulated in liver by hydrocortisone or in uterus by oestrogen. This suggests that the increased radioactivity is not confined to a single species of RNA and that a metabolic stimulation of relevant brain cells had occurred. In addition, the increased incorporation into polysomes of the brain during the training experience suggests that the increased radioactivity is either in messenger RNA or in pre-ribosomal RNA (Adair et al., 1968a; Coleman et al., 1971). Thus, we find that brain responds biochemically in a manner similar to the response found in other tissues. The specificity seems to be in the stimulus that each tissue or cell responds to. We do not find evidence for a unique RNA with a function that does not involve protein synthesis; indeed the RNA we do find is similar to RNA extracted from other tissues. Further work is needed to determine whether this brain RNA is involved in the synthesis of new proteins or in the replenishment of, or an increase in, proteins already present.

The function of these macromolecules in the brain is the major question in this research. Their role could be to replenish chemicals used in nerve activity, similar to the restorative role macromolecules play in all cells, and thus they would be responsible for the maintenance of function and the health of cells. Another possibility is that the changes in macromolecules are related more specifically to new pathway formation by changing connectivity between neurones through the alteration of the probability that a postsynaptic neurone will fire when impulses arrive from presynaptic nerves. The possibility that these macromolecules are encoding the experiential information in their own structure is very unlikely.

Until it is known whether the changes in RNA have anything to do with the learning process *per se*, or with an incidental process, it will be extremely difficult to correlate our results with the formation of long-term memory, although it is extremely tempting to do so. The RNA might code for proteins involved in this process, possibly by rendering permanent the synaptic associations that developed during short-term learning. The protein may be related to the peptide(s) postulated to be involved in the maintenance and retrieval of memory by Flexner and Flexner (1968) and Bohus and de Wied (1966).

Why the core-brain is the site of the greatest (and therefore detectable) change in these molecules is not known. This would make sense if it were correlated with an emotional response, and indeed, we have some evidence that this could be true (Machlus, 1971). If so, it may indicate that the chemical changes detected in this area have nothing to do with the processes that make the changes in connectivity between neurones permanent, and are not related at all to memory storage, a conclusion that would indicate that the magnitude of the RNA and protein synthesis thought to be required for the formation of long-term memory is very small, and is masked by the much larger changes in core-brain. Alternatively, one could postulate that an emotional reaction specific to the learning process affects chemical synthesis in the core-brain. These chemicals affect neuronal connectivity in other parts of the brain, and are thus responsible for the formation of long-term memory. The fact that classical conditioning does not cause similar chemical changes in the core-brain might argue against the idea that core-brain changes are involved in the fixation of neuronal connectivity, but it must be kept in mind that the mice undergoing fifteen minutes of training in the jump-box are considerably overtrained, since most are performing well before ten minutes. The animals we exposed to classical conditioning for up to thirty minutes (Adair *et al.*, 1968b; Coleman, 1969) were probably not overtrained and it may well be that overtraining is necessary to generate sufficient response to detect the chemical changes. Alternatively, there may be real differences in the responses of mice to classical and instrumental experiences. It is important to note that cycloheximide will not interfere with the formation of long-term memory in animals that are overtrained, a fact that suggests that the level of chemical synthesis in these animals is high enough to generate sufficient molecules even in the presence of this inhibitor.

It is the purpose of our research to attempt to understand the significance of the reported effects of behaviour on macromolecules in the nervous system. A detailed discussion of the role of these macromolecules in the learning processes would be very premature; there is no clear evidence that these macromolecules play a direct role in encoding, and cause and effect relationships in this area are almost impossible to prove. The long-range questions we want to ask are as follows. (1) What aspect of the behaviour seems to be important? (2) By what physiological and biochemical processes is the information from outside the animal conveyed to the cells that are responding? (3) What is the significance of the chemical response in terms of the functional role that the macromolecules play in the operations of the cells of the nervous system? If learning is involved, then these data will be of particular interest. However, even if no aspect of the learning process is involved, the fact that behaviour can affect macromolecules should be of great concern to those studying nervous system function. The role these macromolecules play in the nervous system may be only the role they play in the function of all tissues, i.e. that of maintaining cellular health and enabling the cellular machinery to function. If so, it is important to know this in order that the solutions to the problem of the unique functions of the nervous system in regulating behaviour can be sought elsewhere.

The research described in this article was supported by research grants from the U.S. Public Health Service (MH18136, NS07457), the U.S. National Science Foundation (GB-18551), and the Ciba-Geigy Corporation. We are greatly indebted to the numerous collaborators, graduate students and postdoctoral fellows who so diligently carried out the research described in this article and who provided innumerable stimulating discussions, arguments and illuminating thoughts.

References

ADAIR, L. B., WILSON, J. E. and GLASSMAN, E. (1968a). Uridine incorporation into polysomes of mouse brain during different behavioural experiences. *Proc. natn. Acad. Sci., U.S.A.*, **61**, 917–22.

ADAIR, L. B., WILSON, J. E., ZEMP, J. W. and GLASSMAN, E. (1968b). Brain function and macromolecules, III. Uridine incorporation into polysomes of mouse brain during short-term avoidance conditioning. *Proc. natn. Acad. Sci., U.S.A.*, **61**, 606–13.

AGRANOFF, B. W. (1973). Biochemical approaches to learning and memory. In: *Macromolecules and Behaviour* (ANSELL, G. B. and BRADLEY, P. B., Eds.), pp. 143–149. Macmillan, London.

AGRANOFF, B. W., DAVIS, R. E., CASOLA, L. and LIM, R. (1968). Actinomycin D blocks formation of memory of shock-avoidance in goldfish. *Science, N.Y.*, **158**, 1600–1.

ALTMAN, J. and DAS, G. D. (1966). Behavioural manipulations and protein metabolism of the brain: effects of motor exercise on the utilization of leucine-H^3. *Physiol. Behav.*, **1**, 105–8.

APPEL, S. H., DAVIS, W. and SCOTT, S.(1967). Brain polysomes: response to environmental stimulation. *Science, N.Y.*, **157**, 836–8.

ATTARDI, G. (1957). Quantitative behavior of cytoplasmic RNA in rat Purkinje cells following prolonged physiological stimulation. *Expl. Cell. Res.*, **4**, 25–53.

BARONDES, S. H. and COHEN, H. D. (1967). Delayed and sustained effect of acetoxycycloheximide on memory in mice. *Proc. natn. Acad. Sci., U.S.A.*, **58**, 157–64.

BARONDES, S. H. and COHEN, H. D. (1968). Arousal and the conversion of 'short-term' to 'long-term' memory. *Proc. natn. Acad. Sci., U.S.A.*, **61**, 923–9.

BEACH, G., EMMENS, M., KIMBLE, D. P. and LICKEY, M. (1969). Autoradiographic demonstration of biochemical changes in the limbic system during avoidance training. *Proc. natn. Acad. Sci., U.S.A.*, **62**, 692–6.

BOHUS, G. and DE WEID, D. (1966). Inhibitory and facilitatory effect of two related peptides on extinction of avoidance behaviour. *Science, N.Y.*, **153**, 318–20.

BRYAN, R. N., BLISS, E. L. and BECK, E. C. (1967). Incorporation of uridine-^{3}H into mouse brain RNA during stress. *Fedn Proc. Fedn Am. Socs exp. Biol.*, **26**. 709.

COLEMAN, M. S. (1969). Ph.D. Dissertation, The University of North Carolina at Chapel Hill, North Carolina.

COLEMAN, M. S., PFINGST, B., WILSON, J. E. and GLASSMAN, E. (1971). Brain function and macromolecules, VIII. Uridine incorporation into brain polysomes of hypophysectomized rats and ovariectomized mice during avoidance conditioning. *Brain Res.*, **26**, 349–60.

COLEMAN, M. S., WILSON, J. E. and GLASSMAN, E. (1971). Incorporation of uridine into polysomes of mouse brain during extinction. *Nature, Lond.*, **229**, 54–8.

DOUGLAS, R. J. (1967). The hippocampus and behaviour. *Psychol. Bull.*, **67**, 416–42.

EDSTRÖM, J. E. and GRAMPP, W. (1965). Nervous activity and metabolism of ribonucleic acids in the crustacean stretch receptor neuron. *J. Neurochem.*, **12**, 735–41.

FLEXNER, L. B. and FLEXNER, J. B. (1968). Intracerebral saline: effect on memory of trained mice treated with puromycin. *Science, N.Y.*, **159**, 330–1.

FLEXNER, L. B., FLEXNER, J. B. and ROBERTS, R. B. (1967). Memory in mice analyzed with antibiotics. *Science, N.Y.*, **155**, 1377–83.

GLASSMAN, E. (1969). The biochemistry of learning—an evaluation of the role of RNA and protein. *A. Rev. Biochem.*, **38**, 605–46.

HAMBERGER, C. A. and HYDÉN, H. (1945). Cytochemical changes in the cochlear ganglion caused by acoustic stimulation and trauma. *Acta oto-lar.*, suppl. 61, 1–29.

HAMBERGER, C. A. and HYDÉN, H. (1949a). Transneuronal chemical changes in Deiters' nucleus. *Acta oto-lar.*, suppl. 75, 82–113.

HAMBERGER, C. A. and HYDÉN, H. (1949b). Production of nucleoprotein in the vestibular ganglion. *Acta oto-lar.*, suppl. 75, 53–81.

JARLSTEDT, J. (1966a). Functional localization in the cerebellar cortex studied by quantitative determinations of Purkinje cell RNA. I. *Acta physiol. scand.*, **67**, 243–52.

JARLSTEDT, J. (1966b). Functional localization in the cerebellar cortex studied by quantitative determinations of Purkinje cell RNA. II. *Acta physiol. scand.*, **67**, suppl. 271, 1–24.

JOHN, E. R. (1967). *Mechanisms of Memory.* Academic Press, New York.

KAHAN, B., KRIGMAN, M. R., WILSON, J. E. and GLASSMAN, E. (1970). Brain function and macromolecules. VI. Autoradiographic analysis of the effects of a brief training experience on the incorporation of uridine into mouse brain. *Proc. natn. Acad. Sci., U.S.A.*, **65**, 300–3.

KERKUT, G. A., OLIVER, G. W. O., RICK, J. T. and WALKER, R. J. (1970). The effects of drugs on learning in a simple preparation. *Comp. gen. Pharmac.*, **1**, 437–83.

MACHLUS, B. J. (1971). Ph.D. Dissertation, *The Neurobiology Curriculum*, The University of North Carolina, Chapel Hill, North Carolina.

MCGAUGH, J. L. (1968). A multi-trace view of memory storage processes. In: *Attuali Orientamenti della Ricerda Sull Apprendimento e la Memoria* (BOVET, D., BOVET-NITTI, F. and OLIVERO, A., Eds.), vol. CIX. Accademia Nazionale de Lincei, Rome.

MCGAUGH, J. L. and DAWSON, R. G. (1971). Modification of memory storage processes. *Behav. Sci.*, **16**, 46–63.

QUARTERMAIN, D. and MCEWEN, B. S. (1970). Temporal characteristics of amnesia induced by protein synthesis inhibitor: determination by shock level. *Nature, Lond.*, **228**, 677–8.

RAPPOPORT, D. A. and DAGINAWALA, H. F. (1968). Changes in nuclear RNA of brain induced by olfaction in catfish. *J. Neurochem.*, **15**, 991–1106.

SCHLESINGER, K. and WIMER, R. (1967). Genotype and conditioned avoidance learning in the mouse. *J. comp. physiol. Psychol.*, **63**, 139–41.

SCHWARTZ, J. H., CASTELLUCCI, V. F. and KANDEL, E. R. (1971). Functioning of identified neurons and synapses in abdominal ganglion of *Aplysia* in absence of protein synthesis. *J. Neurophysiol.*, **34**, 939–54.

TALWAR, G. P., CHOPRA, S. P., GOEL, B. K. and D'MONTE, B. (1966). Correlation of the functional activity of the brain with metabolic parameters, III. *J. Neurochem.*, **13**, 109–16.

WATSON, W. E. (1965). An autoradiographic study of the incorporation of nucleic-acid precursors by neurones and glia during nerve stimulation. *J. Physiol., Lond.*, **180**, 754–65.

WHITE, R. H. and SUNDEEN, C. D. (1967). The effect of light and light deprivation upon the ultrastructure of the larval mosquito eye. I. Polyribosomes and endoplasmic reticulum. *J. exp. Zool.*, **164**, 461–78.

YOUNG, J. Z. (1965). The organization of a memory system. *Proc. R. Soc.*, B, **163**, 285–320.

ZEMP, J. W., WILSON, J. E. and GLASSMAN, E. (1967). Brain function and macromolecules. II. Site of increased labelling of RNA in brains of mice during a short-term training experience. *Proc. natn. Acad. Sci., U.S.A.*, **58**, 1120–5.

ZEMP, J. W., WILSON, J. E., SCHLESINGER, K., BOGGAN, W. O. and GLASSMAN, E. (1966). Brain function and macromolecules, I. Incorporation of uridine into RNA of mouse brain during short-term training experience. *Proc. natn. Acad. Sci., U.S.A.*, **55**, 1423–31.

Biochemistry and behaviour in the chick*

S. P. R. ROSE
Department of Biology, The Open University, Walton, Bletchley, Bucks., England

P. P. G. BATESON
Sub-Department of Animal Behaviour, Madingley, Cambridge, England

G. HORN
Department of Anatomy, Cambridge, England

The framework within which we are working, and which has governed the choice of experiments presented in this paper, is that which postulates that the learning situation produces an alteration in brain biochemistry, which is correlated with, or causally related to, the changes in behaviour resulting from the training conditions. Our experiments are based on a view of the broad relationships between biochemistry and behaviour similar to that of several other contributors to this meeting. Whilst the observed changes might occur in any aspect of brain biochemistry, for reasons adduced elsewhere (Rose, 1970) we have, in common with most other investigators in this area, chosen to study the changes in production of the macromolecules RNA and protein. The results presented here are part of an attempt to specify behaviourally the conditions associated with such changes by examining the extent to which they are directly linked to the process of learning

---

* Other participants in this interdisciplinary collaborative research are Ann L. Horn, Department of Anatomy, University of Cambridge, J. Haywood and F. Hambley, Brain Research Group, Department of Biology, The Open University.

itself, and to unravel biochemically the sequence of events associated with the environmental trigger which the new learning situation entails.

In our search for an experimental situation which enables these attempts to be made, we have examined the sequence of biochemical changes which occurs during imprinting in the young chick. This situation is one in which the recently-hatched chick, like other precocial birds, will quickly form a social attachment to a conspicuous object as a result of being exposed to it (see Bateson, 1966, for review). This learning process involves the first significant visual experience for the birds and we argued that the consequent cellular changes were likely to be greater than those produced by similar visual experiences later in life. The recently-hatched chick has an additional advantage for *in vivo* work in that the blood–brain barrier has not yet properly developed (Key and Marley, 1962).

Since the experiments described in this paper were essentially exploratory, the experimental design was simplified as much as possible. Domestic chicks were hatched and kept in the dark until they were exposed to a highly conspicuous object at the stage of development when imprinting occurs most readily. The rates at which radioactive lysine or uracil were incorporated into brain regions of these birds were compared with those for a group that was kept in the light but not subjected to the imprinting procedure and those for a group that was kept in the dark. In the preliminary studies no attempt was made to measure imprinting directly by giving the experimental group a choice between the object to which they had been exposed and a dissimilar object. Learning was presumed to have occurred on the grounds that in earlier experiments, chicks exposed to the same imprinting stimulus subsequently preferred it to a dissimilar object (Bateson and Reese, 1969). The methods and results to be described in this paper have been reported in greater detail elsewhere (Bateson, Horn and Rose, 1969, 1972; Rose, Bateson, Horn and Horn, 1970; Haywood, Rose and Bateson, 1970). In later experiments involving control procedures for some of the side-effects of training, direct measures of imprinting have been employed (Horn, Horn, Bateson and Rose, 1971).

Methods

Chicks were hatched in a dark incubator and maintained in the dark until the start of the behavioural procedures, fourteen to nineteen hours after hatching. At this time they were divided into three groups: an experimental group exposed to the imprinting stimulus; light controls, placed in similar pens to the experimentals and illuminated by an overhead light; and dark controls, placed in blacked-out pens. The experimental birds were placed in pens from which they could see a rotating flashing light, the object serving as the imprinting stimulus. At appropriate times before or after exposure, the birds from the three groups were given an intracardiac injection of [^{3}H]lysine or [^{3}H]uracil, assumed to be precursors of protein and RNA respectively. Before the animals were killed, they were tested in an alley for their speed of approach to the flashing light, other behavioural measures (the rate of 'peep' and 'twitter' calls) being taken simultaneously. In later experiments (Horn et al., 1971), the birds were placed in running wheels, and tested by being given a choice between alternative stimuli. In these experiments, the birds had had their supraoptic commissures cut and one eye covered before exposure to the imprinting procedure. Thus only one side of the brain was trained, the other side serving as a control.

After the imprinting and test procedures, the birds were decapitated and the brain crudely dissected into the forebrain 'roof' and 'base', and midbrain regions, the midbrain region including the optic lobes. The hindbrain and cerebellum were discarded. The brain regions, and in some experiments a liver sample, were frozen on dry ice until assay. In the assay procedure the samples were homogenised and portions taken for total counts (pool), trichloroacetic acid (TCA)-insoluble counts and protein determination (see Rose, 1967 for description of method). Radioactivities (disintegrations/min per mg protein) were corrected to a standard body weight of 50 g and in order to eliminate variability between batches the specific radioactivity of the acid-insoluble residue from each sample was divided by the mean for all the brain samples from the dark control birds in that batch. Relative specific radioactivities were calculated by expressing the value for the acid-insoluble counts as a percentage of total counts in the sample. In other experiments no isotope was used, but after killing, the brain regions were homogenised, the cell nuclei separated and the total RNA polymerase activity determined in the presence of [8-^{14}C]adenosine triphosphate, cytidine triphosphate, guanosine triphosphate and uridine triphosphate, ammonium sulphate, magnesium chloride and mercaptoethanol (Hayward et al., 1970).

Results

Incorporation of [^3H]lysine

Because the readiness with which birds can be imprinted depends on maturational age, half the chicks in this first experiment were drawn from the early part and half from the late part of the hatch. The eighteen chicks in each batch were divided equally into experimental (E), light (L_c) and dark (D_c) control groups. It was argued that any effect on protein synthetic rates might take some time after the commencement of the stimulus to express itself. Since the maximum feasible duration from injection of isotope to killing, if relatively simple kinetics of incorporation were to be obtained, was ninety minutes, the experimental and light control birds were tested and then exposed to their respective conditions for sixty minutes, before all three groups were weighed and injected. Experimental and light control birds received a further forty-five minutes of exposure and were

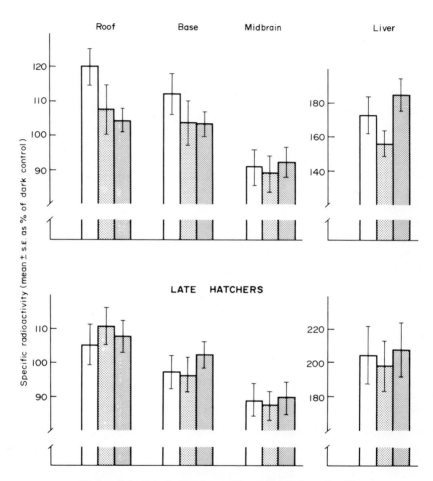

Figure 5.1. Standardised specific radioactivity of acid-insoluble fraction in brain regions and liver following [^{3}H]lysine injection. Birds from the early and late parts of the hatch were subjected to an imprinting stimulus (□) or formed light control (▨) or dark control groups (■), in the experiment described in the text. Vertical bars represent S.E.M. of: early hatching, $E = 17$, $L_c = 18$, $D_c = 17$, birds; late hatching, $E = 10$, $L_c = 15$, $D_c = 15$, birds in each group. (From Bateson *et al.*, 1972.)

returned to a dark incubator for forty minutes. Finally all three groups were tested and killed.

Figure 5.1 shows the standardised specific radioactivity for the acid-insoluble residues. In the early hatching birds, there was a significant difference ($P < 0.05$) between the experimental and the dark control birds in the forebrain roof region; in this region the light control group was intermediate between the two. There were no significant differences in the other brain regions or the liver in the early-hatching birds, and no differences were significant in the late-hatching birds. It may be noted that in the early-hatching groups the pool value was significantly less in the light control than the experimental group in the roof region ($P < 0.05$), while this effect was inverted ($P < 0.05$) in the late-hatching birds. The differences in pool values are not easy to interpret, and it is worth noting that the proportion of unbound lysine in any region could change rapidly as a result of selective changes in cerebral blood flow. But it was encouraging to find that a specific change in the rate of incorporation of precursor into protein occurred in one brain region in the early-hatching experimental birds whilst this change no longer occurred in the late-hatching birds, whose behavioural performance was also sharply differentiated (Bateson et al., 1972). The behavioural difference can be related to the ending of the sensitive period for imprinting (Bateson, 1966) and the apparent lack of an effect on incorporation into protein may be seen as in accord with this behavioural change. In subsequent experiments, therefore, only birds from the early or middle part of the hatch were used.

Incorporation of [^3H]uracil

Two and a half hours after the onset of the imprinting stimulus in the experimental birds, specific changes in the incorporation of [^3H]lysine into protein could be measured. Could an effect of the imprinting procedure on incorporation into RNA also be found? If it could, it would not only enhance the confidence with which we might regard the result with lysine, but it might also prove a more sensitive measure of changed biochemical activity, because the rate of incorporation of precursor into acid-insoluble material was much lower: after ninety minutes the relative specific radioactivity of bound [^3H]lysine was 60–70 per cent, whilst that of bound [^3H]uracil was only 4–6 per cent. In the next experiment, therefore, chicks from each of the experimental and light control groups were tested. The birds from each of the groups (including the dark control) were injected with [^3H]uracil and placed in their respective conditions for 150 minutes before testing again and killing.

Figure 5.2 shows the standardised specific radioactivity for the [^3H]uracil incorporation. All regions of the brain, from both light control and experimental groups, had significantly larger values than those of the dark control groups, while in the midbrain of the experimental group the incorporation was also significantly greater than in that of the light controls. None of the pool values showed significant differences. Thus, in contrast to the specific effects found in the case of the protein incorporation, after 150 minutes of exposure there was a general enhancement of incorporation into RNA. This is consistent with the view that general visual stimulation produces an overall increase in RNA synthesis in the brain. The largest effect was in the midbrain, which contains the optic tectum.

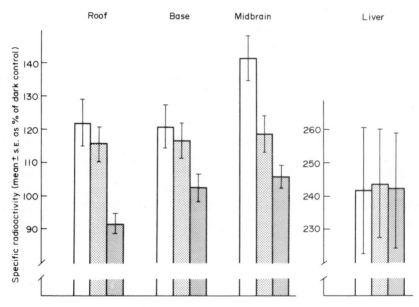

Figure 5.2. Standardised specific radioactivity of acid-insoluble fraction in brain regions and liver following [^{3}H]uracil injection. Birds were subjected to an imprinting stimulus (□) or formed light control (▨) or dark control groups (▪) in the experiments described in the text. Exposure to the respective conditions was 150 minutes. Vertical bars represent S.E.M. of $E = 18$, $L_c = 18$, $D_c = 17$, birds. (From Bateson *et al.*, 1972.)

It was possible that we had 'overexposed' the birds in these experiments and had masked a more specific effect by a general change. To check this possibility a time course of exposure was made. In each case the time from injection to killing was kept constant at 150 minutes, but the period of light exposure or exposure to the imprinting stimulus was varied. The exposure period was arranged symmetrically with respect to the overall incorporation period. Times of exposure to light control and experimental conditions were 0, thirty-eight and seventy-six minutes respectively. In this experiment the birds were not given an initial test before

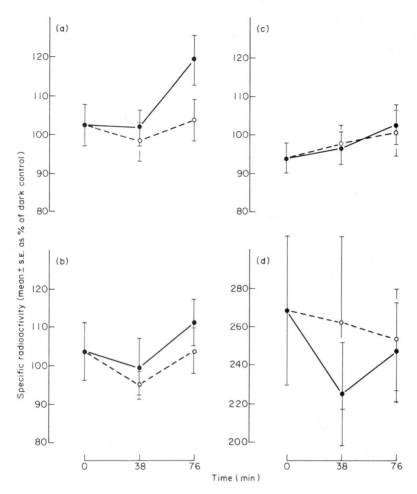

Figure 5.3. Effect of varying time of exposure on [^{3}H]uracil incorporation into acid-insoluble fraction of brain regions and liver. Birds were subjected for 0, thirty-eight or seventy-six minutes to an imprinting stimulus or to light control conditions. Time from injection of isotope to killing remained constant, as described in the text. (a), Forebrain roof; (b), forebrain base; (c), midbrain; and (d), liver. Vertical bars represent S.E.M. of: 0 minutes: $n = 19$, thirty-eight minutes: $E = 12$, $L_c = 12$, seventy-six minutes: $E = 19$, $L_c = 19$, birds. (——●——), Experimental; (---○---), control. (From Bateson et al., 1972.)

exposure, but were all tested immediately before killing. The biochemical results of this experiment are shown in Figure 5.3. The only significant change in incorporation into acid-insoluble material was in the roof region of the experimental birds at seventy-six minutes, which was higher than that into the same region of both light or dark controls. The light control groups also differed significantly from the dark control in both roof and base regions. Thus, in contrast to the experiment of Figure 5.2, when the times of exposure to stimulus were reduced, a significant difference between experimental and control birds appeared in the same brain region as that previously found to show an increased incorporation into protein.

RNA polymerase

The results of the experiments on lysine and uracil incorporation suggested that an increase in RNA synthesis in one brain region preceded increased protein synthesis in the same region. This prompted us to ask whether there might be earlier

Table 5.1

RNA polymerase levels in brain regions of experimental and control birds.

Condition	Forebrain roof (%)	Forebrain base (%)	Midbrain (%)
Experimental	110.3 ± 7.6 ($n = 15$)	124.3 ± 8.6 ($n = 17$)	109.6 ± 8.6 ($n = 17$)
Dark	82.4 ± 7.9 ($n = 17$)	102.4 ± 9.3 ($n = 17$)	97.6 ± 7.3 ($n = 17$)
E/D × 100	133.9	121.3	112.3
$P <$	0.02	0.09	0.30

From Haywood, Rose and Bateson (1970).

observable biochemical changes. If the sequence of biochemical events consequent upon the behavioural stimulus were analogous to that known to operate, for example, in hormonal trigger mechanisms (Tata, 1967), one might anticipate that an enhanced RNA polymerase activity would be detectable before the enhancement of incorporation into RNA and protein. Detection of an effect on an *in vitro* enzyme system would also have the advantage of eliminating problems associated with fluctuations of pool size in *in vivo* incorporation studies.

Experimental chicks were exposed to the imprinting stimulus for thirty minutes, during which time the dark controls remained in their pens. The birds were tested and killed. The brains were dissected and nuclei were prepared from each region separately (Haywood *et al.*, 1970). The results for each dark-control/experimental pair were calculated as percentages of the mean derived from all the results of that pair (Table 5.1). The RNA polymerase activity of the forebrain roof of the experimental birds was 34 per cent higher than that of the dark controls ($P < 0{\cdot}02$); the differences in the other regions were not significant. Thus, after thirty minutes of exposure, an increase in RNA polymerase activity *in vitro* could be detected in the same brain region of the experimental birds in which increases in RNA synthesis

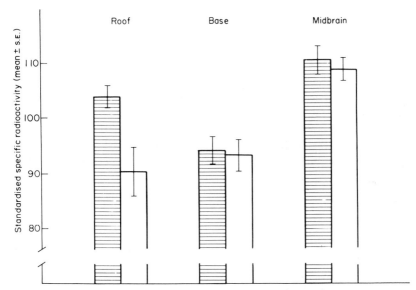

Figure 5.4. Standardised specific radioactivity following [³H]uracil incorporation into acid-insoluble material from trained (▤) and untrained (☐) sides of forebrain roofs, bases and midbrains of split-brain chicks, following experiment described in the text. The trained side was contralateral to the exposed eye. Vertical bars represent S.E.M. of $n = 12$, in each case. (From Horn *et al.*, 1971.)

could be detected at seventy-six minutes and in protein synthesis after 150 minutes. The suggestion that a temporal sequence of events at the biochemical level is operating here is compelling, though not yet conclusive.*

The split-brain animal

The experiments so far devised, whilst they may show a convincing picture of a biochemical sequence of events consequent upon an environmental trigger, do not of course demonstrate unequivocally that this trigger is the learning of the

---

* More recently, we have detected an even earlier change in the level of cyclic AMP in the forebrain roof. This difference is detectable at fifteen minutes (Hambley, Rose and Bateson, 1972).

imprinting stimulus itself; it might be that we were measuring the consequences of a generalised arousal or attention phenomenon, the effects of enhanced motor activity, or some other aspect of the organism's response to its changing environment. One way to test this would be to use one side of the brain as a control for the other. To do this requires the use of the split-brain preparation, and, in these experiments (Horn et al., 1971) the supraoptic commissures of the chick were cut under light anaesthesia one to four hours after hatching. The chicks were returned to their dark incubators for eighteen to twenty-four hours. One eye was then covered with an opaque patch, the birds were injected with [^{3}H]uracil and placed in a modified imprinting situation. One-hundred-and-fifty minutes after injection, they were tested for preference, first with the 'imprinted' eye and then with the patch reversed so that the 'imprinted' eye was covered and the control eye exposed. Only birds which showed no transference of preference were used for biochemical assay (Figure 5.4). Compared with the control side of the brain the forebrain roof on the 'imprinted' side showed a clear and significant ($P < 0\cdot01$) increase in incorporation. No other region showed an effect, and there was no effect on pool activity. Thus some types of nonspecific effect are clearly ruled out by the results of this experiment.

Conclusions

These experiments have clearly shown that the effect of exposure to an imprinting procedure in the young chick is to produce a complex sequence of biochemical events which appear to be specific to a particular brain region. Changes in incorporation rate of precursors into RNA and protein reflect, though they do not accurately measure, changes in synthetic rate. Although we have only measured changes in radioactivity bound to acid-insoluble material, there is good reason to believe that this is likely to be predominantly in RNA and protein from [^{3}H]uracil and [^{3}H]lysine respectively (Bateson et al., 1972). Although such changes might only reflect fluctuations in regional blood flow which would alter the rate of precursor uptake, the fact that changes in the relative specific radioactivity of the bound uracil were also significant goes some way to suggesting otherwise, whilst the existence, in the same brain region, of a specific enhancement of RNA polymerase *in vitro*, would strongly suggest that we are dealing with a real phenomenon related to RNA and protein synthesis.

Meanwhile, of course, we are not claiming that these experiments unequivocally separate out the effects of 'learning' from those of less specific changes. The split-brain experiment is one control which goes some way towards this, but it is still not unequivocal. For instance, the amount of visual stimulus received by the eye exposed to the imprinting stimulus compared to the control is still not controlled for, although in this respect it is encouraging to note that after short exposures the anatomical locus of the observed effect was not in the midbrain, where it might be expected on the basis of a model of nonspecific visual stimulation (cf. Figure 5.2), but in the 'higher' brain region, the forebrain roof. The experiments of Figure 5.2, however, show that some more general, nonspecific effects of exposure also occur, although they seem to be temporally separable from the more specific ones.

Our immediate aim is not to 'prove' that RNA and protein are involved in learning, but to use broad biochemical techniques to identify brain regions which might merit more detailed examination so that the multitude of environmental factors which may influence brain biochemistry may be unravelled. The use of a specific preparation, with a specific environmental stimulus, also enables the temporal sequence of biochemical events triggered by that stimulus to be followed. We believe that the imprinting situation in the young chick is favourable from this point of view, despite the fact that rapid maturational effects are taking place upon which any effects of imprinting must be superimposed, and that the relatively irreversible nature of the imprinting procedure may not be a precise analogue of the less dramatic changes that occur in the more arbitrary learning processes of the adult. In addition, we believe that these experiments are the first in which an extended temporal sequence of biochemical changes following an environmental trigger has been shown to occur, and the first in which changes in RNA polymerase have been observed and the use of split-brain controls adopted.

This work was supported by grants from the Medical Research Council and Science Research Council (to S.P.R.R. and G.H.) and the Agricultural Research Council (to P.P.G.B.). Thanks are due to Mr A. K. Sinha for skilled technical assistance with many of the experiments.

References

BATESON, P. P. G. (1966). The characteristics and context of imprinting. *Biol. Rev.*, **41**, 177–220.

BATESON, P. P. G. and REESE, E. P. (1969). The reinforcing properties of conspicuous stimuli in the imprinting situation. *Anim. Behav.*, **17**, 692–9.

BATESON, P. P. G., HORN, G. and ROSE, S. P. R. (1969). Effect of an imprinting procedure on regional incorporation of tritiated lysine into protein of chick brain. *Nature, Lond.*, **223**, 534–5.

BATESON, P. P. G., HORN, G. and ROSE, S. P. R. (1972). Effects of early experience on regional incorporation of precursors into RNA and protein in the chick brain. *Brain Res.*, **39**, 449–65.

HAMBLEY, F., ROSE, S. P. R. and BATESON, P. P. G. (1972). Effect of early visual experiences on the metabolism of $3':5'$-cyclic monophosphate in chick brain. *Biochem. J.*, **127**, 90P.

HAYWOOD, J., ROSE, S. P. R. and BATESON, P. P. G. (1970). Effect of an imprinting procedure on RNA polymerase activity in the chick brain. *Nature, Lond.*, **228**, 373–4.

Horn, G., Horn, A. L. D., Bateson, P. P. G. and Rose, S. P. R. (1971). Effects of imprinting on uracil incorporation into brain RNA in the 'split-brain' chick. *Nature, Lond.*, **229**, 131–2.

Key, B. J. and Marley, E. (1962). The effect of the sympathomimetic amines on behaviour and electrocortical activity of the chicken. *Electroenceph. clin. Neurophysiol.*, **14**, 90–105.

Rose, S. P. R. (1967). Changes in incorporation of ^{3}H-lysine into protein in the visual cortex during first exposure of rats to light. *Nature, Lond.*, **215**, 253–5.

Rose, S. P. R. (1970). Neurochemical correlates of learning and environmental change. In: *Short-term Changes in Neural Activity and Behaviour* (Horn, G. and Hinde, R., Eds.), pp. 517–51. Cambridge University Press.

Rose, S. P. R., Bateson, P. P. G., Horn, A. L. D. and Horn, G. (1970). Effects of an imprinting procedure on regional incorporation of tritiated uracil into chick brain RNA. *Nature, Lond.*, **225**, 650–1.

Tata, J. R. (1967). The formation and distribution of ribosomes during hormone induced growth and development. *Biochem. J.*, **104**, 1–17.

Behavioural effects of protein synthesis inhibitors: consolidation blockade or negative reinforcement?

D. A. BOOTH and C. W. T. PILCHER

School of Biological Sciences, University of Sussex, Brighton BN1 SQY, England

This paper concentrates on certain behavioural aspects of the topic macromolecules and learning. Such an emphasis is appropriate because neurochemistry, neurophysiology and neuroanatomy are strongly represented in this Symposium and we cannot relate biochemistry to behaviour without attending to behaviour as thoroughly as we attend to neurochemistry and to brain physiology.

The aspect of learning which appears to be of particular interest to most of the participants today is long-term memory retention. In their study of the biochemical aspects of the memory contribution to behaviour, Professors Hydén, Glassman and Rose have all emphasised the necessity to run a suitable variety of behavioural controls to get any basis for the belief that a particular macromolecular correlate of learning is in fact part of laying down the memory trace. Professor Hydén, for example, mentioned that at least some of the protein changes he observes may be involved in arousal, and again, Professor Glassman's diagram of the processes involved in learning locates the RNA incorporation increases seen by his group in an arousal process and not in the consolidation of the long-term information-holding system itself. Professor Rose rightly insists that interpretation of the behavioural relevance of his imprinting correlates is impossible until further controls have been run. Other biochemists here are not immediately concerned to relate their results to the virtually permanent higher forms of memory. Although we can expect all these data to deepen our understanding of the biochemical functioning of neural tissue, there is no basis yet for assuming that they contribute to an understanding of the memory system. It would perhaps be surprising if there were, for it is only over the last few years that well-defined neurochemical effects of physiological stimulation have been observed.

Nevertheless, even when the behavioural controls are available, the results will not by themselves constitute identification of the biochemical character of the memory retention mechanism. It is necessary in addition to demonstrate that disrupting whatever biochemical process has been implicated does indeed prevent the establishment or maintenance of long-term memory. Once again detailed attention to behaviour is essential, for the problem in this case is to justify attribution of a drug-induced behavioural deficit at least in part to loss of memory retention, rather than entirely to disruption of initial learning or of the use of memory.

Barondes and Cohen (1967) have provided the best evidence of this type using mice which had been treated with the protein synthesis inhibitor cycloheximide or its acetoxy derivative. The tasks they used were such that the mouse's performance was right or wrong independently of nonspecific changes in motility, reactivity and motivation. They have also run a wide range of behavioural tests on the long-term retest disruption induced by the antibiotic, and have excluded a number of interpretations that are among the obvious alternatives to retention blockade. Such results have been a substantial reason for believing that the presence of transiently synthesised or rapidly degraded protein or peptide is necessary to set up long-term retention.

In his search for the engram with his remarkable biochemical techniques, Professor Hydén has concentrated in recent years on a motor learning task that has the advantages of including discriminated aspects, being readily amenable to a variety of behavioural controls for non-memory factors and, conceivably, having a relatively localised memory trace. A hungry rat is allowed to reach for food pellets in a topography that obliges it to use its nonpreferred paw. A sufficient number of reaches reverses the paw preference and this motor learning is retained indefinitely. We have studied the behavioural aspects of this task on and off over the years and we are now beginning to look for biochemical factors in retention.

In a recent pilot experiment, cycloheximide solution was placed before and during training on the pia mater, bilaterally over the region of sensorimotor cortex that Peterson and Barnett (1961) have shown to be critical for the forced preference reversal function, that is, the part of the brain within which there is the possibility (though no direct evidence) that much of the motor memory resides. We have confirmed Hydén's finding that the rate of reaching increases with practice, but this occurs whether the rat is forced to use its nonpreferred paw, tending to induce preference reversal, or its preferred paw, with no induced reversal (Booth, 1970). We have some behavioural results that suggest that the relative reaching rates with the two paws are loosely correlated with preference, but it is far from clear whether the acceleration of reaching in initial practice has anything to do with preference-reversal learning. It is also a performance measure that is unsuitable for experiments on behaviour blockade because it is nondiscriminative and liable to disruption by cycloheximide in several ways apart from retention blockade. We therefore interrupted forced reaching with the nonpreferred paw to measure acquisition and retention by direct tests of paw preference. The rat was allowed to use either paw freely to pick up ten pellets in turn. The proportion of left and right paw reaches gives a reliable measure of the direction and degree of paw preference, without detectably influencing later preferences.

In Table 6.1 an initial complete preference for one paw, right or left, is expressed as a score of $+1$, ambidexterity as zero and a completely reversed preference as -1. With saline on the pia, rats showed the usual behaviour after 200 reaches with the nonpreferred paw in our apparatus—namely, a marked reversal of preference and a retention of the reversal for several months. Group means at long-term retest are generally within ± 0.3 of the initial degree of reversal; coincidentally the scores

Table 6.1

Elimination of long-term reversal of paw preference by suprapial cycloheximide during training.

Suprapial solution	Before training	Ten minutes after training	One week after training
Saline	$+0.63$	-0.47	-0.47
Cycloheximide	$+0.66$	-0.53	$+0.30$

were exactly the same in this experiment. When cycloheximide was applied, reversal of preference appeared normal. That is, the performance was definitely established in the memory and remained for some minutes. Furthermore, no gross motor deficit or loss of hunger was evident. Yet there was virtually no sign of memory a week later. This long-term deficit is not simply brain damage, because cycloheximide applied after training does not produce it. The result is consistent with the possibility that, although there is for this task a retention mechanism with a life of at least several minutes that does not depend on new or labile protein, protein synthesis close in time to training is a necessary part of instructing a long-term retention mechanism.

There is a problem with the interpretation of this study, and indeed any other study in which cycloheximide is injected peripherally or in large or deeply intracranial doses. In the course of our group's studies of the effects of amino acids on feeding, we discovered a phenomenon which raises the question of whether failure to perform for long after training under the influence of cycloheximide is really caused by retrograde amnesia.

Table 6.2 shows that a rat injected intraperitoneally with a small dose of cycloheximide has a depressed food intake relative to the day on which it had been given a saline injection. This is the well-known anorexigenic effect of antibiotics. The food presented after injection was given one odour on the cycloheximide day and another odour on the saline day. The design was cross-counterbalanced for injection sequence and odour–injection pairing. In a choice test two days after the second injection, the rats showed a marked acquired aversion for the cycloheximide-paired odour (Booth and Simson, 1973). Indeed these preference scores represent almost complete rejection of the odour associated with cycloheximide effects, in favour of the saline-paired odour.

Le Magnen (1963) and Rozin (1969) have shown that conditioning of this general type sets up aversions not only to odours and tastes but also to places and to visually cued situations, although more weakly. There is therefore the possibility

Table 6.2

Aversion by association with cycloheximide.

N	Dose of cycloheximide (mg/kg i.p.)	Immediate food intakes: CHX day minus saline day (g in 6 h)	Preference test intakes: CHX-paired odour minus saline-paired odour (g in 3 h)
8	0·25	−1·58*	−1·64†
8	0·5	−3·00†	−1·83*

* $P < 0.05$. † $P < 0.01$.

that antibiotics administered near the time of training may negatively reinforce whatever position or cue preference has been acquired by training, whether escape training, active avoidance or approach training. Negative reinforcement may summate over the duration of action of the antibiotic. Thus, injection before cue presentation does not imply backward conditioning. Also, the aversion may grow over several hours after training as the negative reinforcement continues to act on the remembered recent performance: with X-ray induced aversions, the delay between cue and reinforcement may extend to many hours without preventing the acquisition of aversion (Smith and Roll, 1967). Thus, the failure to perform correctly during long-term retest may not be because the animal has forgotten what is correct. It may be rather that the animal is in conflict between, for example, avoiding electric shocks and avoiding antibiotic-induced sickness. Coons and Miller (1960) found the same sort of problem with electroconvulsive shock (ECS) as a supposedly retrograde amnesic agent. Everyone then switched from using active avoidance training to using passive avoidance for ECS studies, although unfortunately the fashion has been for nondiscriminated tasks, with the result that there is still very little evidence that ECS can block retention in animals, as distinct from its effects on retest performance by blocking retrieval and by serving as a punishment.

As biochemists we hope, of course, that the retrograde amnesic effects of antibiotics can be identified, if only for the sake of experimental convenience. Actinomycin D has been found so far either to have a negligible effect in properly controlled retests for as long as they can be delayed before extreme illness sets in (Cohen and Barondes, 1966), to induce various kinds of performance abnormality that cannot be attributed to memory (Squire and Barondes, 1970; Glassman et al., 1970) or to produce a poor performance in a nondiscriminated test (Agranoff et al., 1967) for which motivational or other non-memory deficits have yet to be excluded. Thus, there is no adequate evidence yet that RNA synthesis is necessary for establishing a memory. The result just reported shows that the evidence that memory needs protein synthesis is not adequate either. Cycloheximide and other antibiotics will have to be shown to disrupt long-term (and not short-term) retest performance in tasks which require both discriminated and inhibitory learning, such as alternation or conditioned suppression, in which negative reinforcement would work with memory and not against it. Alternatively, it may be possible to show that cycloheximide or any other antibiotic does not generate negative reinforcement when administered by certain routes which nevertheless allow disruption of macromolecular synthesis in the variable neural elements mediating memory retention. We shall test the suprapial route used in our preference reversal experiment for negative reinforcement of odour preferences.

Sufficient lack of anorexia or distress for apparently normal learning under the influence of cycloheximide does not exclude the possibility of negative reinforcement either in our experiment or in the appetitive task studied by Cohen and Barondes (1968), because learning might not be sensitive to moderate motivational disturbance and in any case it is not yet known whether distress, loss of appetite, or any such behavioural disruption is necessary to produce this type of negative reinforcement (Lovett and Booth, 1970). So the only way to rule out a confusion of negative reinforcement with retention blockade is either to choose a task which cannot confound them or to measure the negative reinforcement effect directly in long-term retest and prove it negligible.

Geller and colleagues (1969, 1970) and Watts and Mark (1971) have shown, using mice and chicks respectively, that cycloheximide impairs passive avoidance in a delayed retest. However, they used nondiscriminated versions of this task, in which the performance is notoriously susceptible to interference from interactions between recent aversive stimulation and the disruptive agent: if ECS is given soon enough after footshock in any environment, the mouse's motor activity is increased, producing retrieval blockade on retest in the passive avoidance environment (Schneider and Sherman, 1968; Nielson, 1968). Quartermain,

McEwen and Azmitia (1970) have demonstrated that this cycloheximide-induced deficit cannot be loss of memory because it is reversed by experience of footshock away from the training box. The results of Potts and Bitterman (1967) and Davis and Klinger (1969) indicate that the long-term shuttle-box avoidance decrements induced in goldfish by inhibition of protein synthesis immediately after training are attributable to an interaction of the same type. Under Potts and Bitterman's conditions the evidence from the discriminated performance measures is consistent with no loss of memory at all. The results of both sets of workers can be attributed to an impairment of the fish's future capacity to be frightened if new protein cannot be made during recovery from any stressful experience. That is, there is no definite evidence for retrograde amnesia or blockade of the consolidation of the conditioned content of fear (as opposed to maintenance of the unconditioned reaction pattern of fear); protein synthesis inhibition after stress outside the shuttle-box might well disrupt initial avoidance acquisition long after the antibiotic has gone. In view of these temporal gradients of motivational deficits with aversive training, it might be best to use tasks which are not only discriminated and inhibitory, but also appetitive or unreinforced.

In conclusion, it is evident that the behavioural analysis of both the neurochemical effects of training and the performance deficits induced by antibiotics is far from complete. We can expect that in the long run the findings to date will help us to understand some aspects of brain function, but we have no definite basis at present for assuming that those functions will include long-term memory retention. The contention that new or labile macromolecules are part of the memory trace remains unsupported. If further behavioural testing along the lines suggested in this paper does establish entirely non-memory deficits, we should perhaps then, if not before, pay more attention to the decreases in macromolecular incorporation observed in trained animals by Professors Hydén, Glassman and Rose: laying down memory by killing off synapses or reducing enzyme levels is as likely *a priori* as growth or new synthesis—indeed it can be argued that it is more likely (Booth, 1970). It is even conceivable that the trace involves not changes in amounts of macromolecules, but short-term conformational changes such as those discussed by Professors Hydén and Kerkut which are stabilised by molecules migrating or undergoing further shape changes.

Mr P. L. Harper and Mr P. C. Simson have collaborated with us in this work, which is supported by an M.R.C. grant.

References

AGRANOFF, B. W., DAVIS, R. E., CASOLA, L. and LIM, R. (1967). Actinomycin D blocks formation of memory of shock-avoidance in goldfish. *Science, N.Y.*, **158**, 1600–1.

BARONDES, S. H. and COHEN, H. D. (1967). Delayed and sustained effect of acetoxycycloheximide on memory in mice. *Proc. natn. Acad. Sci., U.S.A.*, **58**, 157–64.
BOOTH, D. A. (1970). Neurochemical changes correlated with learning and memory retention. In: *Molecular Mechanisms in Memory and Learning* (UNGAR, G., Ed.), pp. 1–57. Plenum Press, New York.
BOOTH, D. A. and SIMSON, P. C. (1973). Aversion to a cue acquired by its association with effects of an antibiotic. *J. comp. Physiol. Psychol.*, in press.
COHEN, H. D. and BARONDES, S. H. (1966). Further studies of learning and memory after intracerebral actinomycin D. *J. Neurochem.*, **18**, 207–11.
COHEN, H. D. and BARONDES, S. H. (1968). Cycloheximide impairs memory of an appetitive task. *Comm. behav. Biol.*, **1**, 337–40.
COONS, E. E. and MILLER, N. E. (1960). Conflict versus consolidation of memory traces to explain 'retrograde amnesia' produced by ECS. *J. comp. Physiol. Psychol.*, **53**, 524–31.
DAVIS, R. E. and KLINGER, P. D. (1969). Environmental control of amnesic agents in goldfish. *Physiol. Behav.*, **4**, 269–71.
GELLER, A., ROBUSTELLI, F., BARONDES, S. H., COHEN, H. D. and JARVIK, M. E. (1969). Impaired performance by post-trial injections of cycloheximide in a passive avoidance task. *Psychopharmacologia*, **14**, 371–6.
GELLER, A., ROBUSTELLI, F. and JARVIK, M. E. (1970). A parallel study of the amnesic effects of cycloheximide and ECS under different strengths of conditioning. *Psychopharmacologia*, **16**, 281–9.
GLASSMAN, E., HENDERSON, A., CORDLE, M., MOON, H. M. and WILSON, J. E. (1970). Effect of cycloheximide and actinomycin D on the behaviour of the headless cockroach. *Nature, Lond.*, **225**, 967–8.
LE MAGNEN, J. (1963). Olfactory identification of chemical units and mixtures and its role in behaviour. In: *Olfaction and Taste* (ZOTTERMAN, Y., Ed.), pp. 337–45. Pergamon, Oxford.
LOVETT, D. and BOOTH, D. A. (1970). Four effects of exogenous insulin on food intake. *Q. J. expl. Psychol.*, **22**, 406–19.
NIELSON, H. C. (1968). Evidence that electroconvulsive shock alters memory retrieval rather than memory consolidation. *Expl Neurol.*, **20**, 3–20.
PETERSON, G. M. and BARNETT, P. E. (1961). The cortical destruction necessary to produce a transfer of a forced-practice function. *J. comp. Physiol. Psychol.*, **54**, 382–5.
POTTS, A. and BITTERMAN, M. E. (1967). Puromycin and retention in the goldfish. *Science, N.Y.*, **158**, 1594–6.
QUARTERMAIN, D., MCEWEN, B. S. and AZMITIA, E. C. (1970). Amnesia produced by electroconvulsive shock or cycloheximide: conditions for recovery. *Science, N.Y.*, **169**, 683–6.

Rozin, P. (1969). Central or peripheral mediation of learning with long CS–US intervals in the feeding system. *J. comp. Physiol. Psychol.*, **67**, 421–9.

Schneider, A. M. and Sherman, W. (1968). Amnesia: a function of the temporal relation of footshock to electroconvulsive shock. *Science, N.Y.*, **159**, 219–21.

Smith, J. C. and Roll, D. L. (1967). Trace conditioning with X-rays as the aversive stimulus. *Psychonom. Sci.*, **9**, 11–12.

Squire, L. R. and Barondes, S. H. (1970). Actinomycin D: effects on memory at different times after training. *Nature, Lond.*, **225**, 649–50.

Watts, M. E. and Mark, R. F. (1971). Separate actions of ouabain and cycloheximide on memory. *Brain Res.*, **25**, 420–3.

Neurochemical aspects of shock-avoidance learning in cockroaches

G. W. O. OLIVER

Department of Pharmacy and Pharmacology, Portsmouth Polytechnic, Portsmouth PO1 2DZ, England

Over the past few years a large amount of interest has centred on the biochemical events underlying the acquisition and retention of memory processes in a wide variety of animals. The invertebrates with their anatomically simplified central nervous system should theoretically provide good experimental material for such studies, provided that they can be conditioned to perform the 'learned task'. Horridge (1962) showed that insects, in particular cockroaches and locusts, could be trained to keep a leg in a new position and theoretically it should be possible to study the electrophysiological and neurochemical changes which occur during the acquisition process. The neurochemical changes have been studied in our laboratories and it is one aspect of these changes I wish to discuss today.

In our earlier papers (Kerkut, Oliver, Rick and Walker, 1970a, b), it was shown that during the acquisition process there is an increased incorporation of uridine into RNA and of leucine into protein. These results indicate that there are changes in both RNA and protein metabolism during learning, and we therefore decided to investigate the protein changes in greater detail and to determine which proteins are involved in the acquisition process. From the work of Kerkut, Pitman and Walker (1969) and Pitman and Kerkut (1970), the two main synaptic transmitters in the cockroach appear to be acetylcholine and γ-aminobutyric acid (GABA). These two transmitter systems were investigated to see if the protein changes could be linked with synaptic transmission.

This paper will only be concerned with the changes which occur in the acetylcholine transmitter system; the changes occurring in the GABA transmitter system are described elsewhere (Oliver, Taberner, Rick and Kerkut, 1971).

Training procedures

Adult male cockroaches, *Periplaneta americana*, were trained by a procedure based on that described by Horridge (1962). The animals were fixed two at a time by elastic bands to a wax block. In general headless insects were used, but in the retention experiments described later whole animals were used because they had to be kept over a period of days. The cockroaches were placed above a bath of saline (Figure 7.1) and electrodes were inserted in their legs so that when the leg of one

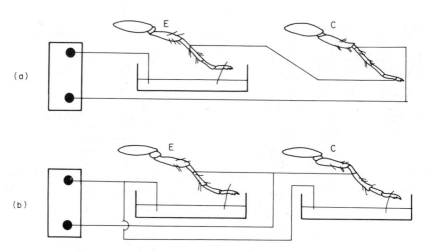

Figure 7.1. The training and retesting circuits. (a), The training circuit used in the conditioning of cockroaches in a shock-avoidance paradigm. When the cockroaches were connected into this circuit, the E animal was able to associate the shock with leg position. The C animal was randomly shocked whenever the E animal received a shock. (b), The retesting circuit. Both E and C animals received a shock when the leg touched the saline, each controlling its own shocking. Any behavioural changes that occurred in the initial training were evident on retesting. (After Horridge, 1962.)

animal touched the saline both animals would receive a shock. The stimulus was of 60 volts and 2 ms in duration, at the rate of one shock a second. A two-channel pen recorder noted when either animal placed its leg in the saline. Draughts were excluded and the temperature was maintained at 20°C, since the rate of learning was sensitive to temperature (Kerkut *et al.*, 1970b). After about forty-five minutes on the training circuit, the two animals were placed in the retest circuit to determine whether any acquisition had taken place in the animals during the initial training period.

Figure 7.2 shows the record of such a training programme. The experimental animal was trained to lift its leg out of the saline and the control animal received a shock each time the experimental animal received a shock regardless of the position of the leg of the control animal. During the initial training period, the experimental animal learned to raise its leg so that after thirty-three minutes the

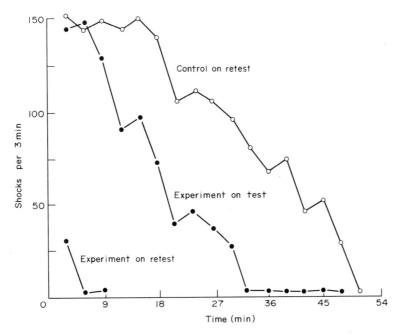

Figure 7.2. Training programme. The experimental animal (●) was given a shock each time its leg touched the saline. It learned in thirty-three minutes to keep its leg out of the saline. Ten minutes later the experimental animal was put on retest and the control animal was also put on test (i.e. given a shock each time its leg touched the saline) (○). The control animal learned in fifty minutes to keep its leg out of the saline. The experimental animal on retest required only a few shocks before it kept its leg out of the saline.

leg was kept out of the saline. This animal was then retested ten minutes later as shown by the line of closed circles. It required only a few shocks, and within six minutes it kept its leg out of the saline. The control animal was placed simultaneously on the retest circuit with the experimental animal. It was fifty-four minutes before it learned to keep its leg out of the saline. Thus the initial training period in which it was a yoked control did not make the animal more susceptible to training; if anything the reverse was true.

Tests in which the position of the leg of the control animal was studied during the training period indicated that the animal received as many shocks whilst the leg was in the saline as it did when the leg was out of the saline. The control animal was thus unable to correlate or associate the position of its leg with the onset of a shock.

Retention of memory

If the experimental animal was given a period of training (as in Figure 7.3), it learned to keep its leg out of the saline after thirty-five minutes. The stimulator was switched off at the end of the first fifty minutes for a period of three hours. During this time the animal placed its leg in the saline. When the stimulator was switched on again, the animal required only a brief period of shocks before it kept its leg out of the saline. The experimental animal therefore retains some of its training for at least twenty-four hours and in many cases up to seventy-two hours.

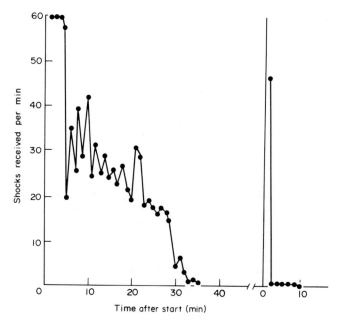

Figure 7.3. Retention of memory. The experimental animal was trained to keep its leg out of the saline. At forty-five minutes, the stimulator was turned off for three hours. The stimulator was then turned on and the animal was re-tested for retention of memory. It required only a few shocks before it kept its leg out of the saline. Animals can retain some memory for flexion up to seventy-two hours after training.

Cholinesterase changes in ganglia

In the following experiments a third type of animal, the 'resting control', was included. It was treated in exactly the same way as the other two but did not receive electric shocks at any time. Thus, it acted as a control for the determination of the effects of handling and shocks on any parameter that was measured. The cholinesterase activity, measured as μmol acetic acid released/hour per 100 μg of protein, was determined using the 'Technicon Autoanalyzer' method of Gage and Litchfield (1966). The experimental details have been given by Kerkut et al. (1970b).

Cockroaches were trained as described for one hour. The ganglia were removed and homogenised for one minute at 0°C in 1 ml of buffer. A 0·5 ml sample was used for the determination of the cholinesterase activity. A further 0·1 ml sample was made up to 1 ml and the protein concentration was estimated using the Technicon Autoanalyzer.

In this series of experiments there were thirty-one animals in each of the three groups, making a total of ninety-three. The cholinesterase activity in the various ganglia are shown in Table 7.1 and Figure 7.4. The levels of activity in the resting

Table 7.1

The cholinesterase levels in the nerve cord of cockroaches undergoing shock-avoidance training.

Ganglia	Acetic acid liberated (μmol/h per 100 μg protein)	
	Mean ± S.E.	No.
Prothoracic		
Resting	1·54 ± 0·21	31
Experimental	1·15 ± 0·05	31
Control	1·44 ± 0·03	31
Mesothoracic		
Resting	1·86 ± 0·23	31
Experimental	1·17 ± 0·05	31
Control	1·47 ± 0·05	31
Metathoracic		
Resting	2·86 ± 0·39	31
Experimental	1·12 ± 0·06	31
Control	2·08 ± 0·15	31
Abdominal (1–6)		
Resting	2·42 ± 0·07	31
Experimental	2·74 ± 0·07	31
Control	2·59 ± 0·10	31

animals were similar to those found by other authors (Colhoun, 1959) in that the lowest activity was in the prothoracic (1·54), followed by the mesothoracic (1·86) and then the abdominal ganglia (2·42), with the highest activity in the metathoracic ganglia (2·86). In the metathoracic ganglia, the activity in the resting animals was 2·86; in the controls (which were shocked) it was 2·08, while in the

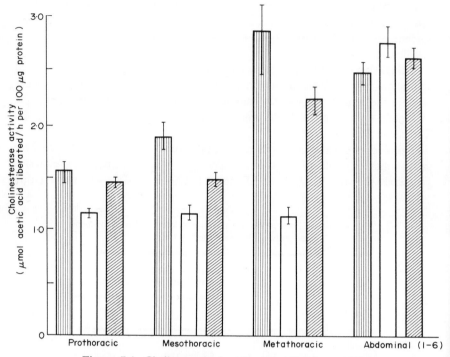

Figure 7.4. Cholinesterase in experimental (□), control (▨), and resting ganglia (▥). Note the difference between the level in the experimental, control, and resting metathoracic ganglia. The level in the experimental ganglia was less than half that in the ganglia from the resting animals.

experimental animals (shocked but learned) it was 1·12. The activity in the experimental ganglia was significantly lower than in the control or resting ganglia ($P < 0.001$). The level in the control ganglia was generally lower than that in the resting ganglia.

Thus, during training there was a reduction in cholinesterase activity in the metathoracic ganglia of the experimental animals. These changes may be correlated to the learning process since it was the metathoracic leg which was conditioned. There were smaller differences between the experimental and control mesothoracic and prothoracic ganglia, though in both cases the experimental ganglia level was lower than that of the control which was lower than the resting level. These changes in the cholinesterase activity of the ganglia may be related to the transfer of learning between the thoracic segments (Kerkut et al., 1970b). There was no such change in the cholinesterase activity in the pooled abdominal ganglia; in this case, the values for the experimental ganglia were higher than those for the resting level, though the differences were not significant ($P = 0.06$ for resting vs. experimental; $P = 0.19$ for resting vs. control).

True and pseudocholinesterases

In the experiments described so far, we determined the total cholinesterase activity in the ganglia. In the next series, the pseudocholinesterase activity was also determined to see if this activity changed. Nerve cords were removed from twelve experimental, twelve control and twelve resting control animals. They were homogenised in 1·5 ml of buffer and divided into three equal portions. The first was used to determine the total cholinesterase activity using acetylcholine as

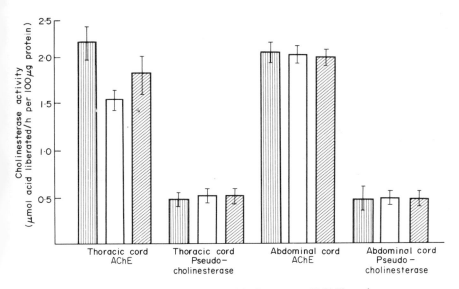

Figure 7.5. Activity of acetylcholinesterase (AChE) and pseudocholinesterase in thoracic and abdominal ganglia. Resting animals (▥) and control animals (▨) showed little difference in the activity of the pseudocholinesterase though there was a marked difference in the thoracic ganglia AChE between the experimental (☐), control, and resting animals.

120 G. W. O. Oliver

substrate in the Autoanalyzer. The second was used to determine the pseudo-cholinesterase activity using butyrylcholine as the substrate. 0·1 ml of the third was made up to 1 ml with buffer and used to determine the protein concentration of the homogenate.

Figure 7.5 shows the acetylcholinesterase and pseudocholinesterase activities in the thoracic and abdominal nerve cords from experimental, control and resting control animals. Although the experimental and resting control ganglia differed significantly in their acetylcholinesterase activities, they were similar in their pseudocholinesterase activities. The two activities were also similar in the

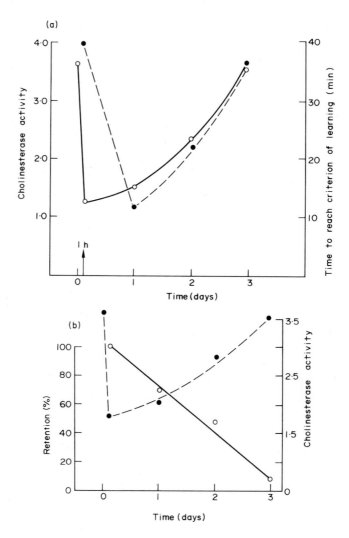

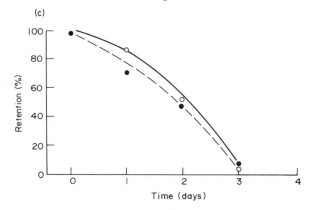

Figure 7.6. Cholinesterase (ChE) activity and the retention of memory. The animals were taken and divided into groups. On day 1 the ChE activity in the metathoracic ganglia of one group was determined. Another group was then trained as experimental animals and their ChE was determined in the metathoracic ganglia. The ChE activity in the ganglia of these trained animals was determined on successive days after training. The time taken for the animals to be retrained to the learning criteria was also determined on successive days. (a), ChE (●) in ganglia, compared with the time required for animals to reach learning criterion (○) on successive days. (b), ChE activity (●) and the percentage retention of memory (○). (c), ChE activity (●) and retention of memory (○) plotted as a change in percentage from the initial value. As the ChE level increased after training, so the memory decreased. Six animals were used at each estimation.

abdominal ganglia of all three groups of animals. Thus it seems that while there is no change in the pseudocholinesterase activity, the activity of the true cholinesterase in the thoracic ganglia of the experimental animals differs significantly from that of the control or resting animals.

Recovery of the cholinesterase activity after training

If the decreased cholinesterase activity is associated with the acquisition of learning, its level should vary according to the degree of memory retention. This postulate was tested in the next series of experiments. Eight groups of animals were treated as follows:

Group 1. These were normal resting animals which were analysed for cholinesterase and protein on day 1 as an indication of the normal resting activity level of cholinesterase in animals which did not undergo training.

Group 2 animals were trained on day 1 for one hour. The cholinesterase activity and protein concentration were determined. This group showed the decrease in cholinesterase after learning.

Group 3 animals were trained on day 1 for one hour. They were retained until day 2 and their level of cholinesterase was determined together with the protein concentration. These results showed the degree of cholinesterase recovery twenty-four hours after the learning session.

Group 4 animals were trained on day 1 for one hour. They were retained until day 2 when they were retested for one hour. These values gave the degree of memory retention after twenty-four hours.

Group 5 animals were trained on day 1 for one hour. They were retained until day 3 when they were analysed for cholinesterase and protein. From these, the degree of cholinesterase recovery after forty-eight hours was measured.

Group 6 animals were trained on day 1 for one hour. They were retained until day 3 when they were retested for one hour. These animals showed the degree of memory retention after forty-eight hours.

Group 7 animals were trained on day 1 for one hour. These animals were retained until day 4 when they were analysed for cholinesterase activity and protein concentration. This gave the degree of cholinesterase recovery after seventy-two hours.

Group 8 animals were trained for one hour on day 1. They were retained until day 4 and then retested for one hour. This gave the degree of memory retention after seventy-two hours.

The results obtained are shown graphically in Figure 7.6. Figure 7.6a shows the cholinesterase levels over a seventy-two hour period. The cholinesterase levels decreased after training but gradually returned to normal resting levels seventy-two hours after training. The percentage retention of memory was calculated as:

$$\frac{\text{time taken to learn during retest}}{\text{time taken to learn during training}} \times 100$$

These values are given in Figure 7.6b together with the cholinesterase activity during the seventy-two hours. As the cholinesterase activity levels returned to normal, the percentage memory retention fell until, at the end of seventy-two hours, the cholinesterase level had returned to the resting value while the retention had decreased to a value close to zero. It is possible to plot the percentage as a fraction of cholinesterase concentration:

$$\frac{\text{resting concentration} - \text{concentration at time } X}{\text{resting concentration} - \text{concentration after training}} \times 100$$

The percentage retention as a factor of cholinesterase was plotted together with the percentage retention as a factor of the learning times (Figure 7.6c). The two curves are very similar, indicating that the retention of memory was closely associated with the cholinesterase concentrations in the metathoracic ganglia.

Effect of drugs on the acquisition of learning

If the cholinesterase activity is associated with the acquisition of learning, drugs modifying cholinesterase activity should also have an effect on the times taken for the animals to learn. The following experiments were designed to test this.

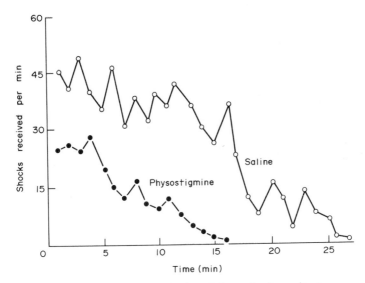

Figure 7.7. The effect of injection of physostigmine on learning. Comparison of saline-injected controls (○) and animals injected with 20 μg of physostigmine (●). The injections were carried out one hour before testing. The saline-injected control learned in twenty-six minutes, whereas the physostigmine-treated animal only took fifteen minutes to learn.

Anticholinesterases were made up in Yamasaki and Narahashi's Ringer solution (1959) and injected as 0·1 ml doses into the haemocoele of the cockroach. The control animals were injected with an equivalent volume of Ringer's solution. The drugs used were edrophonium, neostigmine and physostigmine. Figure 7.7 compares the response of a control (Ringer-injected) animal with that of one injected with 20 μg of physostigmine. The normal control animal learned in thirty minutes whereas the animal injected with physostigmine learned in ten minutes.

Physostigmine therefore facilitated learning. It is possible to prepare a series of dose–response curves which represent various concentrations of the given drugs

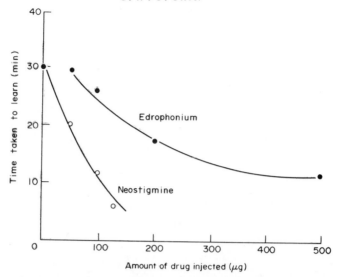

Figure 7.8. Drugs which facilitated learning. The anticholinesterases used made the animals learn more quickly than saline-treated controls. The drugs were injected one hour before the animals were trained. Six animals were injected at each dose level. Here the time taken to reach learning criteria (four or less shocks over any three-minute period) is plotted against dose of drug injected.

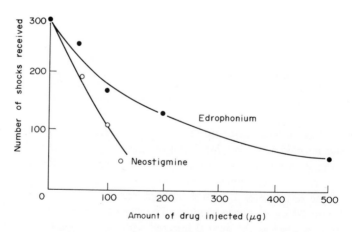

Figure 7.9. Drugs which facilitated learning. The animals were injected with anticholinesterases and the number of shocks received before reaching learning criteria are plotted against the dose of drug injected.

injected into the cockroach and the time taken for the animal to learn to keep its leg out of the saline. In our experiments, cockroaches were assumed to have learned when they received less than four shocks in a three-minute period. The results for neostigmine and edrophonium are shown in Figure 7.8. The fatal dose of physostigmine was too low (30 μg) to obtain any reasonable curves.

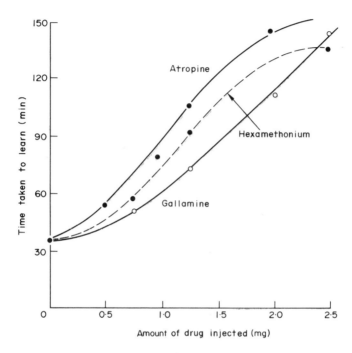

Figure 7.10. The effect of anticholinergic compounds on the time taken for animals to reach learning criteria. These drugs were injected one hour before the animals were trained. Six animals were used at each dose level. All drugs increased the time taken to reach the learning criterion. The drugs in decreasing order of potency were atropine, hexamethonium and gallamine.

In both cases the animals required less time to learn than did the normal Ringer-injected controls. The Ringer-injected animals required about thirty-four minutes to learn but the drug-injected animals required less time to learn, the most effective drug being neostigmine, 150 μg of which enabled the animals to learn in six minutes. Figure 7.9 shows the number of shocks received before the animal learned, plotted against the dose of drug injected. It has been suggested that the drug made the animals more active and enabled them, therefore, to learn more quickly. This was not so. The animals learned more quickly for a given number of shocks.

The effects of the anticholinergic compounds hexamethonium, atropine and gallamine triethiodide (Flaxedil) were also determined. These drugs affect the transmission of nerve impulses at cholinergic synapses by competing with acetylcholine at the receptor site. The net effect of these drugs is to increase the

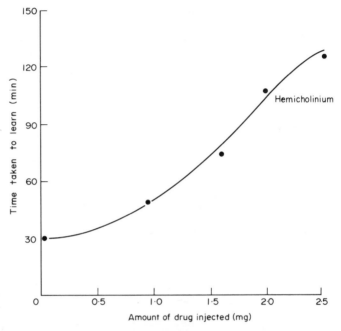

Figure 7.11. Effect of hemicholinium on the time taken to learn. The animals were injected with varying doses of the drug eighteen hours before they were trained. The time taken for the animals to reach the criterion of learning is plotted against the dose of drug injected. Increasing doses of hemicholinium increased the time taken for the animals to reach learning criterion.

synaptic ratio at the synapse, that is, they prevent the passage of the nerve impulse from the presynaptic to postsynaptic fibre.

The experiments were carried out as described previously. The results are shown in Figure 7.10. These drugs all increased the time taken for the animals to learn. Atropine was more potent than hexamethonium, which was, in turn, more potent than gallamine.

A third type of drug, hemicholinium, was injected eighteen hours before training. Again, increases in the dose caused an increase in the time taken for the animals to learn (Figure 7.11). Normal control animals (Ringer-injected) required about thirty minutes to learn whereas a 2 mg dose increased the learning time to 100 minutes or more. Hemicholinium affected the cholinergic transmitter system by reducing the amount of acetylcholine present in the synaptic ending. It prevented

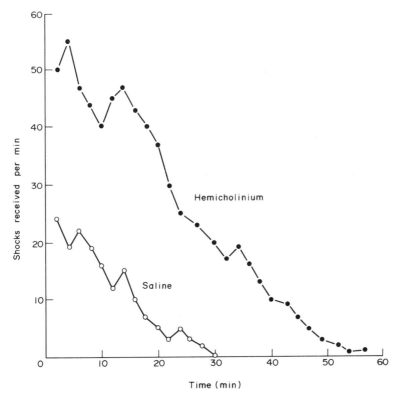

Figure 7.12. The effect of injection of hemicholinium on learning. Saline-injected animals are compared with those injected with 1 mg of hemicholinium eighteen hours before training. The saline control learned in about thirty minutes whereas the drug-injected animals took about fifty-two minutes to learn.

the synthesis of acetylcholine in the nerve and was effective only if given twelve to eighteen hours beforehand.

The anticholinergic substances and the hemicholinium did not inhibit learning by causing paralysis. The animals acted in a similar manner to the normal controls injected with Ringer, except that they received more shocks before reaching the learning criterion. Their learning curves were similar to those of the control animals except that the time axis was elongated (Figure 7.12).

Discussion

The main excitatory transmitter in the cockroach central nervous system appears to be acetylcholine. It is therefore reasonable to assume that the neurochemical changes taking place during the learning of the leg-raising response (Kerkut et al., 1970b) could be reflected by changes in the acetylcholine system. The results described here show that there was a rapid fall in the cholinesterase activity during the thirty to sixty minutes of training. They also show that shock alone can decrease the cholinesterase activity: activities in the control and resting animals were $2 \cdot 08 \pm 0 \cdot 06$ and $2 \cdot 86 \pm 0 \cdot 39$, respectively. However, by far the largest decreases

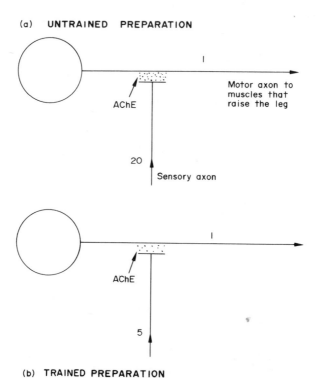

Figure 7.13. Acetylcholinesterase (AChE) changes at the synapse. It is suggested that normally twenty or so action potentials are required presynaptically to bring about one postsynaptic action potential (synaptic ratio of 20:1). If the cholinesterase activity is reduced, the synaptic ratio can change so that it then requires only five presynaptic potentials to set up one postsynaptic potential (synaptic ratio of 5:1). The AChE activity could control and alter the pathways through the neuropil.

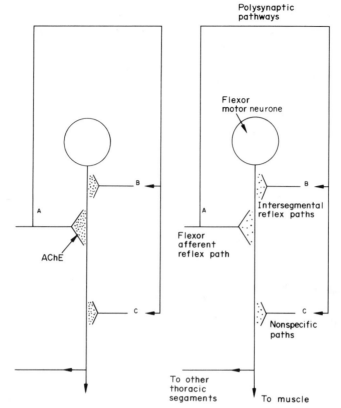

BEFORE LEARNING
(a)

AFTER LEARNING
(b)

Figure 7.14. Effect of changes in the synaptic ratio on the choice of pathways in the neuropil. (a), Diagram of flexor motor neurone with motor axon to the flexor muscle and connections to the walking reflex in other segments. It received afferent information A from the sensory nerves in its own leg, B from reflexes in other segments, and C through excitation from diffuse background activity. The synapses were cholinergic and excitatory, and had AChE in the synaptic clefts. (b), After learning, the AChE in the synaptic clefts A, B, and C was reduced. This led to a change in the synaptic ratio at these synapses. If the leg was extended it got a shock and pathways A and B brought about a maintained flexion. If synapse C became fully facilitated (synaptic ratio of 1 or so), the background activity came through and kept the leg in a flexed position. The alteration in the AChE in the polysynaptic pathways brought about changes in the synaptic ratio and hence a change in the flow of action potentials through the pathways, so making facilitated routes where there had previously been a high resistance polysynaptic network. 'Lack of use' allowed the AChE to rise and hence the synaptic ratio returned to 20:1 and the pathway became highly resistant again.

were found in the experimental animal which had learned to associate leg position with shock; here the cholinesterase activity was $1\cdot12 \pm 0\cdot06$.

Experiments investigating the mechanism by which these decreases occur have indicated that they could be the result of substrate (acetylcholine) inhibition, the presence of a blood-borne anticholinesterase (Menn and McBain, 1968) or allosteric changes in the cholinesterase enzyme due to changes in the ionic environment of the synapse. At the moment we are able to provide evidence in favour of substrate inhibition only, but we are investigating the other possibilities.

One of the functions of a synapse is to prevent an action potential from passing. Most synapses require several presynaptic action potentials for a postsynaptic action potential to be elicited. This can be described by the synaptic ratio, a synaptic ratio of 20:1 meaning that it requires twenty presynaptic potentials before one postsynaptic potential occurs. The synaptic ratio in a cholinergic system depends on the release and breakdown of the acetylcholine. If one could alter either the amount of acetylcholine released per action potential or the effectiveness of the cholinesterase, one could change the synaptic ratio of the system. Thus the model suggested here for the cockroach is as follows. Normally the pathway for the flexor reflex of the leg has a synaptic ratio of say 20:1, that is, it requires twenty action potentials in the sensory nerve before there is an action potential in the flexor motor neurone. With repeated stimulation and specific afferent reinforcement (Kerkut *et al.*, 1970b) the cholinesterase at the synapse on the flexor motor neurone would be reduced in activity, and the synaptic ratio would be reduced to 5:1 or even 1:1 (Figure 7.13). The afferent input connects through interneurones on other flexor motor neurones in that segment and to the motor neurones in the other segments through the walking reflexes. Due to specific afferent reinforcement, the synaptic ratio along the pathways leading to the flexor motor neurones in the metathoracic segment would be changed so that the limb is lifted out of the saline and maintained in that position by the activity of the interneuronal pathways (Figure 7.14).

This simplified scheme indicates a way in which the change in the behaviour could be related to the change in the cholinesterase activity. It also indicates how physostigmine, neostigmine and edrophonium facilitate learning by lowering the synaptic ratio much more quickly. Conversely, hexamethonium, atropine, gallamine and hemicholinium cause an inhibition of learning by increasing the synaptic ratio. In these cases the effective concentration of acetylcholine at the synapse is decreased and the animals require more shocks before the specific afferent reinforcement can bring the cholinesterase down to reduce the synaptic ratio to the value required for this scheme. However, it must not be imagined that this is the whole story. Other experiments on the inhibitory transmitter GABA (Oliver *et al.*, 1971) indicate that there are decreases in the enzyme activity of glutamate decarboxylase and hence decreases in the transmitter GABA. Thus, the whole story may be much more complex than has been indicated here.

References

COLHOUN, E. H. (1959). Physiological events in organophosphorus poisoning. *Can. J. Biochem. Physiol.*, **37**, 1127–34.

GAGE, J. C. and LITCHFIELD, M. H. (1966). An automated determination of cholinesterase activity in microsamples and low activity media. *Technicon International Symposium*, pp. 92–102.

HORRIDGE, G. A. (1962). Learning of leg position of the ventral nerve cord in headless insects. *Proc. R. Soc.*, B, **157**, 33–52,

KERKUT, G. A., OLIVER, G. W. O., RICK, J. T. and WALKER, R. J. (1970a). Chemical changes during learning in an insect ganglion. *Nature, Lond.*, **227**, 722–3.

KERKUT, G. A., OLIVER, G. W. O., RICK, J. T. and WALKER, R. J. (1970b). The effects of drugs on learning in a simple preparation. *Comp. gen. Pharmac.*, **1**, 437–84.

KERKUT, G. A., PITMAN, R. M. and WALKER, R. J. (1969). Iontophoretic application of Acetylcholine and GABA onto insect central neurones. *Comp. Biochem. Physiol.*, **31**, 611–33.

MENN, J. J. and MCBAIN, J. B. (1968). Possible occurrence of natural cholinesterase inhibitors in the German cockroach, *Blatella germanica*. *Ann. ent. Soc. Am.*, **61**, 1578–80.

OLIVER, G. W. O., TABERNER, P. V., RICK, J. T. and KERKUT, G. A. (1971). Changes in GABA level, GAD and ChE activity in the CNS of an insect during learning. *Comp. Biochem. Physiol.*, **38B**, 529–35.

PITMAN, R. M. and KERKUT, G. A. (1970). Comparison of the actions of iontophoretically applied acetylcholine and gamma aminobutyric acid with the EPSP and IPSP in cockroach central neurons. *Comp. gen. Pharmac.*, **1**, 221–30.

YAMASAKI, T. and NARAHASHI, T. (1959). The effects of potassium and sodium ions on the resting and action potentials of the cockroach giant axon. *J. Insect Physiol.*, **3**, 146–58.

Neurochemical correlates of behavioural change: a problem in dynamics

J. T. RICK

Department of Psychology, University of Birmingham, Birmingham B15 2TT, England

Metabolism and behavioural change are both essentially dynamic systems. Studies in either area are concerned with ongoing processes, with events rather than things. Thus, attempts to derive meaningful relationships between biochemical and behavioural events must first incorporate adequate control for the dynamics of the situation. Without such control, any measured concomitance may well be simply fortuitous. In this paper I am going to argue that dynamic control is more easily imposed during the active loss of an acquired response, that is during extinction, than during the acquisition of that response, that is during learning. If this is so, it follows that investigations of extinction offer greater scope for the clarification of macromolecular involvement in behavioural change.

Firstly, how does extinction differ from forgetting? Psychologists use the term 'extinction' to describe the removal of reinforcement that previously followed, and maintained, a specific behavioural response. The outcome of this procedure is for the subject to cease behaving specifically in response to the conditioned stimulus. The fact that the response is actively suppressed rather than forgotten can be demonstrated either by the reintroduction of the reinforcement, which is followed by the immediate return of the response, or by the two extinction phenomena, first described by Pavlov (1927), of disinhibition and spontaneous recovery.

The commonly used design for achieving dynamic control in learning experiments is to connect two animals so that one receives the conditioning stimuli of the other, but because of some asymmetry in the design, cannot utilise this input for further action. Such an animal is termed a yoked control. The yoked animal's behaviour may well change during the experiment, but any changes that do take place are assumed to be incidental to the imposed conditions and not to systematically reflect them. The assumption that the changes taking place in the control animal in the yoked design are necessarily unsystematised has been questioned. Church (1964) points to the possibility of a systematic effect of random error when there is a temporal relationship between a response in the yoked control and the conditioning event or when individual differences in the effectiveness of the event are suspected. I shall return to this criticism later and, in passing, I am not questioning the involvement of RNA and protein synthesis in the acquisition of a new response (see Agranoff, Glassman and Kerkut, this volume). The point I hope to make is that the design is more applicable to studies of extinction than to studies of acquisition.

The limitation of the design arises primarily from the fact that the behavioural change in learning is dependent on a specific pattern of imposed stimulation and that, therefore, the experimenter has to control the stimulation to which both the experimental and yoked animals are exposed. Since macromolecular changes can only be measured after the event, the acquisition process must be a relatively rapid one and this normally precludes any learning that requires more than one training session. In order to attain rapid acquisition it is usual to use an aversive training procedure incorporating electric shock, a form of stimulation which in itself significantly increases RNA synthesis. For example, in our work with cockroaches the shock increased RNA synthesis in the ganglia of the yoked control animal as compared to the resting, unshocked control by over 20 per cent (Kerkut, Oliver, Rick and Walker, 1970). This incremental effect on RNA synthesis following shock, in the light of Church's criticism (1964), imposes a constraint on the interpretation, rather than the validity of the data (for a discussion of this point, see Campbell and Church, 1969, p. 522). Given that RNA metabolism is involved in learning, one has still to consider how specific is this macromolecular involvement?

Let us turn to the process of extinction. Extinction follows the removal of reinforcement and is the active suppression of the previously reinforced response. Since reinforcement is being removed, and with it an imposed stimulus pattern, stimulus control is less constraining than it is during acquisition. In nearly all experiments in which a specific behaviour is maintained by reinforcement, withdrawal of the reinforcement causes the specific behavioural pattern to disappear usually within a period of less than one hour. I am not implying that all other types of nonspecific responses, notably autonomic, are equally sensitive to the removal of reinforcement (Eysenck, 1968), but rather that specific behavioural change in extinction is rapid relative to its counterpart in acquisition. Extinction is rapid whether the behaviour is originally maintained by reward or by punishment and whether the acquired level of responding is reached after one or numerous training sessions; the extinction of many types of acquired responding is therefore equally accessible to biochemical study. A few exceptions to the rapid extinction of the behavioural response have appeared in the literature, but they are mainly restricted to avoidance techniques incorporating shock levels that are barely sub-tetanising (Solomon, Kamin and Wynne, 1953) and, in the majority of reports, reinforced behaviours obtained in the laboratory are quickly suppressed on the removal of the stimulus control. Lastly, since one does not have to balance specific stimulation of reinforcement between the experimental and control animals, there is little constraint on the different types of yoked control animal that can be employed. A summary of these various characteristics of acquisition and extinction of a reinforced response are given in Table 8.1.

Having decided that studies of extinction of a reinforced response present fewer practical difficulties than those of its acquisition in attempting to identify the

Table 8.1

A comparison of the characteristics of behavioural change in the acquisition and extinction of a reinforced response. Note that points 2 and 3 mitigate against the use of an acquisition paradigm in the study of neurochemical correlates of behavioural change employing a yoked control design.

Reinforced response	
Acquisition	Extinction
1. Active behavioural change.	1. Active behavioural change.
2. Specific stimulation pattern.	2. No specific stimulation pattern.
3. Rapid only in specific circumstances—usually involving shock stimulation.	3. Normally rapid.

neurochemical aspects of behavioural change, one has then to determine the extent to which neurochemical correlates of extinction are identifiable, and, in particular, the extent to which macromolecular biosynthesis is involved. There are three main approaches to the second problem and all have enabled evidence to be found for the involvement of RNA in extinction.

Glassman and his co-workers have demonstrated increased biosynthesis of RNA in mouse brain during extinction of an avoidance response which is similar to that found during the acquisition of the response (Coleman, Wilson and Glassman, 1971). Glassman stresses that the increased incorporation of radioactive uridine into RNA during the acquisition of the response seems to take place only in the diencephalic region of the mouse brain. The increased labelling of RNA in both acquisition and extinction may therefore reflect the emotional state of the animal in the experimental environment rather than the biochemical activity directly concerned with the behavioural change. This is an interpretation of the data which cannot be dismissed lightly, for it is consistent with both a well formulated psychological theory of extinction in terms of frustrative non-reward (Amsel, 1962) and a recent topographical study of uridine incorporation into rat brain RNA as a result of novel electric shock (Gardner, DeBold, Firshein and Heermans, 1970). By methods similar to those used by Glassman's group, these workers found increased incorporation as a result of unavoidable electric shock only in the basal brain structures and not in cortex. However, pre-trained mice on subsequent exposure to the avoidance context fail to show enhanced RNA biosynthesis (Adair, Wilson and Glassman, 1968) which seems to rule out an interpretation based on emotional reactivity, and, to return to the experiment of Coleman *et al.* (1971), it is pertinent that the one mouse which failed to extinguish the response was chemically identical to the yoked control.

Extinction has also been facilitated by injection of RNA from the brains of extinguished donors (Braud, 1970). Braud has replicated an experiment in which extracts rich in RNA prepared from the brains of goldfish that had acquired and then extinguished an avoidance response were injected intracranially into other fish. The recipients extinguished the response significantly faster than fish injected with extracts prepared from the brains of naïve donors.

The third approach to implicate RNA involvement in this form of behavioural change is pharmacological. Matthies (1969) has demonstrated that orotic acid, a precursor of brain uridine phosphates which are incorporated in RNA, increases extinction of a conditioned response in rats by up to 200 per cent, while having little or no effect upon the rate of acquisition. He also showed that the effect does not occur if the incorporation of orotic acid into uridine phosphates is blocked by 4-aza-uracil. We have obtained the same result using the cockroach (Rick, Oliver and Kerkut, 1972). Cockroaches were arranged so that when they lowered the metathoracic leg they were shocked. Over a period they gradually maintained the leg in a flexed position. Intact animals, headless animals and isolated segments in which the ganglion controlling the leg movements was isolated from the rest of the nervous system were used. Figure 8.1 gives the mean times for initial learning, extinction and relearning. It can be seen from this that the isolated segment does not strictly extinguish since its relearning time is not different from that of the initial learning. In reaching the criterion of extinction, keeping the leg extended for more than 90 per cent of a three-minute period, the ganglion has essentially forgotten, rather than suppressed, the originally acquired response. In contrast, relearning in the intact and headless animals was relatively rapid after extinction, indicating that these animals had suppressed rather than forgotten the acquired response. Three doses of orotic acid, 250 μg, 500 μg and 1 mg, were injected into groups of all three preparations twenty-four hours before acquisition. A dose–response curve against extinction time for the headless groups is shown in Figure

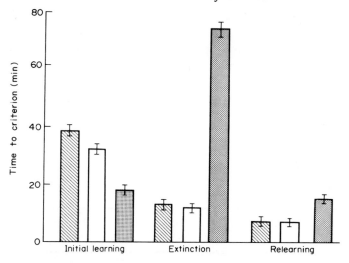

Figure 8.1. The effects of nerve lesions on learning, extinction and relearning times in the cockroach. The time of relearning does not differ significantly from initial learning in the isolated segment. (▨), Intact; (▦), isolated segments; (☐), headless.

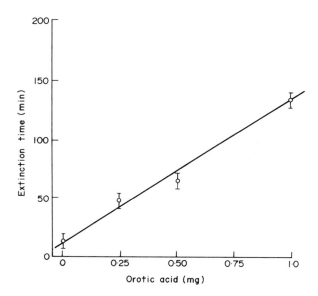

Figure 8.2. The effect of orotic acid on the extinction time of an avoidance response in headless cockroaches. The drug was administered twenty-four hours prior to testing.

8.2 and the initial learning, extinction and relearning times for each of the preparations at all dose-levels used is given in Table 8.2. From these data it can be seen that while there is a significant increase in the extinction time with dose of orotic acid, initial learning and relearning times are not so affected. This specific effect of orotic acid on extinction was also obtained by Matthies (1969) and, although the specificity is difficult to interpret in terms of RNA synthesis related to be-

Table 8.2

The learning, extinction and relearning times for an avoidance response in the cockroach under three doses of orotic acid using intact and lesioned nervous systems. Note the dose–response effect of the drug on extinction times. Data are given as means ± S.E. N = number of animals/condition.

Orotic acid, μg	Initial learning, min	Extinction time, min	Relearning, min	N
Isolated				
0	18.0 ± 2.0	73.7 ± 0.5	15.9 ± 1.8	15
250	16.5 ± 2.5	79.7 ± 9.3	16.2 ± 2.3	6
500	19.3 ± 1.8	164.8 ± 10.4	15.0 ± 1.7	6
1000	14.4 ± 1.3	246.2 ± 9.1	15.8 ± 1.2	6
Headless				
0	32.0 ± 1.4	12.2 ± 1.1	7.1 ± 1.9	12
250	30.0 ± 0.8	48.3 ± 8.0	11.5 ± 0.6	6
500	31.9 ± 0.6	65.0 ± 1.9	12.0 ± 0.8	8
1000	30.5 ± 0.9	136.8 ± 4.1	11.3 ± 0.9	6
Intact				
0	39.0 ± 2.4	13.7 ± 2.0	6.6 ± 1.9	15
250	38.5 ± 8.8	53.8 ± 7.0	11.0 ± 2.1	6
500	32.5 ± 5.8	61.0 ± 7.6	9.5 ± 1.3	6
1000	28.0 ± 4.6	114.8 ± 6.8	7.2 ± 1.5	5

havioural change, it does indicate the involvement of RNA metabolism in extinction.

To conclude, I have argued that the major problem facing attempts to define neurochemical correlates of behavioural change is that of controlling for the dynamic character of the events involved. The yoked control design has gone some way to overcome this difficulty in experiments dealing with the acquisition of a conditioned response, but, owing to the biochemical repercussions of the imposed stimulus patterns that are required for rapid acquisition, the design is likely to prove more useful when dealing with extinction.

The author acknowledges a grant from the Mental Health Research Fund and thanks Professor P. L. Broadhurst for his helpful comments on the draft of this paper.

References

ADAIR, L. B., WILSON, J. E. and GLASSMAN, E. (1968). Uridine incorporation into polysomes of mouse brain during different behavioural experiences. *Proc. natn. Acad. Sci., U.S.A.*, **61**, 917–22.

AMSEL, A. (1962). Frustrative non-reward in partial reinforcement and discrimination learning. *Psychol. Rev.*, **69**, 306–28.

BRAUD, W. G. (1970). Extinction in goldfish: facilitation by intracranial injection of RNA from the brains of extinguished donors. *Science, N.Y.*, **168**, 1234–6.

CAMPBELL, B. A. and CHURCH, R. M. (1969). *Punishment and Aversive Behaviour*. Appleton-Century-Crofts, New York.

CHURCH, R. M. (1964). Systematic effect of random error in the yoked control design. *Psychol. Bull.*, **62**, 122–31.

COLEMAN, M. S., WILSON, J. E. and GLASSMAN, E. (1971). Incorporation of uridine into polysomes of mouse brain during extinction. *Nature, Lond.*, **229**, 54–5.

EYSENCK, H. J. (1968). A theory of the incubation of anxiety/fear responses. *Behav. Res. Ther.*, **6**, 309–21.

GARDNER, F. T., DEBOLD, R. C., FIRSHEIN, W. and HEERMANS, JR., H. W. (1970). Increased incorporation of ^{14}C-Uridine into rat brain RNA as a result of novel electric shock. *Nature, Lond.*, **227**, 1242–3.

KERKUT, G. A., OLIVER, G. W. O., RICK, J. T. and WALKER, R. J. (1970). The effects of drugs on learning in a simple preparation. *Comp. gen. Pharmac.*, **1**, 437–83.

MATTHIES, H. (1969). The role of RNA precursor in memory processes, p. 295. *Fourth Int. Congr. Pharmac.* (Abstracts). Schwabe, Basel.

PAVLOV, I. P. (1927). *Conditioned Reflexes* (translated by G. V. ANREP). London, Oxford.

RICK, J. T., OLIVER, G. W. O. and KERKUT, G. A. (1972). Acquisition, extinction and reacquisition of a conditioned response in the cockroach: effects of orotic acid. *Q. Jl expl Psychol.*, **24**, 282–6.

SOLOMON, R. L., KAMIN, L. J. and WYNNE, L. C. (1953). Traumatic avoidance learning; the outcomes of several procedures with dogs. *J. abnorm. soc. Psychol.*, **48**, 291–302.

Modifications of brain chemistry in relation to behaviour

Chairman: S. V. Perry
Department of Biochemistry, Medical School, Birmingham

Biochemical approaches to learning and memory

B. W. AGRANOFF

Mental Health Research Institute, University of Michigan, Ann Arbor, Michigan 48104, USA

For a number of years it has been thought that permanent memory is formed by a biphasic process (Gerard, 1955; Hebb, 1949) involving macromolecules (Hebb, 1949; Katz and Halstead, 1950; Hydén, 1960). In our laboratory we have obtained preliminary evidence of a multiphasic memory process in which macromolecular cellular processes are selectively involved in the formation of long-term memory but not in the formation of short-term memory.

It may be useful first to visualise a model neurone as it is conceived at present. The perikaryon contains the nucleus in which the principal DNA and RNA synthesis resides, although it seems that replication does not occur in neurones after the neonatal period. Ribosomes are present in profusion in the perikaryon, but not beyond the axon hillock. This is paradoxical, since larger particles, such as mitochondria and synaptic vesicles, are seen in the presynaptic region and often throughout the axon. These particles together with some identified proteins are known to be synthesised in the perikaryon and transported down the axon by a pumping process that is independent of protein synthesis. Since neurones communicate via chemical synapses, we must bear in mind that mechanisms for synaptic regulation that are genetically programmed should in principle require axonal flow of the information in the form of new protein to presynaptic sites.

We have examined the effects of several inhibitors of DNA, RNA and protein synthesis on the biphasic memory process. These inhibitors are antibiotics developed in nature through selection and mutation, as biostatic effectors in the armamentarium of the organisms that secrete them. Arabinosyl cytosine blocks DNA synthesis for several hours with few other effects. Actinomycin D blocks

RNA synthesis rather selectively, although in general, it is more toxic than other antibiotics and may have long-term effects, days or weeks after its injection. Protein synthesis is blocked by a number of agents, including puromycin, and glutarimide derivatives such as acetoxycycloheximide and cycloheximide. More recently, we have studied a third glutarimide, anisomycin.

Our experimental subject is the common goldfish. This animal has many suitable behavioural qualities, including the ability to rapidly acquire learning of a shock-avoidance task, and to retain this learning for days to weeks. From the biochemical standpoint, its brain is easily accessible by intracranial injections. We

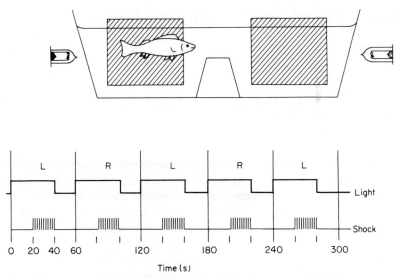

Figure 9.1. Diagrammatic representation of shuttle-box for training goldfish. Shock-avoidance coupled to a light stimulus. (From Agranoff, Davis and Brink, 1966.)

have developed a simple technique whereby 10 μl of solution are injected through a 30-gauge needle fitted to a Hamilton syringe directly through the skull of a hand-held goldfish. The 70–80 mg brain of a 10 g goldfish bathes in sufficient cranial fluid to permit rapid penetration of the injected agent. The cranial fluid–brain barrier is much more permeable than the blood-brain barrier, and less drug enters the rest of the body than when subcutaneous or intraperitoneal injections are used.

The behavioural task we have used is conditioned shock-avoidance to a light stimulus (Agranoff and Klinger, 1964) (Figure 9.1). Fish were placed in individual boxes consisting of two similar sides separated by a barrier rising to within one inch of the surface. Shock-producing electrodes and photodetector beams were present on either side of the barrier, and a signal light was placed at either end of the apparatus. At the beginning of a trial, the signal light (the conditioned stimulus,

CS) was turned on at the end of the box nearest the fish. Twenty seconds later, intermittent electrical shock (the unconditioned stimulus, US) was initiated through the water. After a few shocks, the fish swam over the barrier into the darkened (and presumably safe-appearing) end of the apparatus. The light and shock remained on in the starting side of the apparatus for forty seconds, at which time both light and shock were terminated. After twenty seconds of darkness, the second trial began with onset of light on the side of the apparatus into which the fish swam to avoid (the first twenty seconds of the trial), or to escape the shock. The response of the animals was recorded automatically. Fish did not generally swim over the barrier spontaneously or upon onset of the light signal, but did so after receiving the punishing shocks. Pairing of light and shock led to acquisition of a conditioned response. That is, the fish showed an increasing tendency to cross the barrier during the first twenty seconds of a trial, thereby avoiding the shock. On the bases of preliminary experiments, we adopted a paradigm in which groups of fish were each given twenty trials on the first day of an experiment, returned to 'home' storage tanks and given ten additional training trials three days later (day 4). We observed approximately two, four and six avoidances for trials 1–10, 11–20 (on day 1) and 21–30 (on day 4) respectively. The fish thus exhibited both acquisition and stable memory. If trials 21–30 were given on day 1 instead of on day 4, the response rate was almost sixty per cent. Fish with high response rates on day 1 generally had correspondingly higher responding rates on day 4. The use of a regression equation permitted us to combine results of fish showing different levels of responding. This was particularly useful in comparing groups trained at different times of the year, since a seasonal variability was encountered.

Results of an experiment in which puromycin was injected at various times after the first training session are shown in Table 9.1 (Agranoff, Davis and Brink, 1966). Injection of 170 μg of the drug intracranially immediately after training resulted in a performance on day 4 that was indistinguishable from that of untrained animals, while those that were returned to home tanks and injected one hour after the end of training had avoidance scores that were indistinguishable from those of animals that had not been injected. We concluded that puromycin interfered with performance of a trained task and that the effect was time-dependent. The effect is similar to that seen in animals after electroconvulsive shock (ECS) and other convulsant treatments, from which a consolidation of memory is inferred—a growing insusceptibility to disruption during a post-training period. The present experiments were characterised by an important difference. In our studies, there was no evidence of unconsciousness or other signs of neurological disturbance during the period of action of the disruptive agent. During the period of time that memory had either been disrupted or had failed to form in a permanent way, there was no detectable impairment in function. Further experiments established a dose–response relationship of the drug and intermediate points in the appearance of insusceptibility to the agent (the consolidation curve).

Injection of protein synthesis inhibitors before training had little effect on acquisition, but on retraining three days later, severe deficits were seen. This suggests a biphasic memory process: short-term memory formation (acquisition) does not require normal ongoing macromolecular synthesis, while long-term memory does. Fish injected either before or just after training and retrained at various later times (six hours to two days) showed a gradual decrease in response rates. That is, the memory associated with acquisition (short-term memory) appeared to decay slowly without conversion to a permanent form. The puromycin-disruptible process could be delayed by allowing fish to remain in the training apparatus after

Table 9.1

Effect of puromycin injected after training on memory.

No.	Trials day 1		Treatment	Trials day 4		Retention score (A–P)
	1–10	11–20		21–30 A	21–30 P	
72	2·3	3·4	Uninjected	5·3	5·3	0
36	2·5	3·8	Puromycin dihydrochloride 170 μg, immediate	2·7	5·4	−2·7
35	2·5	4·6	Puromycin dihydrochloride 170 μg, 60 min delay	5·5	5·6	−0·1

A: Score achieved; P: score predicted.

(From Agranoff, Davis and Brink, 1966.)

their session. This gave rise to the suggestion of an 'environmental trigger', of possible importance to avoidance learning in other species as well (Davis and Agranoff, 1966). Other protein inhibitors and an RNA synthesis blocker produced similar results. The cleaved fragments of puromycin produced neither amnesia nor inhibition of protein synthesis. A DNA blocker had no effect. Since our subjects are poikilotherms, we were able to establish that the rate of memory formation, judged by disruptibility, was temperature-dependent. Cooling the fish by 10° immediately after training for a two-hour period had no effect on subsequent retraining but prolonged the period of susceptibility to disruptive agents (Davis, Bright and Agranoff, 1965).

In assessing the significance of these results, let us consider whether the observed effects are related to memory or to some aspect of physiology or behaviour that could affect performance. A crude index of performance is the ability of the fish to escape after shock, since no previous training is required. No measurable effect of puromycin or acetoxycycloheximide on this innate response was seen. More important is the fact that these agents have a lesser effect on performance on day 4 when they are injected a few hours after initial training. Such a result unequivocally rules out the possibility that lingering effects of the drug account for the reduced performance. The type of learning or the aspect of learning that is blocked by these agents is not known. That the fish had been trained to avoid shocks and had not been simply activated by the shock was ruled out by experiments in which light and shock were given randomly. No avoidance learning was seen under these circumstances.

It remains possible that elements of sensitisation, conditioned fear, etc., are selectively blocked by the drug. Yet to determine which aspect of learning and memory is blocked seems to be less important than to find the molecular basis of the behavioural effect. We do not know, for example, whether the protein blockers are exerting their effect on performance by virtue of their known action or by some unknown mechanism. Their action as macromolecular blockers is suggested by the following observations. Firstly, both puromycin and the glutarimide antibiotics block memory, although they possess very different chemical structures. The only known effects these two classes of agent share is the inhibition of protein synthesis. Secondly, the doses of these agents that maximally inhibit protein synthesis, are those that also maximally block memory formation. Thirdly, the time course of the puromycin inhibition of protein synthesis in the goldfish closely resembles its effectiveness in blocking memory, judged by varying the time of injection before training on day 1.

A possible alternative mechanism for the action of puromycin on memory, based on the drug's potentiation of convulsions, was proposed several years ago (Cohen and Barondes, 1967). While puromycin, in doses that block memory in the fish or in the mouse, did not produce observable convulsions, it lowered the threshold dose of the convulsant, pentylenetetrazol. At the time, it was also thought that the glutarimide blockers did not produce amnesia, but this was shown to be incorrect (Barondes, 1970) and the connection between the convulsion-potentiating effect of puromycin and the memory block is therefore unknown. We have found that puromycin aminonucleoside, a hydrolysis product of puromycin, shares the convulsion-potentiating property of puromycin, but has no effect on protein synthesis or on memory (Agranoff, 1970).

If the agents are exerting their effects through inhibition of protein synthesis, which proteins are most directly involved? Protein (enzyme) turnover, growth processes, axonal flow and countless other major physiological functions intimately involve ongoing protein synthesis, and any or all of these may be directly involved in memory formation. While this question cannot be answered at present, we can address ourselves to the general question of whether there is failure of novel protein synthesis resulting in a memory block, or whether the agents act by lowering the steady-state level of some existing protein which mediates the memory process. In the second instance, we would also postulate that the relevant protein turns over rapidly, since injection of the drug produces an effect shortly thereafter. We might expect that injection of the protein inhibitor at various times before training would cause even further reductions in the concentrations of proteins that turn over rapidly. In fact, we find no greater inhibition after a pretrial injection, and we are therefore inclined to favour the failure of induction or growth during some critical period after training as the mechanism of action of the blocking agents. The action of actinomycin D in our experiments suggests that RNA as well as protein is implicated in the steps that lead to permanent memory formation.

More direct proof of macromolecular involvement in memory formation would doubtless come from studies with radioactive precursors administered during learning in the absence of blocking agents. In studies of both RNA and protein synthesis, we have not observed differences between experimental and control animals, but laboratories such as that of Dr Glassman (Glassman and Wilson, 1973) have shown that RNA labelling increases in animals during training. It is significant that protein labelling changes have not been seen in these experiments, for if the reported labelling increase is related to the known function of RNA, one would expect to observe greater changes in protein synthesis than in RNA synthesis.

Other current questions relate to physiological and behavioural considerations. Cannot a block in protein synthesis produce some sort of interference with memory instead of its destruction? If antibiotic-induced amnesia is temporary, we would be forced to think in terms not of memory loss but of a defect in some retrieval mechanism. A problem here is that we cannot quantify a unit of memory. The usual training task involves multiple components of behaviour, so that it is not surprising that an animal which seems completely amnesic may show some recovery of memory when given learning cues. We have not, however, observed recovery of memory in the goldfish after antibiotic treatment.

A variant of this argument states that an injected drug has stimulus effects. For example, puromycin might produce a 'headache' in the goldfish which then acts as an unconditioned stimulus. The fish injected with the drug is, by this line of reasoning, punished. Therefore, on retraining, it does not demonstrate the avoidance behaviour. We have concerned ourselves with this possibility, since it is an alternative explanation to the 'consolidation' interpretation of retrograde amnesia. Evidence from two sorts of experiments is in favour of consolidation of memory and opposes interference with memory. Firstly, pretrial injection of puromycin produces amnesia. To explain its stimulus effects under these circumstances, we must either postulate backward conditioning (the US before the CS) or a delayed aversive effect. Neither idea is attractive. Secondly, when puromycin is injected into fish that have been anaesthetised after training, there is nevertheless the expected amnesic effect (Agranoff, 1971). It remains possible that an aversive response can be produced in anaesthetised subjects (Berger, 1970).

We conclude that the most parsimonious interpretation of our results is that macromolecular synthesis is involved in the formation of long-term memory. Why then have we been unsuccessful in finding anything concomitant with labelled RNA or protein precursors in the absence of the blocking agents? Perhaps it is because the relevant changes are too small to be detected by the methods we use. In fact, as has been suggested (Agranoff, 1967), gross changes in brain labelling may represent epiphenomena of learning in memory rather than concomitants of the specific information storage processes.

References

AGRANOFF, B. W. (1967). Agents that block memory. In: *The Neurosciences: A Study Program* (QUARTON, G. C., MELNECHUK, T. and SCHMITT, F. O., Eds.), pp. 756–64. Rockefeller University Press, New York.

AGRANOFF, B. W. (1970). Protein synthesis and memory formation. In: *Protein Metabolism of the Nervous System* (LATHJA, A., Ed.), pp. 533–43. Plenum Press, New York.

AGRANOFF, B. W. (1971). Effects of antibiotics on long-term memory formation in the goldfish. In: *Animal Memory* (HONIG, W. K. and JAMES, P. H. R., Eds.), pp. 243–58. Academic Press, New York.

AGRANOFF, B. W., DAVIS, R. E. and BRINK, J. J. (1966). Chemical studies on memory fixation in goldfish. *Brain Res.*, **1**, 303–9.

AGRANOFF, B. W. and KLINGER, P. D. (1964). Puromycin effect on memory fixation in the goldfish. *Science, N.Y.*, **146**, 952–3.

BARONDES, S. H. (1970). Cerebral protein synthesis inhibitors block 'long-term' memory. *Int. Rev. Neurobiol.*, **12**, 177.

BERGER, B. D. (1970). Learning in the anesthetized rat. *Fedn Proc. Fedn Am. Socs exp. Biol.*, **29**, 749.

COHEN, H. D. and BARONDES, S. H. (1967). Puromycin effect on memory may be due to occult seizures. *Science, N.Y.*, **157**, 333–4.

DAVIS, R. E. and AGRANOFF, B. W. (1966). Stages of memory formation in goldfish: evidence for an environmental trigger. *Proc. natn. Acad. Sci., U.S.A.*, **55**, 555–9.

DAVIS, R. E., BRIGHT, P. J. and AGRANOFF, B. W. (1965). Effect of ECS and puromycin on memory in goldfish. *J. comp. Physiol. Psychol.*, **60**, 162–6.

GERARD, R. W. (1955). Biological roots of psychiatry. *Science, N.Y.*, **122**, 225–30.

GLASSMAN, E. and WILSON, J. E. (1973). RNA and brain function. In: *Macromolecules and Behaviour* (ANSELL, G. B. and BRADLEY, P. B., Eds.), pp. 81–92. Macmillan, London.

HEBB, D. O. (1949). *The Organization of Behaviour*. Wiley, New York.

HYDÉN, H. (1960). The neuron. In: *The Cell: Biochemistry, Physiology and Morphology* (BRACHET, J. and MIRSKY, A. E., Eds.), Vol. 4, pp. 215–323. Academic Press, New York.

KATZ, J. J. and HALSTEAD, W. C. (1950). Protein organization and mental function. *Comp. Psychol. Monog.*, **20**, 1–38.

Molecular mechanisms in central nervous system coding

G. UNGAR

Department of Anesthesiology, Baylor College of Medicine, Houston, Texas 77025, USA

The essential function of the nervous system is to process information. Information pouring in from the external and internal environment is continuously screened, integrated, stored and retrieved in order to dictate the appropriate behaviour. For this reason, the nervous system has a network of richly interconnected neurones; the human brain, for example, has 10^{10} neurones, each connected to 10^4 other neurones by synapses which, like the switches in a computer, direct the nerve impulses through an intricate maze of pathways.

Like all information processing machines, the brain has to convert the real world into a system of signals forming a code. The neural code has been the object of intensive investigations in the last ten years, but most of the effort was directed towards the coding by electrical patterns. An electric code, however, could not account for long-term storage of information. It seems, furthermore, that the only elements of information encoded in the electrical patterns concern the intensity of the stimulus recorded in terms of frequencies, as shown by Adrian (1928) a long time ago. It is probable that the essential information is encoded in the structure of the brain. This was expressed almost 150 years ago by Johannes Müller (1826) in his 'law of specific energies' (which could more properly be called today the law of specific information). According to this law, the quality of the information is independent of the nature of the stimulus but is determined entirely by the central connections of the pathway stimulated. In other words, if the optic nerve is hit with a hammer, light will be seen, or as Du Bois–Reymond put it: "If we could cross the optic nerve with the acoustic nerve, we could hear the lightning and see the thunder." The same basic idea was further developed by Sherrington (1906) in his emphasis on the 'local sign' in reflex action.

There is good evidence to support the idea that the fundamental coding of the nervous system is in its 'labelled lines,' that is, in the differentiation of its centres and pathways. This organisation takes place during embryonic development and

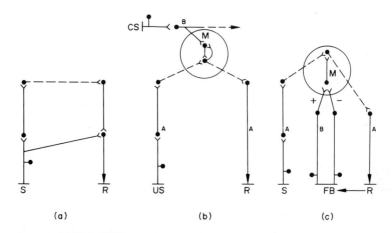

Figure 10.1. Establishment of new connections during learning. (a), Diagram of innate, reflex or instinctive behaviour; response (R) to stimulus (S) through prewired pathways. (b), Creation of a classical conditioned reflex. Response to unconditioned stimulus (US) through innate pathway A. If conditioned stimulus (CS) travelling through pathway B is presented under appropriate conditions, simultaneous firing of neurones belonging to both pathways activates modifiable neurones (M) which will link together A and B. When connection is consolidated, CS elicits R. (c), Conditioned avoidance. For example, light stimulus (S) in most rodents elicits flight to dark (R), through innate pathway A. If, on entering the dark, the animal receives an electric shock, the information is returned to the brain through feedback circuit (FB) which, by blocking the normal response, produces dark-avoiding behaviour.

stems ultimately from a blueprint laid down in the genetic code. I will come back to this point in the discussion of the molecular nature of the neural code.

In most higher vertebrates, the nervous system is fully developed at birth or shortly after. The young animal is ready to respond to certain stimuli in a stereotyped fashion. These innate responses, going from simple reflexes to complex instinctive patterns of behaviour, result from the rigidly determined connections that form the 'prewired' pathways (Figure 10.1a). The problem now is to reconcile with this rigid determinism the possibility of putting out new patterns of behaviour, of responding to stimuli not foreseen by our genetic inheritance and of storing new information for future reference. The importance of learning and memory is obvious: they assure greater flexibility and better adaptation to a wide range of unexpected environmental conditions.

Figure 10.1b shows how learning can take place by the creation of new connections between existing pathways, as illustrated by classical conditioning. The unconditioned stimulus and the corresponding response are carried by an innate pathway (A) from US to R. The conditioned stimulus is conducted through another innate pathway (B) not originally connected with A. However, when pathways A and B fire simultaneously or almost simultaneously in the appropriate sequence, the two pathways become connected. This probably takes place through specialised cells (M), called modifiable neurones by Brindley (1967) or memory neurones by Szilard (1964). The process shown in the encircled area occurs simultaneously in widely dispersed areas of the brain at a number of hierarchic levels. Figure 10.1c illustrates the conditioned avoidance type of learning in which the response is modified through positive or negative feedback, returning information to the brain on the outcome of the response.

These circuit diagrams may explain how the new connections are established but they leave open the question of their consolidation. In other words, they account for short-term memory but not for the persistence of acquired information. The 'reverberating circuit' hypothesis was shown to be untenable because complete arrest of electrical phenomena in the brain (by hypothermia or electroconvulsive shock) fails to affect long-term memory. The idea of synaptic growth, proposed by Ramón y Cajal (1909–11) and still widely held, is unlikely because it would be both too slow and too permanent to be compatible with what is known of the learning process.

The general tendency today is to regard learning as the result of an ill-defined process of 'synaptic facilitation'. This may consist of increased availability of transmitters at the presynaptic neurone or of receptors at the postsynaptic side. Jacobson (1969) proposes the term 'synaptic validation' which is supported by the findings of Cragg (1968) that only about 10 per cent of the morphologically detectable synapses are functional; the remaining 90 per cent could, therefore, be made functional by the process just described.

These synaptic changes associated with learning imply, of course, the existence of chemical correlates. This has been supported by the elegant experiments of Hydén (1967), followed by many others showing changes in brain RNA and protein. Further evidence for the importance of these chemical changes is the possibility of interfering with learning by means of drugs that inhibit RNA or protein metabolism.

The results of these experiments have been interpreted in two different ways. According to the most commonly held view, the changes would be nonspecific, that is, they would indicate merely a heightened metabolism and an increased need for transmitters or receptors, and the newly synthesised molecules would not represent a record of the information acquired.

The other view, which I propose to defend here, is that some of these molecules are specifically coded and are part of the neural code. These coded substances are, however, present in such low concentrations that they are drowned by the 'chemical noise' of increased metabolism. This would explain why the chemical studies have been inconclusive.

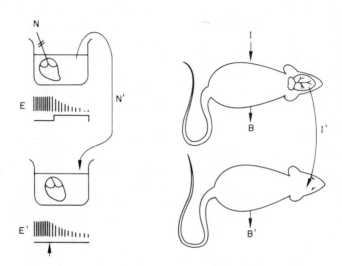

Figure 10.2. Comparison between physiological and behavioural bioassays. Left, Diagram of Loewi's experiment to demonstrate chemical transmission of vagal effect on the heart. N, Vagal stimulation; E, Effect on heart; N', Chemical equivalent of vagal stimulation; and E', its effect on heart. Right, Diagram of behavioural bioassay. I, Information put into animal during training; B, Resulting behaviour; I', Chemical equivalent of information; and B', its behavioural effect.

In the past, under similar circumstances, the problem was solved by the use of bioassays. Hormones, vitamins and neurotransmitters were first demonstrated by virtue of their biological activities, not their chemical or physical properties. Figure 10.2 shows the diagram of the original experiment by which Loewi (1921) demonstrated the chemical transmission of the action of the vagus (N) on the heart. The effect produced by vagal stimulation of a donor heart (E) could be transferred to a recipient heart by means of the bathing fluid (E'). The same principle could be applied to the problem of coding. An input of information (I) produces a behavioural change in the donor animal. When this is well consolidated, an extract of the donor brain is injected into recipient animals. If, without having been given the actual information, these recipients show the same or a closely similar behavioural change (B′), it is probable that the brain extract contained the information in chemical form (I′).

Experiments of this type have now been successfully performed in at least twenty-eight laboratories and the number of publications is well over a hundred. There have been some unsuccessful attempts, especially at the early stages of the research when the conditions were little known. This problem is discussed in several recent reviews and I shall describe only one of the bioassay methods, one that has enabled us to identify a coded molecule (Ungar, 1971a, b; Ungar and Chapouthier, 1971; Ungar, Galvan and Clark, 1968).

Training of the donor animals was based on the innate preference of rodents for dark enclosures. This preference can be reversed by submitting the animals to electric shocks when they take refuge in the dark. Dark avoidance develops after a few trials but we found that training must be continued for at least five days. At this time, the donors were killed and a crude extract of their brain was injected into recipients that had been previously tested for dark preference. These animals were never shocked; they were given the choice between the lighted and dark compartments for three minutes and the time spent in each was recorded.

During a period of slightly over two years, about 4000 donor rats were trained and 115 extracts were prepared from their brains. Figure 10.3 shows the results of the tests performed with these extracts injected into groups of mice. Each mouse was tested for the time spent in the dark-box (DBT), once before injection (column S) and four times during the forty-eight hours following the injection (E). Other groups of mice were injected with thirty-four control extracts taken from untrained rats (C). The vertical lines indicate the standard deviation. The probability of column E representing the same population as columns S or C is <0.001.

Using this method as a bioassay, we started isolating the active material from 5 kg of trained-rat brain. First we made an RNA extract of the brain from which the active substance was dialysed out at low pH. This step gave us 1–5 mg of material per g of brain. By passing this through a gel filtration column (Sephadex G-25) we obtained an active fraction of 5–10 μg/g. This was further purified by thin-layer chromatography under a variety of conditions until we obtained a spot (R_F 0·55) that could not be resolved into further components. The presence of this spot could not be detected in the same amount of an identically purified extract of untrained brain (Figure 10.4).

We knew from the beginning that the active substance was a peptide since it had a comparatively low molecular weight, its activity was destroyed by trypsin, and the spot containing it was stained by ninhydrin. We determined, therefore, its amino acid content, first qualitatively by a microdansylation method (Neuhoff, von der Haar, Schimme and Weise, 1969), then quantitatively. It was found to have fifteen amino acid residues, split in the middle by trypsin between lysine and serine. The N-terminal group was serine. The sequence of amino acids was determined by high resolution mass spectrometry with the help of my colleague Dr D. M. Desiderio. Table 10.1 shows the fragments identified by their masses and the way they fall into place to give the whole sequence (A). The uncertainties at positions 2, 5 and 11 are due to the possibility of the loss of amide groups during

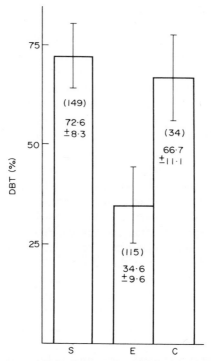

Figure 10.3. Summary of tests in mice injected with brain extracts from 4000 rats. DBT, Percentage of time spent in dark compartment during 180-second tests ±S.D.; S, Screening values obtained before injection; E, Values obtained in mice injected with brain extracts from trained rats; and C, Effect of extracts from untrained rats. Figures in parentheses indicate number of extracts, each from pooled brains of twenty to one hundred rats.

the ionisation process. To resolve the problem, a peptide with all three hydroxyl groups free (B) was synthesised by Dr B. Weinstein of the University of Washington. It had only 2 per cent of the biological activity of the natural peptide. The fully amidated compound (C), made by Dr W. Parr, of the University of Houston, showed 10 per cent activity. Finally, Dr Parr made peptide D which had the full activity and which showed the same chromatographic behaviour as the natural product (Ungar, Desiderio and Parr, 1972).

I gave the name scotophobin to this peptide (from the Greek *skotos*, dark and *phobos*, fear). I plan to label it and devise a radioimmunoassay for its detection. This would replace the bioassay which has been the most difficult and least reliable step in the whole procedure. All bioassays suffer from this defect but it becomes particularly marked when the test is based on the measurement of behaviour with its multiple and complex determinants.

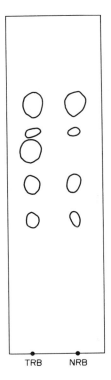

Figure 10.4. Thin-layer chromatogram of preparations obtained from trained-rat brain (TRB) and untrained-rat brain (NRB). Solvent system: *n*-butanol, ethanol, acetic acid, water (80:20:10:30). The ninhydrin-stained spot at R_F 0·55 contained all the biological activity.

We have started to prepare another behaviour-inducing substance which in our early experiments was found to be capable of transferring habituation to a sound stimulus (Ungar and Oceguera-Navarro, 1965). It is also a peptide, inactivated by chymotrypsin. We have already collected about 3 kg of donor brain. We also plan to identify the peptides first described by Zippel and Domagk in their colour discrimination experiments with goldfish (Zippel and Domagk, 1969). About

Table 10.1

Determination of the amino acid sequence of scotophobin.

	1	2	3	4	5	6	7	8	9	10	11	12	13	14	15
	SER	ASX	ASN	ASN											
			ASN	ASN	GLX										
					GLX	GLN									
						GLN	GLY								
							GLY	LYS							
							GLY	LYS	SER						
									SER	ALA					
										ALA	GLX				
											GLX	GLN			
												GLN	GLY		
												GLN	GLY	GLY	
													GLY	GLY	TYRNH$_2$
(A)	SER	ASX	ASN	ASN	GLX	GLN	GLY	LYS	SER	ALA	GLX	GLN	GLY	GLY	TYRNH$_2$
(B)	SER	ASP	ASN	ASN	GLU	GLN	GLY	LYS	SER	ALA	GLU	GLN	GLY	GLY	TYRNH$_2$
(C)	SER	ASN	ASN	ASN	GLN	GLN	GLY	LYS	SER	ALA	GLN	GLN	GLY	GLY	TYRNH$_2$
(D)	SER	ASP	ASN	ASN	GLN	GLN	GLY	LYS	SER	ALA	GLN	GLN	GLY	GLY	TYRNH$_2$
	1	2	3	4	5	6	7	8	9	10	11	12	13	14	15

The di- and tri-peptides were identified by their masses by high-resolution mass spectrometry. Sequence A, deduced from the data, contained uncertainties at positions 2, 5 and 11. Sequence B had 2 per cent of the biological activity of natural scotophobin, sequence C had 10 per cent and sequence D had 100 per cent activity.

20 000 goldfish brains will be required for the isolation of each of these peptides. It is obvious that many more of these behaviour-inducing substances will have to be identified before we can understand their real significance. My working hypothesis, in the meantime, is that scotophobin is one of the many codewords in which information is processed by the brain.

Speculations on a possible molecular code of acquired information have been made either in the context of the field theory or against the background of the connectionist view. McConnell (1965), Landauer (1964), Robinson (1966) and others tend to regard the molecular code as independent of the neural pathways. These hypotheses are proud to be 'non-neurological' and envisage the molecular codewords as 'tape-recorder molecules' which encode experience in some entirely novel and unknown manner. To use Hebb's metaphor (1949), they float in the bowlful of porridge that, in the field theory, represents the structure of the brain.

It is difficult to accept the idea that the highly differentiated organisation of the brain—perhaps the most complex structure, with the highest information content, existing on earth—has no part in information processing. Most hypotheses such as those proposed by Halstead (1951), Szilard (1964), Rosenblatt (1967), Best (1968) and others place the molecular code in the framework of neural organisation. So does the hypothesis I first put forward in 1968 (Ungar, 1968). This hypothesis is based on the concept of chemospecific pathways, developed by Sperry (1963), Gaze (1970), Jacobson (1969) and others, according to which the differentiation of the pathways in the CNS takes place by a process of chemical recognition. The cells intended to be connected together recognise each other by the chemical labels they bear. The many experimental data collected on the embryonic development of the optic and somatosensory pathways cannot at present be interpreted in any other way. One can therefore assume that, before any learning can take place, the brain is provided with a genetically determined coding system. Parenthetically, one should note that this system may be an extreme refinement of the molecular recognition between all cells of the same type. Moscona and Moscona (1963) have shown that this depends on the presence of specific recognition molecules and that it can be inhibited by puromycin.

The problem now is to find out how the innate neural code can be used for the processing of acquired information. According to what I said earlier, learning requires the formation of new connections between existing pathways. In Szilard's hypothesis (1964), this is accompanied by what he called 'transprinting,' that is, the passage of the specific molecular label from one neurone to another. Figure 10.5 shows this possibility as it would occur in Pavlovian conditioning. Before conditioning, stimulus S_A would elicit a stereotyped response R_A because of the inborn connections of the pathway marked by label A. During conditioning, when the conditioned stimulus (travelling on pathway B) and the unconditioned stimulus (A) are presented in close temporal proximity, the new connection formed results in the transprinting of the labels in the memory neurone. The two labels then form a complex AB which represents a permanent record of the connection so that S_B will now elicit the response previously produced by S_A only.

Paul Weiss (1965) suggested that acquired information may use the innate alphabet to form new words. It may perhaps be more correctly stated that it uses the innate vocabulary to form new sentences, the innate vocabulary being represented by the codewords of the preformed pathways. Scotophobin could then be

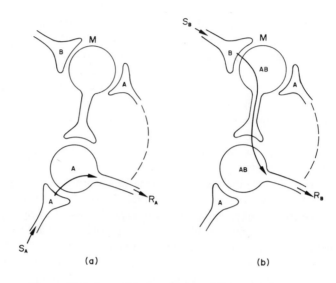

Figure 10.5. A possible functioning of the molecular code. The classical conditioning situation illustrated in Figure 10.1b is shown (a), before, and (b), after consolidation of the acquired behaviour. The two pathways involved are assumed to be labelled by peptides A and B. The newly formed connection between the pathways is explained by the merger of their two labels, perhaps in the modifiable neurones (M), which serve as connecting elements. The resulting composite peptide AB represents the codeword for the new connection.

regarded as a sentence or a composite word, encoding the connections through which nerve impulses travel to produce the dark-avoiding behaviour.

The neural code would operate to direct the differentiation of the CNS during embryonic development, and throughout life to record the creation of new synaptic connections corresponding to the acquisition of new information. This hypothesis can be submitted to experimental verification in the foreseeable future but the main task ahead of all of us interested in solving the problem of brain function is to accumulate more material and identify more of the coded molecules.

One can represent the brain as a computer capable of reprogramming itself in the light of new input of information. The important correction to make to the computer model is that the brain functions by chemical means: it obtains the energy that drives it from metabolic processes, its switches (the transmitters) are chemical and, finally, its programming is done by a molecular code. This chemical computer may function by simulating the universe, to each of us our particular universe, and our relations with it.

References

ADRIAN, E. D. (1928). *The Basis of Sensation*. Christophers, London.
BEST, R. M. (1968). Encoding the memory in the neuron. *Psychol. Rep.*, **22**, 107.
BRINDLEY, G. S. (1967). The classification of modifiable synapses and their use in models for conditioning. *Proc. R. Soc.*, B, **168**, 361–76.
CRAGG, B. G. (1968). Are there structural alterations in synapses related to functioning? *Proc. R. Soc.*, B, **171**, 319–23.
GAZE, R. M. (1970). *The Formation of Nerve Connections*. Academic Press, New York.
HALSTEAD, W. C. (1951). Brain and intelligence. In: *Cerebral Mechanisms in Behavior* (JEFFRESS, L. A., Ed.), p. 244. Wiley, New York.
HEBB, D. O. (1949). *The Organization of Behavior*. Wiley, New York.
HYDÉN, H. (1967). Behavior, neural function and RNA. *Prog. Nucl. Acid Res.*, **6**, 187–218.
JACOBSON, M. (1969). Development of specific neuronal connections. *Science, N.Y.*, **163**, 543–47.
LANDAUER, T. K. (1964). Two hypotheses concerning the biochemical basis of memory. *Psychol. Rev.*, **71**, 167–79.
LOEWI, O. (1921). Über die humorale Übertragbarkeit der Herznervenwirkung. *Pfluegers Arch. Ges. Physiol.*, **189**, 239–42.
MCCONNELL, J. V. (1965). A tape recorded theory of memory. *Worm Runner's Digest*, **7** (2), 3.
MOSCONA, M. H. and MOSCONA, A. A. (1963). Inhibition of adhesiveness and aggregation of dissociated cells by inhibitors of protein and RNA synthesis. *Science, N.Y.*, **142**, 1070–1.
MÜLLER, J. (1826). *Zur vergleichenden Physiologie des Gesichtsinnes des Menschen und der Tiere*. Knobloch, Leipzig.
NEUHOFF, V., VON DER HAAR, F., SCHIMME, E. and WEISE, M. (1969). *Hoppe-Seyler's Z. physiol. Chem.*, **350**, 121.
RAMÓN Y CAJAL, S. (1909–11). *Histologie du système nerveux de l'homme et des vertébres*. Maloine, Paris.
ROBINSON, C. E. (1966). A chemical model of long-term memory and recall. In: *Molecular Basis of Some Aspects of Mental Activity* (WALAAS, O., Ed.), Vol. I, p. 29. Academic Press, New York.

ROSENBLATT, F. (1967). Recent work on theoretical models of biological memory. In: *Computer and Information Sciences* (TOU, J., Ed.), Vol. II. Spartan Books, Washington D.C.

SHERRINGTON, C. S. (1906). *Integrative Action of the Nervous System*. Yale University Press, New Haven.

SPERRY, R. W. (1963). Chemoaffinity in the orderly growth of nerve fiber patterns and connections. *Proc. natn. Acad. Sci., U.S.A.*, **50**, 703–10.

SZILARD, L. (1964). On memory and recall. *Proc. natn. Acad. Sci., U.S.A.*, **51**, 1092–9.

UNGAR, G. (1968). Molecular mechanisms in learning. *Perspect. Biol. Med.*, **11**, 217.

UNGAR, G. (1971a). Chemical transfer of acquired information. In: *Methods in Pharmacology* (SCHWARTZ, A., Ed.), Vol. I, p. 479. Appleton-Century-Crofts, New York.

UNGAR, G. (1971b). Chemical transfer of information. In: *Handbook of Neurochemistry* (LATHJA, A., Ed.), Vol. VI, p. 241. Plenum Press, New York.

UNGAR, G. and CHAPOUTHIER, G. (1971). Mécanismes moléculaires de l'utilisation de l'information par le cerveau. *L'Année Psychologique*, p. 153.

UNGAR, G., DESIDERIO, D. M. and PARR, W. (1972). Isolation, identification and synthesis of a specific-behaviour-inducing brain peptide. *Nature, Lond.*, **238**, 198–202.

UNGAR, G., GALVAN, L. and CLARK, R. H. (1968). Chemical transfer of learned fear. *Nature, Lond.*, **217**, 1259–61.

UNGAR, G. and OCEGUERA-NAVARRO, C. (1965). Transfer of habituation by material extracted from brain. *Nature, Lond.*, **207**, 301–2.

WEISS, P. (1965). Specificity in the neurosciences. *Neurosci. Res. Progr. Bull.*, **3**, 5.

ZIPPEL, H. P. and DOMAGK, G. F. (1969). Versuche zur chemischen Gedachtnisübertragung von farbdressierten Goldfischen auf undressierte Tiere. *Experientia*, **25**, 938–40.

Specific and nonspecific RNA synthesis in relation to behavioural changes

P. MANDEL, R. DI CARLO,* S. SIMLER and H. RANDRIANARISOA

Centre de Neurochimie du CNRS, 11 rue Humann, 67-Strasbourg, France

There is need for clarification of the relationship between RNA or proteins and behaviour, which has been reported by several authors (Quarton, Melnechuk and Schmitt, 1967; Glassman, 1969). It seems highly probable that specific biochemical and/or biophysical changes, correlated with environmental stimulation or learning, occur in the brain. These changes might involve alterations in the rate of synthesis of some pre-existing molecules involved in overall cellular activity or the synthesis of new molecular species.

Two possible means by which macromolecules like RNA or proteins may be involved in behaviour can be considered: (1) indirect involvement: the macromolecules may be involved in the synthesis of enzymes producing energy or involved in active transport, in the synthesis of different cellular constituents and structures, and in various metabolic pathways, (2) direct involvement: the macromolecules may be triggers directly responsible for behavioural states through their role as receptors or storage molecules, or as effectors which may act on these receptors. These effectors should be distinguished from the information-storing molecules.

If learning is related to production of new receptor molecules, we must be able to identify these molecules and study their synthesis, and if precursor molecules are normally present, the changes in their conformation.

* Present address: Istituto di Farmacologia, Università di Torino, Italy.

RNA and learning

The hypothesis of the involvement of RNA in memory and learning was formulated by Hydén (1960). Using very elegant techniques, Hydén and his co-workers (Hydén and Egyhazi, 1962, 1964; Hydén and Lange, 1965; Hydén, 1967) demonstrated that learning caused either an increase in the amount of RNA or a shift to a DNA-like base ratio of the RNA in neuronal nuclei. Changes in the amount and synthesis rate of RNA in various behavioural and learning situations have been reported by several authors (Watson, 1965; Zemp, Wilson, Schlesinger, Boggan and Glassman, 1966; Zemp, Wilson and Glassman, 1967; see also review by Glassman, 1969), and production of RNA species specific to learning has been claimed by Machlus and Gaito (1969). Although all these experiments were done very carefully, some errors cannot be excluded. Rather than experimental details we will discuss the implications of the working hypothesis, the methodological limitations and the problem of nonspecific changes following learning and memory storage.

Since RNA synthesis is a transcription phenomenon, only RNA molecules complementary to the cellular DNA can be produced. However, if we assume that for every learning or memory phenomenon a new RNA species is synthesised, we expect that specific nucleotide sequences for this RNA exist in the DNA of the individuals who learn, and in the parental DNA, the former being produced by replication of the latter. Thus, the inference we should·draw from the hypothesis that specific RNA molecules ensure the storage of information would be that all that we will learn and remember from this meeting was already coded in our own and in our parents' DNA. This is an obligatory conclusion of the concept that the memory engram is a new messenger RNA, and seems difficult to accept.

Methodological limitations

If we ascribe the storage of a memory to synthesis of a specific new RNA molecule, the question is: are we able, with the usual methods, to detect the appearance of this molecule ? This is of fundamental importance for deeper research in this field. According to generally accepted data, every cell contains and produces a few thousand proteins, some corresponding to common biochemical pathways, some being specific. In an area of the central nervous system where several cell types are close to each other, several thousand different proteins are present. This implies that several thousand messenger RNAs can be expected. Since transcription in the different cells is asynchronic, taking into account the half-life values of the mRNA, it is reasonable to accept that at least 1000 mRNA species are synthesised per hour, the usual labelling delay during learning experiments. Thus, if as a result of learning one or two new RNA species appear, it seems unlikely that they can be detected with the methods available, the methods which were in fact used. The direct analytical method for the determination of the changes of the four RNA nucleotides is not satisfactory since with four ciphers it is obviously impossible to detect one RNA molecule among a thousand others. The isolation and the determination of the primary structure of these new molecules has never been achieved, the amount of available material being extremely low.

The use of isotopic tracers might facilitate the detection of changes in RNA neosynthesis but there are limitations due to the complexity of the kinetics which should be taken into account.

Hybridisation methods

Newly induced RNA molecules present in the brain of learning animals, but not in naïve animals, could in theory be pulse labelled and detected by direct or competitive hybridisation experiments. In fact, Machlus and Gaito (1968a, b, 1969) reported the detection of RNA species unique to a behavioural task. Unfortunately, because of the limitations of the methods used, the detection of a significant difference seems unrealistic. More recently, Von Hungen (1970) failed to replicate the hybridisation experiments which were reported. Very large excesses of short-term pulse labelled RNA are required to approach saturation of the complementary DNA (Bondy and Roberts, 1968; Stevenin, Samec, Jacob and Mandel, 1968; Wyatt and Tata, 1968) and very large amounts of competitive RNA are required for effective competition (Church and McCarthy, 1968; Shimada and Gorbman, 1970). The specific radioactivity of mRNA which can be obtained in brain is rather low; the differences between duplicates are, under these conditions, of about five per hundred and the goal is to find a difference of one per thousand (one new messenger among a thousand others). Moreover, a high degree of redundancy of DNA cistrons coding for RNA (Britten and Kohne, 1968; Stevenin et al., 1968; Stevenin, Mandel and Jacob, 1969) increases the difficulties in interpreting hybridisation experiments.

This redundancy is suggested by the hybridisation data reported in Figure 11.1. Since 0·15 per cent of brain DNA was hybridised by ribosomal RNA, there were 3000 cistrons for every ribosomal RNA (18S and 28S). The hybridisation data of the total and cytoplasmic RNA, respectively 1, 2 and 0·8 per cent of the DNA, suggested an average value of 30 000 to 300 000 transcribed cistrons of brain cells if we assumed that the average molecular weight of the peptide chains was 10 000–100 000. This implies a high redundancy of messenger-type RNA and a coding of some messenger RNA molecules by repetitive cistrons. In fact, Britten and Kohne (1968) using the DNA reassociation method discovered a large number of repeated sequences in eukaryotic DNA. Thus, the detection of a unique molecule of a messenger or of any new RNA by hybridisation experiments appears laborious and extremely difficult. It is even more difficult in brain than in other tissues since it is very hard to obtain highly labelled RNA in neuronal cells. The hybridisation of RNA from single copy chains is not easily distinguished from that of RNA which is the product of repeated chains, and depends strongly on the

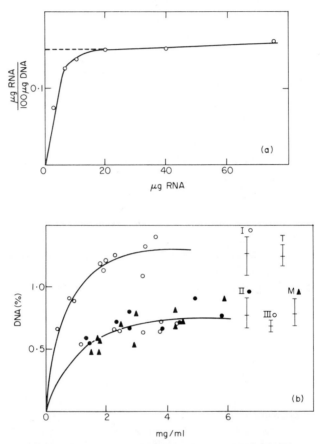

Figure 11.1. Saturation of DNA (a) with ribosomal RNA and (b) with total (T), microsomal (M▲), giant-size (I○) and ribosomal RNA (II● = 28S; III○ = 18S). It appears that ribosomal RNA hybridises with 0.15 per cent of the DNA, total RNA with 1.27 per cent (1.09–1.40) and microsomal RNA with, at a maximum, 0.8 per cent.

ionic strength and annealing temperature (Church and McCarthy, 1968). It should also be pointed out that only 70 per cent of the transcribed DNA present in the brain nuclei was transferred to the cytoplasm (Figure 11.1). This means that 30 per cent of the synthesised RNA was nucleus-restricted and would be degraded in this organelle. Thus, in experiments using for instance [^{3}H]uridine as a precursor, about 30 per cent of the labelled UMP and CMP of RNA molecules would not be translated in terms of proteins. After a short pulse much of the label would be in this type of RNA which was not functioning as messenger RNA, and might be a cause of errors in the interpretation of changes following learning experiments.

In addition, in normal hybridisation experiments, and even more in the competitive hybridisation experiments which are more desirable for the detection of new messengers, changes in precursor pool can cause differences in labelling of populations of RNA species; this can lead to data which might erroneously be interpreted as induction of new species of RNA. This is especially important for evaluating hybridisation results concerning behaviour and brain RNA metabolism since the training or the stress situation might produce an increase in the incorporation of the labelled molecules used in the intracellular heterogeneous pool of free nucleoside diphosphates, the direct RNA precursors. In experiments performed on amphetamine-treated rats, we found a large increase in the labelling of the α-phosphate of ATP after labelling with ^{32}P although the amount of brain ATP remained constant (*vide infra*). Since the α-phosphate was incorporated into the RNA molecule, changes in the specific activities of different RNA types could be expected to result simply from alterations in the free nucleotide pools.

RNA polymerase activity

Increases in RNA polymerase activity have been reported as effects of various hormones (Weill, Busch, Chambon and Mandel, 1963; Doly, Ramuz, Mandel and Chambon, 1965; Tata, 1967a; for references see Tata, 1967b). Since an increase in RNA synthesis in brain during learning has been reported, an attempt has been made to correlate this increase with the activation of RNA polymerase. In this meeting, a significant increase in the level of RNA polymerase activity was reported in the forebrain roof of the chicken in imprinting experiments by Rose, Bateson and Horn (1973).

In fact, RNA polymerase activity is quite high in brain. The figures for brain cells are approximately two or three times greater than those for liver (Table 11.1), and twice as high in neurones as in glia cells, when the measurements are performed in the presence of 0·4 M ammonium sulphate. However, in the presence of ammonium sulphate, the whole potential activity is measured. The actual enzymatic activity measured at 37°C without ammonium sulphate, is altered by degradation of the product by nucleases (Chambon, Ramuz, Mandel and Doly, 1968; Munoz and Mandel, 1968). Thus, the RNA synthesised is mainly ribosomal in nature, the messenger RNA being much more labile. This is why experiments without ammonium sulphate should be performed at 17°C, a temperature at which ribonuclease activity is negligible. But under these conditions the activities measured are relatively low and a part of this activity may correspond to the nucleus-restricted nonfunctional RNA. Moreover, the RNA polymerase activity measured is in principle related to the biosynthesis of all cellular RNA, that is, of several thousand molecular types. Thus if a significant increase in RNA polymerase activity is found, it would probably correspond to an overall increase of RNA synthesis related to a general stimulation of cellular activity, rather than to the additional synthesis of one or two RNA species.

Table 11.1

Aggregate RNA polymerase activity.

Organ	nmol [^{32}P]GTP incorporated/mg DNA			
	37°C, 10 min		17°C, 20 min	
	$-(NH_4)_2SO_4$	$+(NH_4)_2SO_4$	$-(NH_4)_2SO_4$	$+(NH_4)_2SO_4$
Brain	2·6	12·0	1·2	7·0
Liver	2·0	5·5	0·75	2·5

(From Munoz and Mandel, 1968.)

Nonspecific RNA synthesis during learning

It seems reasonable to assume that the usual learning experiments involve stress or some kind of emotion. In order to evaluate the effect of stress on RNA metabolism we studied a rather extreme caricatural situation, very far from learning but able to offer clues as to the extent of the phenomenon. Our investigations concerned the effect of amphetamine and of audiogenic seizure on RNA metabolism. Amphetamine is one of the most powerful sympathomimetic amines with respect to stimulation of the central nervous system. Changes in the size and labelling of the free nucleotide pools and of different precursor pools were studied. There were no significant quantitative changes in the free nucleotide and nucleic acid content of the brains of mice treated with ($\pm$)-amphetamine sulphate at the dose of 15 mg/kg i.p. Comparison of the distribution of the free nucleotides in control and amphetamine-treated mice indicated only a slight decrease of ATP (about 10 per cent) (Table 11.2).

On the other hand, the specific activities (S.A.) of phosphocreatine and of the α-, β- and γ-phosphates of ATP in the brain of mice killed six hours after an injection of [^{32}P]PO$_4^{3-}$ (1 mCi/100 g body weight i.p.) and treated with ($\pm$)-amphetamine sulphate at the dose of 15 mg/kg i.p. (Table 11.3) were increased with increasing time of exposure to amphetamine.

Table 11.2

Cerebral nucleoside triphosphate distribution in mice treated with (±)-amphetamine sulphate (15 mg/kg i.p.) 2 h before death. Results are expressed in μmol per 100 g fresh weight of brain and are means ± S.D.

	Controls	Amphetamine treatment
ATP	210·0 ± 7·3	189·0 ± 13·2
GTP	24·8 ± 1·6	23·0 ± 1·58
UTP	20·0 ± 1·4	18·3 ± 1·38

After injection of [^{3}H]uridine into the brain of mice treated with (±)-amphetamine at the level of 7·5 mg/kg, no significant difference in the S.A. of total RNA and the different RNA fractions could be found (Table 11.4). When the values of the radioactivity of RNA were related to the S.A. of the UMP precursors, an increase in the relative S.A. was observed. In the brains of mice treated with (±)-amphetamine at the higher dose (15 mg/kg), a clear increase in the S.A. was observed. The average increases in the S.A. and in the relative specific activity were +49 per cent and +105 per cent respectively.

The specific activities of the different fractions of cerebral RNA separated on sucrose density gradient were all increased in the brain of mice treated with

Table 11.3

Specific activity (c.p.m./μmol PO$_4$) of α-, β-, and γ-phosphates of ATP in the brain of mice killed six hours after an injection of [^{32}P]PO$_4^{3-}$ and treated or not with (±)-amphetamine sulphate (15 mg/kg i.p.) one, three or six hours before death.

Amphetamine treatment (delay before death)	α-phosphate	β-phosphate	γ-phosphate	Phosphocreatine
Control	0·230	0·867	0·868	1·060
Amphetamine 1 h	0·275	0·885	1·010	1·086
Control	0·343	1·188	1·193	1·105
Amphetamine 3 h	0·462	1·310	1·440	1·245
Control	0·226	0·688	0·583	0·910
Amphetamine 6 h	0·352	1·019	0·970	1·235

Table 11.4

RNA/UMP relative specific activity in the different cerebral RNA fractions of mice killed 4 h after i.v. injection of [^{3}H]uridine and treatment with ($\pm$)-amphetamine sulphate (15 mg/kg i.p.) 2 h before death.

Treatment	Fraction I tRNA	Fraction II 6–10 S RNA	Fraction III 18 S rRNA	Fraction IV 28 S rRNA	Fraction V >28 S RNA
Controls (16)	0·089	0·195	0·194	0·269	0·457
Amphetamine (16)	0·268	0·379	0·300	0·421	1·029

The number of animals appears in brackets.

amphetamine. The increase in S.A. in the amphetamine-treated mice in comparison with controls was more marked for tRNA, 6–10 S RNA and >28 S RNA.

Effect of audiogenic seizure on RNA metabolism

In these experiments a very high stress-emotional state as well as motor activity was produced. Seizures were induced in a special strain of Swiss mice inbred for their very high susceptibility to audiogenic seizure (Lehmann and Busnel, 1964).

Table 11.5

RNA of the brain hemispheres and RNA/DNA ratio in mice (1) treated with ($\pm$)-amphetamine sulphate (15 mg/kg i.p.) and (2) after audiogenic seizures.

Treatment	RNA μg RNA-P/100 mg protein	RNA/DNA
Controls	121·4 ± 7·49	0·903
Audiogenic seizures		
after 3 s clonic jerks	122·73 ± 7·47	0·939
after 20 min	132·06 ± 5·85	0·926
after 1 h	114·60 ± 8·239	0·920
after 18 h	120·84 ± 10·05	0·947
Amphetamine treatment		
after 2 h	130·05 ± 8·62	0·925
after 4 h	133·92 ± 22·83	0·945
after 7 h	118·72 ± 3·88	0·932
after 18 h	121·50 ± 6·77	0·925

After the acoustic stimulus, the animals pass through a latency phase, a running phase, a clonic-jerking phase, a tonic phase and a clonic phase. The mice were killed at the end of the clonic-jerking phase, since in this phase the most important effect on brain RNA turnover was observed in our preliminary studies. The labelling of the nucleotides was studied in order to determine whether the difference in labelling of RNA is due to a modification in the transformation of the radioactive markers to the immediate precursors, or to a different rate of RNA synthesis.

No quantitative changes in brain RNA content were found in mice killed immediately after the clonic-jerking phase of audiogenic seizures or four hours later as well as after amphetamine treatment. The RNA/DNA ratio does not indicate any significant difference (Table 11.5).

Table 11.6

RNA/UMP relative specific activity in the different cerebral RNA fractions of mice killed 4 h after i.v. injection of [^{3}H]uridine and submitted to audiogenic stimulation.

	Fraction I tRNA	Fraction II 6–10 S RNA	Fraction III 18 S rRNA	Fraction IV 28 S rRNA	Fraction V >28 S RNA
Controls	0·090	0·231	0·254	0·287	0·554
Audiogenic stim.	0·261 (+190%)	0·664 (+187%)	0·761 (+199%)	0·767 (+167%)	1·748 (+215%)

The percentage variations in comparison with controls appear in brackets.

When [^{3}H]uridine was injected, a clear increase in the incorporation of the radioactive precursor was observed in the total RNA and in the different fractions >28 S, 28 S, 18 S, >4 S and between <18 S and >4 S. The increase was more evident when the RNA specific activity was related to that of the free uridine nucleotide precursors of the RNA (Table 11.6). Since the absolute quantities of brain RNA do not change it has to be admitted that in parallel with the activation of RNA biosynthesis increased degradation occurs. Thus the turnover is increased and brain homeostasis is ensured. The data obtained after auditive as well as pharmacological stimulation confirm the existence of a correlation between the level of functional activity of the central nervous system and RNA metabolism.

Environmentally determined changes in protein synthesis

Talwar, Chopra, Goel and D'Monte (1966) and Singh and Talwar (1969) found an increase in lysine incorporation in visual cortex proteins when comparing flashing light-exposed monkeys and rabbits with controls. Rose (1967) observed an increase in the incorporation of tritiated lysine into TCA-insoluble material after exposure of litter-mate rats to light. Rose (1969) also found an increase in the incorporation of lysine in the forebrain roof while studying the effect of imprinting in newly hatched birds. On the other hand, Altman and Das (1966) and Altman, Das and Chang (1966) using autoradiographic techniques, and Metzger, Cuenod, Grynbaum and Waelsch (1967) by biochemical methods, failed to find any change in the incorporation of radioactive amino acids into brain proteins following visual stimulation.

Recently Hydén (1969) and Singh and Talwar (1969) found increases in soluble acidic brain proteins similar to Moore's S-100 protein. Changes in the S-100 proteins were observed by Hydén (1969) mainly in the hippocampal region, where, according to the author, this protein is present in neurones, although in other brain areas it seems to be a glial protein (Perez, Olney, Cicero, Moore and Bahn, 1970).

As in the case of RNA, the question arises as to whether the changes in the rate of protein synthesis are a direct consequence of learning or memory storage. The possibility that we are dealing with an alteration representing one step between the arrival of information at the brain and functional activity at the synaptic level cannot yet be excluded. Our recent experiments suggest the hypothesis that the S-100 protein might have a role in the movement of cations, and their distribution in glial cells.

Evidence using RNA or protein synthesis blocking agents

In experiments using RNA or protein synthesis blocking agents two problems have to be considered: (1) the cause–effect relationship; (2) the specificity of the inhibitory effect. In a reaction sequence:

$$A \to B \to \text{information storage or physiological effect}$$

one may generally assume from the fact that blocking the reaction $A \to B$ and finding that at the same time the physiological effect of B is suppressed, B is responsible for this effect. However, the possibility of a reaction sequence $B \to C \to D \to$ physiological effects, cannot be excluded. The inhibition of the reaction $A \to B$ implies only that B is involved in a manner which has to be clarified (in the physiological or behavioural effect), but not that it is directly responsible for it. Although the experiments performed with puromycin and cycloheximide strongly suggest that an inhibition of protein synthesis blocks long-term memory, we cannot exclude the possibility that the effect is due to an inhibition of the synthesis of several short half-life protein molecules which are involved somehow or somewhere in a sequence of reactions involved in the memory-fixation processes, but not directly responsible for information storage. In fact, the time-scale of protein synthesis does not seem to be compatible with a direct role of a specific protein molecule synthesis in information storage.

Following the first experiments by Dingman and Sporn (1961) showing that 8-azaguanidine injected intracisternally in rats produces increased numbers of errors in animals placed for the first time in a new maze, Agranoff and Klinger (1964), Agranoff, Davis and Brink (1965) and Davis and Agranoff (1966) found that in goldfish trained in shuttle-boxes and injected intracranially with puromycin immediately after the training trials, there is a time-dependent and dose-dependent loss of memory retention. Similar effects were obtained with acetoxycycloheximide (AXM), another protein synthesis inhibitor (Brink, Davis and Agranoff, 1966). This experiment suggests that these antimetabolites alter some process necessary for retention of information, and therefore prevent memory formation. However, the experiments with puromycin in mice (Flexner, Flexner and Roberts, 1966), which confirm Agranoff's experiments on goldfish (1970) are confused by the data of Flexner and Flexner (1968). The results obtained in mice with AXM and puromycin appear quite complex and difficult to interpret (Flexner and Flexner, 1965; Flexner, Flexner and Roberts, 1966). It was also demonstrated that, within the same animal species, different tasks are differentially susceptible to the amnesic effect of inhibitors of protein synthesis (Geller and Jarvik, 1970). Thus, the interpretation of the amnesic effects is not easy. Furthermore, since it is well known that the specificity of an inhibitor decreases as the number of experiments performed increases, it is also necessary to control in order to prevent these inhibitors from altering basic processes such as membrane permeability, ion transport and electrogenesis.

It has been argued that puromycin produces electrical abnormalities in the brain (Cohen, Ervin and Barondes, 1966) and that it increases the susceptibility of mice to seizures (Cohen and Barondes, 1967). These effects rather than inhibition of protein synthesis might be responsible for its amnesic effect.

Selective damage of neuronal mitochondria by puromycin was reported (Gambetti, Gonatos and Flexner, 1968a, b). It is likely that some other lesions induced by puromycin are related not to the inhibition of protein synthesis, but to the released peptides and the possible damage of such potent pharmacological agents (Gambetti, Gonatos and Flexner, 1968b; Longnecker and Farber, 1967). The possible role of inhibition of 3'-5'-AMP cyclic phosphodiesterase and the concomitant increase of tissue concentration of cyclic AMP also remains to be studied (Hofert, Gorski, Mueller and Boutwell, 1962; Appleman and Kemp, 1966). Cycloheximide also inhibits RNA and DNA synthesis (McMahon, 1971), and it was suggested that it alters the conformation of nascent peptides (Lee and Evans, 1971). Some side-effects which were reported, such as acceleration of glyconeogenesis (Elson, Shrago and Yatvin, 1971), should point to other possible side-effects. Cycloheximide has been shown to produce changes in mitochondria and microbodies in rat liver (Molnar, Riede, Seebass and Rohr, 1971).

General discussion

Investigations of learning and memory centre around RNA, probably because of the mechanisms discovered in molecular biology for which the terms genetic memory, immunological memory and informational macromolecule, were used. Many analogies with antibody formation are made in order to explain memory, but in fact even now we do not understand the mechanism of antibody formation, and we cannot try to explain one unknown process by another about which we are equally ignorant.

Several investigations suggest that macromolecules, particularly RNA, undergo changes when information is registered, or retained, in the nervous system. However, the relationship between these chemical changes and the behavioural trials remains unknown. At least, the time-scale for registration in short-time behavioural memory seems incompatible with the much longer time necessary for synthesis of RNA molecules. The results reported appear to be correlated rather with some global brain process that occurs concomitantly with learning. The amount of learning-specific RNA can hardly be detected by the method used.

Several hypotheses can be suggested to explain the changes in RNA observed during training. (1) The changes in RNA are due to the activity associated with the training experiments. In fact stress and visual and olfactory stimulation produce alterations in RNA or polysomes similar to that reported during learning or memory behaviour. Even careful experiments (Glassman and Wilson, 1970) cannot exclude such possibilities. (2) The changes are due to an increase in the biosynthesis of messenger RNA and proteins, or peptides of a short half-life which may play an important role in the regulation of the effectiveness of transmitters and connection mechanisms of the synaptic level. These macromolecules are not necessarily the behaviour trigger responsible for the information storage. A great number of peptides are involved in neuroendocrine regulation. It has also been postulated that some peptides present in nerve membrane are involved in active transport (Mandel and Ledig, 1966), while the possibility of a more direct role of peptides in memory has been suggested (Bohus and de Wied, 1966; Flexner and Flexner, 1968).

The complex neuronal network, with the specific pathways and centres for sensory perception, makes probable the localisation of the process of memory fixation at the synaptic level. In this area RNA and protein synthesis, unless in mitochondria, probably does not occur (Morgan, 1970). Proteins supposed to be involved in the behavioural changes have to arrive at the synaptic cleft by the axonal flow which seems too slow in terms of information, registration or retention. Even the fast transport (200–300 mm/day) (Grafstein, 1969) does not seem to be in the time-scale of memory trace fixation. However, a synthesis of proteins in the postsynaptic region associated with long-term memory cannot be excluded.

The experiments using antimetabolites, although very suggestive, are not unequivocal since a direct cause–effect relationship cannot be demonstrated in this way, and since the specificity of the inhibitor is always under discussion. Moreover, under circumstances where protein synthesis in brain is highly inhibited, many side-effects should be expected if we take into account the fact that brain synthesises protein at a more rapid rate than any other tissue in the body with the exception of the liver (Lajtha and Toth, 1966).

Thus, the only safe conclusion is that RNA and protein synthesis must be going on normally in order to form permanent memory. The manner by which these macromolecules may contribute to the formation of permanent memory is still hypothetical.

It seems reasonable that if macromolecules play a direct role in information storage proteins localised close to the synapses are the best candidates for this task. With regard to instinctive behaviour, such genetically determined proteins should already exist, thus explaining behaviour independent of the individual experience. With regard to learned behaviour, the proteins would pre-exist and would undergo conformational changes subsequent to the experience of the animal. Oscillatory conformational changes of these proteins regulated by alterations in the electrical fields might fit with the postulated time-scale of memory fixation and the basic, ionic phenomena of the transmission of neuronal influx. Glycoproteins localised at the synaptic membranes might be involved in information storage as has been postulated (Bogoch, 1968) although the mechanism may be more complex than was initially thought (Barondes, 1970).

More sensitive techniques and helpful models are necessary in order to find out the specific molecular mechanisms of learning and information storage. The molecular basis of genetically determined natural facilities for learning (Bovet, Bovet-Nitti and Oliverio, 1969; Bovet, 1970; Oliverio, 1971) may be a good tool for approaching the problem of macromolecules and behaviour.

References

AGRANOFF, B. W. (1970). Current questions in brain and behavior. In: *Biochemistry of Brain and Behaviour* (BOWMAN, R. E. and DATTA, S. R., Eds.), pp. 347–58. Plenum Press, New York.

AGRANOFF, B. W., DAVIS, R. E. and BRINK, J. J. (1965). Memory fixation in the goldfish. *Proc. natn. Acad. Sci., U.S.A.*, **54**, 788–93.

AGRANOFF, B. W. and KLINGER, P. (1964). Puromycin effect on memory fixation in the goldfish. *Science, N.Y.*, **146**, 952–3.

ALTMAN, J. and DAS, G. D. (1966). Behavioural manipulations and protein metabolism of the brain: effects of motor exercise on the utilisation of ^{3}H-leucine. *Physiol. Behav.*, **1**, 105–8.

ALTMAN, J., DAS, G. D. and CHANG, J. (1966). Behavioural manipulations and protein metabolism of the brain: effects of visual training on the utilisation of ^{3}H-leucine. *Physiol. Behav.*, **1**, 111–15.

APPLEMAN, M. M. and KEMP, R. G. (1966). Puromycin: a potent metabolic effect independent of protein synthesis. *Biochem. biophys. Res. Commun.*, **24**, 564–8.

BARONDES, S. H. (1970). Brain glycomacromolecules and interneuronal recognition. In: *Neurosciences: Second Study Program* (SCHMITT, F. O., Ed.), pp. 747–60. Rockefeller University Press, New York.

BOGOCH, S. (1968). *The Biochemistry of Memory with an Inquiry into the Function of the Brain Mucoids.* Oxford University Press, New York.

BOHUS, B. and DE WIED, D. (1966). Inhibitory and facilitatory effect of two related peptides on extinction of avoidance behaviour. *Science, N.Y.*, **153**, 318–20.

BONDY, S. C. and ROBERTS, S. (1968). Hybridizable ribonucleic acid of rat brain. *Biochem. J.*, **109**, 533–41.

BOVET, D. (1970). Approche biochimique et biopsychologique de la mémoire et de l'apprentissage. In: *La mémoire* (BOVET, D., FESSARD, A., FLORÈS, C., FRIJDA, N. H., INHELDER, B., MILNER, B. and PIAGET, J., Eds.) Presses Universitaires Françaises, Paris.

BOVET, D., BOVET-NITTI, F. and OLIVERIO, A. (1969). Genetic aspects of learning and memory in mice. *Science, N.Y.*, **163**, 139–49.

BRINK, J. J., DAVIS, R. E. and AGRANOFF, B. W. (1966). Effects of puromycin, acetoxycycloheximide and actinomycin D on protein synthesis in goldfish brain. *J. Neurochem.*, **13**, 889–96.

BRITTEN, R. J. and KOHNE, D. E. (1968). Repeated sequences in DNA. *Science, N.Y.*, **161**, 529–40.

CHAMBON, P., RAMUZ, M., MANDEL, P. and DOLY, J. (1968). The influence of ionic strength and a polyanion on transcription *in vitro*. I. Stimulation of the aggregate RNA polymerase from rat-liver nuclei. *Biochim. biophys. Acta*, **157**, 504–19.

CHURCH, R. B. and MCCARTHY, B. J. (1968). Related base sequences in the DNA of simple and complex organisms. II. The interpretation of DNA–RNA hybridization studies with mammalian nucleic acids. *Biochem. Genet.*, **2**, 55–73.

COHEN, H. D. and BARONDES, S. H. (1967). Puromycin effect on memory may be due to occult seizures. *Science, N.Y.*, **157**, 333–4.

COHEN, H. D., ERVIN, F. and BARONDES, S. H. (1966). Puromycin and cycloheximide: different effects on hippocampal electrical activity. *Science, N.Y.*, **154**, 1557–8.

DAVIS, R. E. and AGRANOFF, B. W. (1966). Stages of memory formation in goldfish: evidence for an environmental trigger. *Proc. natn. Acad. Sci., U.S.A.*, **55**, 555–9.

DINGMAN, W. and SPORN, M. B. (1961). The incorporation of 8-azaguanine into rat brain RNA and its effect on maze learning by the rat. *J. Psychiat. Res.*, **1**, 1–11.

DOLY, J., RAMUZ, M., MANDEL, P. and CHAMBON, P. (1965). Soluble DNA dependent RNA polymerase from prostate nuclei. *Life Sci.*, **4**, 1961–6.

ELSON, C., SHRAGO, E. and YATVIN, M. (1971). Acceleration of glyconeogenesis in *Tetrahymena pyriformis* following inhibition of protein synthesis by cycloheximide. *Fedn Proc. Fedn Am. Socs exp. Biol.*, **30**, p. 1231, Abstr. 1045.

FLEXNER, L. B. and FLEXNER, J. B. (1965). Effects of AXM and an AXM-puromycin mixture on cerebral protein synthesis and memory in mice. *Proc. natn. Acad. Sci., U.S.A.*, **55**, 369–74.

FLEXNER, L. B. and FLEXNER, J. B. (1968). Intracerebral saline: effect on memory of trained mice treated with puromycin. *Science, N.Y.*, **159**, 330–1.

FLEXNER, L. B., FLEXNER, J. B. and ROBERTS, R. B. (1966). Stages of memory in mice treated with AXM before or immediately after learning. *Proc. natn. Acad. Sci., U.S.A.*, **56**, 730–5.

GAMBETTI, P., GONATOS, N. K. and FLEXNER, L. B. (1968a). The fine structure of puromycin-induced changes in mouse entorhinal cortex. *J. Cell. Biol.*, **36**, 379–90.

GAMBETTI, P., GONATOS, N. K. and FLEXNER, L. B. (1968b). Puromycin: action on neuronal mitochondria. *Science, N.Y.*, **161**, 900–2.

GELLER, A. and JARVIK, M. E. (1970). The role of consolidation in memory. In: *Biochemistry of Brain and Behaviour* (BOWMAN, R. E. and DATTA, S. R., Eds.), pp. 245–77. Plenum Press, New York.

GLASSMAN, E. (1969). The biochemistry of learning: an evaluation of the role of RNA and protein. *A. Rev. Biochem.*, **38**, 605–46.

GLASSMAN, E. and WILSON, J. E. (1970). The effect of short experiences on macromolecules in the brain. In: *Biochemistry of Brain and Behaviour* (BOWMAN, R. E. and DATTA, S. R., Eds.), pp. 279–99. Plenum Press, New York.

GRAFSTEIN, B. (1969). Axonal transport: communication between soma and synapse. In: *Advances in Biochemical Psychopharmacology* (COSTA, E. and GREENGARD, P., Eds.), Vol. 1, pp. 11–25. Raven Press, New York.

HOFERT, J., GORSKI, J., MUELLER, G. C. and BOUTWELL, R. K. (1962). The depletion of liver glycogen in puromycin-treated animals. *Archs Biochem. Biophys.*, **97**, 134–7.

HYDÉN, H. (1960). The neuron. In: *The Cell* (BRACHET, J. and MIRSKY, A., Eds.), Vol. IV, pp. 215–325. Academic Press, New York.

HYDÉN, H. (1967). Biochemical changes accompanying learning. In: *The Neurosciences* (QUARTON, G. C., MELNECHUK, T. and SCHMITT, F. O., Eds.), pp. 765–72. Rockefeller University Press, New York.

HYDÉN, H. (1969). Properties and response of brain cell proteins at establishment of new behaviour. *FEBS Meeting Madrid*, Abstr., pp. 42, 79.

HYDÉN, H. and EGYHAZI, E. (1962). Nuclear RNA changes of nerve cells during a learning experiment in rats. *Proc. natn. Acad. Sci., U.S.A.*, **48**, 1366–72.

HYDÉN, H. and EGYHAZI, E. (1964). Changes in RNA content and base composition in cortical neurons of rats in a learning experiment involving transfer of handedness. *Proc. natn. Acad. Sci., U.S.A.*, **52**, 1030–5.

HYDÉN, H. and LANGE, P. W. (1965). A differentiation of RNA response in neurons early and late in learning. *Proc. natn. Acad. Sci. U.S.A.*, **53**, 946–52.

LAJTHA, A. and TOTH, J. (1966). Instability of cerebral proteins. *Biochem. biophys. Res. Commun.*, **23**, 294–8.

LEE, S. G. and EVANS, W. R. (1971). Mechanism of cycloheximide inhibition of protein synthesis in *Euglena gracilis*. *Fedn Proc. Fedn Am. Socs exp. Biol.*, **30**, p. 1112, Abstr. 343.

LEHMANN, A. and BUSNEL, R. G. (1964). A study of the audiogenic seizure. In: *Acoustic Behaviour of Animals* (BUSNEL, R. G., Ed.), pp. 244–74. Elsevier, Amsterdam.

LONGNECKER, D. S. and FARBER, E. (1967). Acute pancreatic necrosis induced by puromycin. *Lab. Invest.*, **16**, 321–9.

MACHLUS, B. and GAITO, J. (1968a). Detection of RNA species unique to a behavioral task. *Psychon. Sci.*, **10**, 253–4.

MACHLUS, B. and GAITO, J. (1968b). Unique RNA species developed during a shock-avoidance task. *Psychon. Sci.*, **12**, 111–12.

MACHLUS, B. and GAITO, J. (1969). Successive competition hybridization to detect RNA species in a shock-avoidance task. *Nature, Lond.*, **222**, 573–4.

MANDEL, P. and LEDIG, M. (1966). Amidated phosphopeptides in nervous tissue. *Biochem. biophys. Res. Commun.*, **24**, 275–9.

MCMAHON, D. (1971). Cycloheximide is not a specific inhibitor of protein synthesis. *Fedn Proc. Fedn Am. Socs exp. Biol.*, **30**, p. 1112, Abstr. 345.

METZGER, H. P., CUENOD, M., GRYNBAUM, A. and WAELSCH, H. (1967). The effect of unilateral visual stimulation on synthesis of cortical proteins in each hemisphere of the split-brain monkey. *J. Neurochem.*, **14**, 183–8.

MOLNAR, J. J., RIEDE, U. N., SEEBASS, C. and ROHR, H. P. (1971). Ultrastructural morphometric studies on the rat liver cell after cycloheximide-induced protein synthesis inhibition. *Fedn Proc. Fedn Am. Socs exp. Biol.*, **30**, p. 547, Abstr. 2117.

MORGAN, I. (1970). Protein synthesis in brain mitochondrial and synaptosomal preparations. *FEBS Letters*, **10**, 273–5.

MUNOZ, D. and MANDEL, P. (1968). Etude comparée de l'activité RNA polymérasique de divers tissus du Rat. *C. r. Séanc. Soc. Biol.*, **162**, 2283–6.

OLIVERIO, A. (1971). Genetic variations and heritability in a measure of avoidance learning in mice. *J. comp. physiol. Psychol.*, **74**, 390–7.

PEREZ, V. J., OLNEY, J., CICERO, T. J., MOORE, B. W. and BAHN, B. A. (1970). Wallerian degeneration in rabbit optic nerve: research on cellular localization of the S-100 and 14-3-2 proteins. *J. Neurochem.*, **17**, 511–19.

QUARTON, G. C., MELNECHUK, T. and SCHMITT, F. O., Eds. (1967). *The Neurosciences, a Study Program*. Rockefeller University Press, New York.

ROSE, S. P. R. (1967). Changes in incorporation of ^{3}H lysine into protein in the visual cortex during first exposure of rats to light. *Nature, Lond.*, **215**, 253–5.

ROSE, S. P. R. (1969). Neurochemical correlates of learning and environmental change. *FEBS Letters*, **5**, 305–12.

Rose, S. P. R., Bateson, P. P. G. and Horn, G. (1973). Biochemistry and behaviour in the chick. In: *Macromolecules and Behaviour* (Ansell, G. B. and Bradley, P. B., Eds.), pp. 93–104. Macmillan, London.

Shimada, H. and Gorbman, A. (1970) Long lasting changes in RNA synthesis in the forebrains of female rats treated with testosterone soon after birth. *Biochem. biophys. Res. Commun.*, **38**, 423–30.

Singh, U. B. and Talwar, G. P. (1969). Identification of a protein fraction in the occipital cortex of the monkey rapidly labelled during the exposure of the animal to rhythmically flickering light. *J. Neurochem.*, **16**, 951–61.

Stevenin, J., Mandel, P. and Jacob, M. (1969). Relationship between nuclear giant-size dRNA and microsomal dRNA of rat brain. *Proc. natn. Acad. Sci., U.S.A.*, **62**, 490–7.

Stevenin, J., Samec, J., Jacob, M. and Mandel, P. (1968). Détermination de la fraction du génome codant pour les RNA ribosomiques et messagers dans le cerveau du rat adulte. *J. molec. Biol.*, **33**, 777–93.

Talwar, G. P., Chopra, S. P., Goel, B. K. and D'Monte, B. (1966). Correlation of the functional activity of the brain with metabolic parameters. III. Protein metabolism of the occipital cortex in relation to light stimulus. *J. Neurochem.*, **13**, 109–16.

Tata, J. R. (1967a). The formation and distribution of ribosomes during hormone-induced growth and development. *Biochem. J.*, **104**, 1–17.

Tata, J. R. (1967b). Hormones and the synthesis and utilization of ribonucleic acids. *Progr. in Nucleic Acid Res. and Molecular Biol.* Vol. 5, pp. 191–250.

Von Hungen, K. (1970). Hybridization of rat brain RNA: failure to confirm reports of new species of RNA induced with learning. *Proc. Am. Soc. Neurochem.*, **1**, 76.

Watson, W. E. (1965). An autoradiographic study of the incorporation of nucleic acid precursors by neurons and glia during nerve stimulation. *J. Physiol.*, **180**, 754–65.

Weill, J. D., Busch, S., Chambon, P. and Mandel, P. (1963). The effect of estradiol injections upon chicken liver nuclei ribonucleic acid polymerase. *Biochem. biophys. Res. Commun.*, **10**, 122–6.

Wyatt, G. R. and Tata, J. R. (1968). The hybridization capacity of ribonucleic acid produced during hormone action. *Biochem. J.*, **109**, 253–8.

Zemp, J. W., Wilson, J. E. and Glassman, E. (1967). Brain function and macromolecules. II. Site of increased labelling of RNA in brains of mice during a short-term training experience. *Proc. natn. Acad. Sci., U.S.A.*, **58**, 1120–5.

Zemp, J. W., Wilson, J. E., Schlesinger, K., Boggan, W. O. and Glassman, E. (1966). Brain function and macromolecules. II. Incorporation of uridine into RNA of mouse brain during short-term training experience. *Proc. natn. Acad. Sci., U.S.A.*, **55**, 1423–31.

Neuronal interactions, learning and memory

Chairman: J. T. Eayrs
Department of Anatomy, Medical School, Birmingham

Anatomical evidence for plasticity in the central nervous system in the adult rat

G. RAISMAN

Department of Human Anatomy, University of Oxford, Oxford OX1 3QX, England

In this paper, I shall consider some anatomical aspects of the reactions of neurones to injury which provide evidence for a form of positive or plastic reaction under these circumstances. Such reactions form a useful model in which the new formation of synaptic connections in the adult central nervous system can be studied, although the evidence must not be assumed to apply directly in the very different conditions obtaining in the study of the effects of experience and learning.

When a neurone is damaged, the form of the subsequent reaction depends upon several factors, the most important being the location of the neurone and the species of animal. In considering specifically the effects of injury involving section of axons, a distinction has to be made between the central and peripheral nervous system, and between cold-blooded species such as fish or amphibia and the warm-blooded mammalian species. When an axon is sectioned, the part detached from the cell body (the distal segment) undergoes irreversible degeneration leading to total degradation (orthograde degeneration). In the peripheral nervous system, the proximal stump of the axon (i.e. the part attached to the cell body) starts to grow and ultimately, its original connections may be regenerated. In the central nervous system of cold-blooded animals, regeneration has also been shown to occur in several systems, and it may lead to what can be quite a faithful reconstitution of the original connections (Gaze, 1970). In the brain and spinal cord of mammals, however, effective regeneration of connections by cut axons does not occur. The reason for this failure of regeneration has long puzzled investigators, and is still unknown, although the observations included here may offer some clues (Guth and Windle, 1970).

Apart from the regenerative reaction of cut axons, a further positive reaction has been shown to occur in the peripheral nervous system. This is generally called collateral sprouting, and involves the formation of new sprouts from the intact axons in the vicinity of the denervated region. These sprouts have been shown to take over the territories and to some extent the functions of the cut axons (Weddell, Gutmann and Gutmann, 1941; Edds, 1953) although when the originally cut axons regenerate they appear to displace the sprouts (Guth and Bernstein, 1961) or to render them functionless (Mark, Marotte and Johnstone, 1970). These reactions are of considerable potential interest in future studies of the effect of experience on the nervous system, as they afford evidence for factors which can induce the formation of new connections in the adult; they also illustrate a situation in which there appears to be some kind of selectivity—in this case between collateral sprouts and regenerating axon tips—which results in a definite rearrangement of functional relationships.

It has been thought for some time that a form of collateral sprouting may occur in the central nervous system of mammals (McCouch, Austin, Liu and Liu, 1958). Light microscopic studies of the reaction of dorsal root fibres to loss of adjacent dorsal roots (Liu and Chambers, 1958) or the reaction of retinal fibres to loss of corticofugal axons in the ventral part of the lateral geniculate nucleus or the lateral nucleus of the optic tract (Goodman and Horel, 1966) have supported the view that deafferentation can lead to collateral sprouting. Furthermore, the ultrastructural work of Hamori (1968) on the dorsal lateral geniculate nucleus suggests that after destruction of the retinal fibres, the surviving axon terminals increase their number of synaptic contacts, probably because the surviving axons have occupied sites denervated as a result of the original lesion. My work confirms the occurrence of collateral sprouting in the mammalian central nervous system, and also offers evidence that new synapses can be formed. These conclusions are based on recent experimental ultrastructural studies of the chronically deafferented septal nuclei (Raisman, 1969a) which have shown that characteristic changes in the configuration of synaptic contacts may occur after a lesion in the central nervous system of the adult rat. These changes, which are currently under further investigation, suggest that one of the results of deafferentation of central nervous tissue may be to induce new synapse formation as a result of which surviving axon terminals may innervate sites which have been deafferented. It is also suggested that the occurrence of collateral sprouting in the central nervous system of mammals might be important as a factor discouraging the regeneration of the originally cut axons. If therefore the readiness with which the mammalian central nervous system can form collateral sprouts is taken as an index of its synaptic plasticity, it may be the very existence of this form of plasticity which militates against regeneration of the type found in cold-blooded animals (Bernstein and Bernstein, 1969).

Results

Several factors have combined to make the septal nuclei a suitable site for this type of study. There are two extrinsic fibre pathways—the fimbrial fibres from the hippocampus and the medial forebrain bundle fibres from the hypothalamus— which may be destroyed separately and completely by lesions placed well away from the septum and which do not therefore directly cause damage to the septum itself. The two pathways converge upon the septal neuropil where they

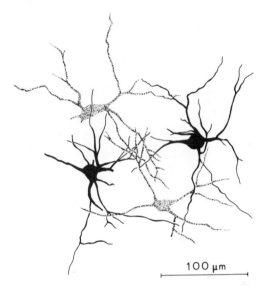

Figure 12.1. A *camera lucida* drawing of a group of four cells from the medial septal nucleus in the rat, stained by the Golgi–Kopsch technique, to show the intermingling of the main dendrites. (Finer dendritic branches and dendritic spines are not shown.)

give rise to a large proportion of the synapses, and where, because of the intermingling of the septal neuronal dendrites (Figure 12.1), their terminal fields are closely interspersed. Selective lesions of one or other pathway result in orthograde degeneration of terminals, which can be recognised by their electron-dense reaction (Figures 12.3, 12.5) two days after operation, when the majority of degenerating terminals are still in contact with their postsynaptic elements. By examination of the medial septal nucleus two days after such lesions (Raisman, 1969b) it was shown that the fimbrial fibres terminate exclusively on dendritic shafts or spines, accounting for about a third of all the axodendritic synapses (Figures 12.2, 12.3, 12.10b), while the medial forebrain bundle fibres account for a further one-fifth

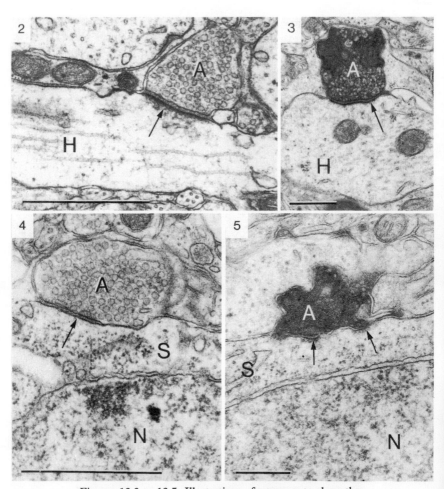

Figures 12.2 to 12.5. Illustrations of synapses to show the difference between normal and degenerating synapses and the distinction between terminations upon dendrites and upon cell somata. Figure 12.2. Normal axodendritic synapse. Figure 12.3. Degenerating axodendritic synapse. Figure 12.4. Normal axosomatic synapse. Figure 12.5. Degenerating axosomatic synapse. Calibration bar = 1 μm. A, Axon terminal; H, dendritic shaft; S, portion of cell body; N, nucleus; ↑, synaptic contact region.

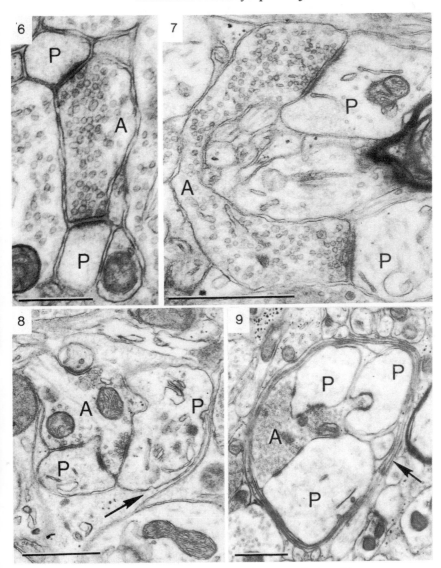

Figures 12.6 to 12.9. Illustrations of axon terminals making multiple synaptic contacts in the medial septal nucleus of the rat after a chronic lesion of the fimbria. A, Axon terminal; P, postsynaptic profile; ↑, astroglial envelope which is formed by a single layer in Figure 12.8 and multiple layers in Figure 12.9. Calibration bar = 0.5 μm in Figure 12.6, 1 μm in Figures 12.7, 12.8 and 12.9.

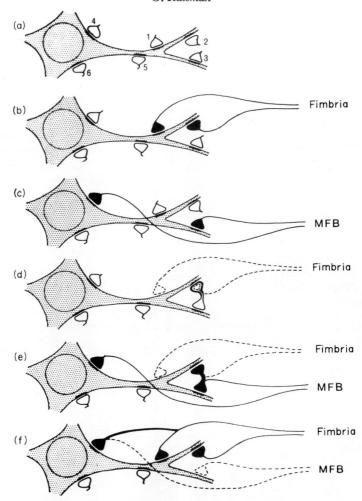

Figure 12.10. A summary of the findings and an interpretation of the effects of lesions in the afferent pathways to the septum. (a), Normal septal neuropil. Terminals numbered 1, 2, 3 and 5 are axodendritic, terminals numbered 4 and 6 axosomatic. (b), An acute lesion of the fimbria enables a proportion of the axon terminals to be identified by means of the electron-dense reaction associated with orthograde degeneration (1 and 2, filled in black). (c), An acute lesion of the medial forebrain bundle (MFB) enables a further proportion of the axodendritic terminals (3) and some of the axosomatic terminals (4) to be identified. (d), A chronic lesion of the fimbria, allowing a survival time sufficient for the removal of degenerating axons and terminals (discontinuous lines) results in an increased number of axodendritic synapses in

of the synapses on dendrites, but differ absolutely from the fimbrial fibres by forming additional contacts upon cell bodies, where they constitute approximately one quarter of all the axosomatic synapses (Figures 12.4, 12.5, 12.10c).

In a second series of experiments, lesions of the pathways were made but a survival time of at least fifty days was allowed. By this time all the orthograde degenerating axon terminals had been completely removed from their synaptic contact sites as a result of astrocytic phagocytosis, and the degenerating fragments were completely degraded. At such survival times, it was found that a chronic lesion of the fimbria had resulted in an increase in the number of axon terminals which made synaptic contact with more than one postsynaptic element in the plane of the section (Figures 12.6, 12.7, 12.10d). A possible explanation is that the surviving axon terminals had extended their distribution so as to reinnervate the vacant sites. That the axon terminals making these multiple contacts could belong to medial forebrain bundle fibres was proved by showing that a proportion of them undergo orthograde degeneration after a second, acute lesion of the medial forebrain bundle (Figure 12.10e). The hypothesis that the effects of chronic deafferentation could include this sort of reinnervation gains support from the observation that after a chronic lesion of the medial forebrain bundle (causing partial deafferentation of the cell bodies), a second, acute lesion of the fimbria, which enables the fimbrial fibre terminals to be identified by the reaction of orthograde degeneration, shows that the fimbria has now extended its distribution to occupy sites on cell bodies (Figure 12.10f). These sites are not normally occupied by fimbrial fibres, and the fact that they have been chronically deafferented to a major degree by the first lesion suggests that their deafferentation acts as a stimulus for reinnervation.

The experiments in this series do not afford much information on the intermediate stages of the proposed plastic reaction, and a further series examining the time course of the effect between two days and two months survival is designed to

---

which the axon terminal makes contact with more than one postsynaptic element (2, 3). (e), An acute lesion of the medial forebrain bundle in an animal with a chronic lesion of the fimbria enables a proportion of the axon terminals making multiple synaptic contacts to be identified (by means of the electron-dense reaction of orthograde degeneration) as belonging to axons in the medial forebrain bundle (2 and 3, filled in black). (f), In an animal with a chronic lesion of the medial forebrain bundle, a second, acute lesion of the fimbria gives rise to degeneration of axon terminals making axosomatic contacts (4). Heavy lines indicate the proposed plastic changes by means of which the medial forebrain bundle terminals in (e) have taken over axodendritic sites denervated by the fimbrial lesion, and the fimbrial fibres in (f) have taken over axosomatic sites vacated as a result of the chronic lesion of the medial forebrain bundle.

throw light on such problems as the fate of the synaptic thickenings and the rate of development of new synaptic contacts. It has been noticed, however, that the astrocytes, whose processes have been shown to phagocytose the degenerating axon terminals have also been found to produce abnormal, often multiple, wrappings around the multiple synapses (Figures 12.8, 12.9), suggesting that astrocytic elements in the tissue may play an important part not only as scavengers of debris but also in detecting the presence of deafferented neuronal sites, and to stimulate and guide newly growing sprouts towards them.

Conclusions

The results of these experiments with the septal nuclei of the adult rat support the view that the central nervous system of warm-blooded animals may not be as completely inert in the face of injury as has often been supposed, but that a form of collateral sprouting, possibly similar to that known to occur in the peripheral nervous system may occur under favourable conditions. They also stress the potential importance of signals from deafferented sites as promoters of growth, to the extent that sprouting may be induced from the terminals of neighbouring axons even though those axons are not damaged and do not normally innervate the sites in question. In the septum the formation of adventitious axosomatic synapses by the fimbrial fibres implies that the constraints normally operating during the establishment of septal connections are no longer effective in this situation. While there is as yet no evidence that the effects seen in the septum necessarily occur in all sites, they do suggest that the existence of heterotypic reinnervation cannot be excluded in the central nervous system. Furthermore such a process would result in the reoccupation of denervated sites, and presumably therefore the removal of a growth stimulus, an effect which might go some way to explaining why cut axons in the brain fail to reconstitute their former connections.

While these findings indicate that the central nervous system may be capable of considerable synaptic rearrangement, it must be borne in mind that the changes described have been provoked by means of a destructive lesion in the brain. They therefore provide evidence for plasticity only in the post-traumatic situation in which the region under consideration has suffered a major loss of terminals. They do not, of course, provide any direct evidence that such a rearrangement of synapses occurs in the intact brain as a result of experience, learning or memory.

References

BERNSTEIN, J. J. and BERNSTEIN, M. E. (1969). Ultrastructure of normal regeneration and loss of regenerative capacity following Teflon blockage in goldfish spinal cord. *Expl Neurol.*, **24**, 538–57.

EDDS, M. V. JR. (1953). Collateral nerve regeneration. *Q. Rev. Biol.*, **28**, 270–6.

GAZE, R. M. (1970). *The Formation of Nerve Connections.* Academic Press, New York.

GOODMAN, D. C. and HOREL, J. A. (1966). Sprouting of optic tract projections in the brain stem of the rat. *J. comp. Neurol.*, **127**, 71–88.

GUTH, L. and BERNSTEIN, J. J. (1961). Selectivity in the re-establishment of synapses in the superior cervical sympathetic ganglion of the cat. *Expl Neurol.*, **4**, 59–69.

GUTH, L. and WINDLE, W. F. (1970). The enigma of central nervous regeneration. *Expl Neurol.*, Suppl. 5, 1–43.

HAMORI, J. (1968). Presynaptic-to-presynaptic axon contacts under experimental conditions giving rise to rearrangement of synaptic structures. In: *Structure and Functions of Inhibitory Neuronal Mechanisms* (VON EULER, C., SKOGLUND, S. and SÖDERBERG, U., Eds.), pp. 71–80. Pergamon Press, Oxford.

LIU, C. N. and CHAMBERS, W. W. (1958). Intraspinal sprouting of dorsal root axons. *Archs Neurol. Psychiat.*, **79**, 46–61.

MARK, R. F., MAROTTE, L. R. and JOHNSTONE, J. R. (1970). Reinnervated eye muscles do not respond to impulses in foreign nerves. *Science, N.Y.*, **170**, 193–4.

McCOUCH, G. P., AUSTIN, G. M., LIU, C. N. and LIU, C. Y. (1958). Sprouting as a cause of spasticity. *J. Neurophysiol.*, **21**, 205–16.

RAISMAN, G. (1969a). Neuronal plasticity in the septal nuclei of the adult rat. *Brain Res.*, **14**, 25–48.

RAISMAN, G. (1969b). A comparison of the mode of termination of the hippocampal and hypothalamic afferents to the septal nuclei as revealed by the electron microscopy of degeneration. *Exp. Brain Res.*, **7**, 317–43.

WEDDELL, G., GUTMANN, L. and GUTMANN, E. (1941). The extension of nerve fibres into denervated areas of skin. *J. Neurol. Psychiat., Lond.*, **4**, 206–25.

Synaptic plasticity in the hippocampal formation

T. V. P. BLISS

National Institute for Medical Research, Mill Hill, London NW7 1AA, England

A. R. GARDNER-MEDWIN

Department of Physiology, University College, London WC1E 6BT, England

and T. LØMO

Institute of Neurophysiology, University of Oslo, Norway

The possibility that the hippocampal formation may play a significant role in the elaboration of the memory trace has intrigued a number of authors (Douglas, 1967; Elazar and Adey, 1967; Grastyan and Karmos, 1962; Milner, 1970; Vinogradova, Semyonova and Konovalov, 1970; see also the papers by Hydén, 1973 and Glassman and Wilson, 1973). From a neurophysiological point of view, a first step in establishing whether any particular part of the brain is directly involved in the processes underlying memory (that is, whether it is involved in the storage, and not merely the transmission of learned information) is to look for evidence of synaptic plasticity. For a study of this sort, the hippocampus offers the important advantage of having a relatively simple and stereotyped neuronal organisation. As a result, identified monosynaptic pathways can be investigated, thus greatly facilitating the analysis of any long-term effects observed. We present here some details of experiments, a full account of which is in preparation, showing that brief tetanic stimulation of one such monosynaptic pathway, the perforant path

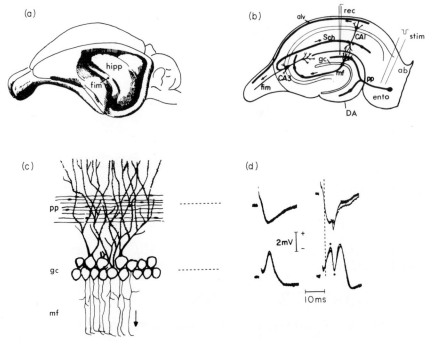

Figure 13.1. Anatomy of the hippocampal formation (a–c) and the population potentials evoked in the dentate area by stimulation of the perforant path (d). (a), Lateral view of the dorsal hippocampal surface in the rabbit after removal of overlying cortical tissue. hipp = Hippocampus, fim = fimbria. (b), Sagittal section through the hippocampal formation, showing the major cell populations and connections. ab = Angular bundle, alv = alveus, CA1, CA3 = pyramidal cell layer, fields CA1 and CA3, DA = dentate area, ento = entorhinal area, gc = granule cell body layer, mf = mossy fibres, pp = perforant path, Sch = Schaffer collaterals. (c), Enlarged view of part of the dentate area. The perforant path synapses occupy the middle third of the granule cell apical dendrites. (d), Population potentials evoked in the dentate area by weak (left) and strong (right) shocks to the perforant path. Horizontal broken lines indicate the depth, relative to the granule cells, at which each potential was recorded. The vertical broken line (right) is drawn 1 ms after the onset of the synaptic wave, the time at which measurements of the amplitude of the synaptic wave (population EPSP) are made. The two dots (lower right) span the peak-to-peak amplitude of the population spike.

input to the dentate area, can result in long-lasting increases in the synaptic effectiveness of the stimulated fibres.

Synapses with this sort of property, in one guise or another, feature in many theoretical discussions of learning (Hebb, 1949; Eccles, 1953; Brindley, 1969; Gardner-Medwin, 1969; Marr, 1970). Our immediate aim has been to establish that there exists in the mammalian cortex an identifiable set of synapses possessing this property (Bliss and Lømo, 1970; Bliss and Gardner-Medwin, 1971). It should be emphasised, however, that we have no evidence one way or the other that the effect we have demonstrated has anything to do with learning.

Anatomy of the dentate area

The dentate area forms the most ventral part of the hippocampal formation. A view of the exposed dorsal surface of the hippocampus in the rabbit is shown in Figure 13.1a. The granule cell population of the dentate area forms a densely packed C-shaped layer interlocking with the pyramidal cell layer of the hippocampus (Figure 13.1b). The apical dendrites of the granule cells extend into the molecular layer as far as the hippocampal fissure. Within the molecular layer there is a strict localisation of afferent fibres so that axon terminals from any given source are restricted to specific regions of the dendritic tree (Ramón y Cajal, 1911; Lorente de Nó, 1934; Blakstad, 1956; Raisman, Cowan and Powell, 1965). An important excitatory input is the perforant path, whose cells of origin lie in the entorhinal area. This relay is the first link in a trisynaptic excitatory chain, comprising granule cells and CA3 and CA1 pyramidal cells, which links the entorhinal area to the hippocampus and its efferent pathways (Figure 13.1b). The lightly myelinated perforant path fibres occupy the middle third of the molecular layer, making numerous synapses-en-passage on dendritic spines (Figure 13.1c); these synapses account for thirty-seven per cent of the total in this region of the dendritic tree (Nafstad, 1967).

Population potentials

If a stimulating electrode is advanced through the angular bundle to weakly excite the perforant path fibres which run beneath, a characteristic evoked response is recorded by a microelectrode placed in the dentate area (Figure 13.1d, left). This is a postsynaptic population potential, arising from the synchronous activation of many granule cells. It is correlated in time with monosynaptically evoked intracellular excitatory postsynaptic potentials (EPSPs), and on this and other evidence it has been called the 'extracellular EPSP' (Lømo, 1971). As can be seen from Figure 13.1d, the polarity of the potential depends on the depth of the recording electrode. In the region of the perforant path synapses, the potential is maximally negative, as a result of the inward flow of synaptic current. It reverses and becomes positive as the cell body layer, which acts as a passive source of current, is approached. With stronger volleys, the slope and amplitude of the population EPSP increase as more perforant path fibres are recruited. If the stimulus strength is increased further, a graded spike appears, superimposed on the population EPSP. This component of the evoked potential, which is negative in the cell body layer and positive in the synaptic layer, corresponds in time with unit discharges, and is called the 'population spike'. Its size is a function of the number of granule cells discharged, and also of the synchrony of discharge. The number of cells discharged by a given perforant path input will depend on the balance of inhibitory and excitatory activity along all afferent paths and on intrinsic factors, such as firing threshold. The population spike therefore provides a measure of the overall state of excitability of the granule cell population. The population EPSP, on the other hand, as recorded in the synaptic layer, is relatively uninfluenced by activity elsewhere and consequently can be taken as a measure of the functional state of the perforant path synapses alone.

Experimental arrangements and results

The experiments were performed either on rabbits anaesthetised with urethane–chloralose, or on awake unrestrained rabbits with implanted electrodes. In both cases, the basic experimental protocol was the same. Standard test shocks were delivered to the perforant path at regular intervals of two to six seconds to sample the amplitude of the population EPSP (measured at an early fixed latency; see Figure 13.1d, broken line) and the latency and amplitude of the population spike. When control values had remained stable for some time, a conditioning train of tetanic stimuli, usually ten to fifteen times per second for a few seconds, was given and the after effects of this brief episode on the various parameters of the evoked response were observed. A second pair of electrodes was in many cases positioned in the dentate area of the opposite side, or in various configurations on the same side, in order to control for generalised changes in the excitability of the granule cells.

The result of an acute experiment of this sort is shown in Figure 13.2. A microelectrode was advanced into the cell body layer of the dentate area on the left side to record the population potential evoked by the tungsten stimulating electrode positioned caudally among the perforant path fibres. A recording and stimulating pair was positioned in similar locations on the other side. The two sets of graphs show the effects of conditioning on the amplitude and latency of the population spike and also, for the left side, on the amplitude of the EPSP. Two conditioning, trains were given (ten times per second for ten seconds at the test strength), first to the right side, and later to the left (Figure 13.2, arrows). During conditioning, frequency potentiation developed, a phenomenon characteristic of this pathway at

Cortical synaptic plasticity

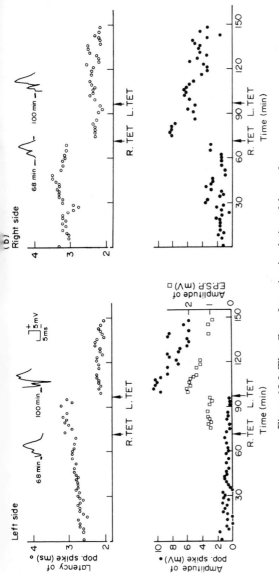

Figure 13.2. The effect of tetanic stimulation of the perforant path in an anaesthetised rabbit. Plots of latency-to-onset (○) and peak-to-peak amplitude (●) of the evoked population spike on the left side (a) and right side (b), as a function of time. Each point was derived from a computed average of twenty consecutive responses evoked by single test shocks given simultaneously to both sides at three-second intervals. At the times marked by arrows, conditioning tetanic stimulation (ten times per second for ten seconds at the same strength as the test shocks) was given, first to the right side and then to the left. Note that in each case the resulting potentiation was confined to the tetanised side. The amplitude of the population EPSP on the left side, measured 1 ms after the onset of synaptic positivity, is also plotted in (a) (□), for a period before and after conditioning. Insets show averaged population potentials before (68 minutes) and after (100 minutes) the two conditioning episodes.

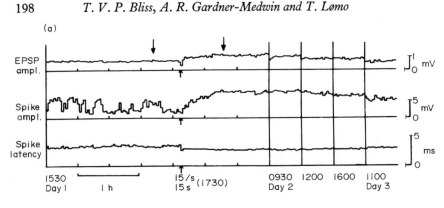
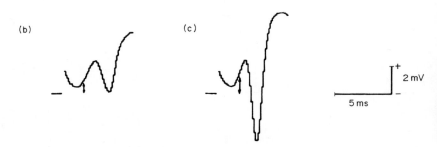

Figure 13.3. Effect of tetanic stimulation of the perforant path in an awake rabbit. (a), Plots of the amplitude of the extracellular EPSP (measured 0·8 ms after onset) and of the peak-to-peak amplitude and latency-to-onset of the population spike, as functions of time, showing potentiation of the response lasting over twenty-four hours after a single episode of tetanic stimulation (fifteen times per second for fifteen seconds at same strength as test shocks). Each point was derived from a computed average of sixteen consecutive responses evoked by single test volleys given every six seconds. Two such averages are shown in (b) and (c), obtained before and after conditioning, at the times indicated by the arrows above (a). Time scale is the same throughout, but broken at the vertical lines.

stimulus frequencies of ten to fifteen times per second (Lømo, 1966). Afterwards, the response to single test shocks was greatly potentiated, with an increase in the amplitude of the population spike (Figure 13.2, filled circles), a reduction in spike latency (open circles) and, on the left side but not on the right, an increase in the extracellular EPSP (Figure 13.2a, open squares). In each case these changes were confined to the conditioned side. The striking nature of the potentiation can be seen in the two sets of averaged responses (Figure 13.2, insets), computed from twenty consecutive test responses before and after the two conditioning trains.

The time course of the effect in this experiment was significantly different for each of the three parameters measured. On the left side, the EPSP declined to its preconditioning control value over a period of thirty to forty minutes, while the population spike, though also declining, was still greatly potentiated fifty minutes after conditioning. The reduction in spike latency, on the other hand, persisted without decrement for the duration of the experiment (Figure 13.2a). On the right side, the population spike returned to its control value within sixty to seventy minutes, but again there was no decrement in the latency effect (Figure 13.2b). In other acute experiments, in which several trains were given at intervals of thirty to sixty minutes, it was often the case that the first one or two episodes resulted in a relatively short-lasting potentiation; the effect of subsequent trains was then as much to stabilise the response as to produce further potentiation. In several such experiments the population response remained at an elevated level for several hours after the last conditioning train.

The experiments with unanaesthetised, chronically prepared animals followed essentially the same pattern, with the advantage that it was possible to follow the after effects of conditioning for much longer periods of time (Figure 13.3). Here the potentiation produced by a single buzz (fifteen times per second for fifteen seconds) lasted more than twenty-four hours. Averaged responses evoked by the test stimulus before and after conditioning can be compared in Figures 13.3b and 13.3c. In only one animal out of seven prepared satisfactorily for chronic recording did we fail to find potentiation lasting one hour or more after single conditioning trains. With repeated trains, much longer effects can often be produced. In a later experiment with the rabbit showing the effects in Figure 13.3, potentiation lasting for several weeks occurred after a series of conditioning trains at strengths greater than the test shocks.

A particularly noticeable feature of the chronic experiments was the great variation in the amplitude of the population spike, apparent even in averaged records (see Figure 13.3) and the marked reduction in this variability after conditioning. It is not immediately obvious why the variation about the mean value should be so large, nor why it should be so greatly reduced by conditioning. Clearly, however, the phenomenon may well have some functional importance, in increasing the reliability of transmission through the perforant path–granule cell relay.

Mechanism of the effect

It is clear from a more detailed analysis of these experiments that there are two distinct mechanisms contributing to the long-lasting potentiation of the evoked perforant path response. The first is an increase in the efficiency of synaptic coupling between perforant path and granule cells and the second is a generalised increase in the excitability of the stimulated granule cell population.

Enhanced synaptic coupling, resulting in an increased flow of evoked synaptic current, is the simplest explanation for increases in the amplitude of the extracellular EPSP. The mechanism for this could be either presynaptic (e.g. increased release of transmitter, either from the same or an enlarged population of terminal

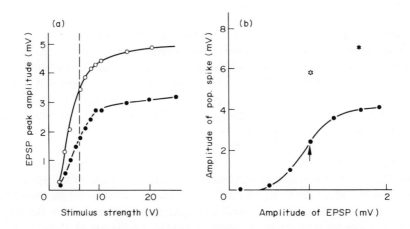

Figure 13.4. Changes in transfer characteristics produced by tetanic stimulation. (a), Stimulus–response curves obtained from an anaesthetised preparation before (●) and forty minutes after (○) conditioning with tetanic stimulation at one hundred times per second for four seconds. Note increase in the slope of the initial part of the curve without change in threshold. Broken line indicates strength used for conditioning (6 V). (b), Synaptic input-output curve obtained in the experiment illustrated in Figure 13.2a. The amplitude of the evoked population spike is plotted against EPSP amplitude for a series of shocks of increasing strength. The point marked by an arrow corresponds to the test strength. Twenty minutes (★) and forty minutes (☆) after conditioning (ten times per second for ten seconds) the test shock evoked an averaged response characterised by the filled and open stars respectively.

endings) or postsynaptic (e.g. increased receptor sensitivity). We have no evidence enabling us to distinguish between these or other possibilities. One point, however, can be made. The stimulus–response curves plotted in Figure 13.4a show that long-term potentiation can be obtained even if the postsynaptic cells do not discharge during conditioning. In this experiment weak shocks were used to evoke a pure extracellular EPSP, without any superimposed population spike. The same strength was used during conditioning, which consisted of a four-second buzz at one hundred times per second (a frequency at which a population spike, if present, is very rapidly blocked). It is therefore highly unlikely that any appreciable number of granule cells were discharged during conditioning. Nevertheless a large, long-lasting increase in the amplitude of the extracellular EPSP occurred, as can be seen by comparing the slope of the stimulus–response curve before the conditioning train (Figure 13.4a, filled circles) with that obtained forty minutes after the train (open circles). A further point worth noting from this pair of curves is that, to a first approximation, the increase in slope is confined to that part of the post-conditioning curve lying to the left of the broken vertical line intersecting the abscissa at 6 V, which was the strength used for testing and conditioning. This is what would be expected if the effect were confined to granule cells innervated by those fibres activated during the conditioning train (that is, those recruited by shocks of 6 V or less), and was not generalised to fibres recruited by shocks stronger than 6 V.

Increases in synaptic efficiency alone are not sufficient to explain the results of experiments in which potentiation of spike amplitude occurred without change in the amplitude of the extracellular EPSP, or in which the increase in spike size was disproportionately large. Figure 13.4b (from the same experiment as that of Figure 13.2) illustrates the point. The graph may be regarded as an input–output curve for the perforant path–granule cell system, where the input is represented by the amplitude of the EPSP and the output by the size of the population spike. The points were obtained from stimulus–response curves before conditioning. Each point is associated with a particular stimulus strength, the point corresponding to the strength used for testing (and conditioning) being indicated by an arrow. Twenty minutes after conditioning, the test shock evoked a response corresponding to the filled star; conditioning therefore resulted in an increase in both the extracellular EPSP and the population spike, but the increase in the latter was considerably greater than that predicted by the synaptic input–output curve on the basis of the postconditioning value of the EPSP. The open star shows the situation twenty minutes later; the EPSP had declined to its control value, yet the spike remained at an elevated level (see Figure 13.2a). This extra component of spike potentiation, which was seen in the majority of experiments for which sufficient data was available for an assessment of this sort to be made, may be attributed to an increase in the overall excitability of the conditioned population of granule cells.

References

BLAKSTAD, T. W. (1956). Commissural connections of the hippocampal region in the rat, with special reference to their mode of termination. *J. comp. Neurol.*, **105**, 417–538.

BLISS, T. V. P. and GARDNER-MEDWIN, A. R. (1971). Long-lasting increases of synaptic influence in the unanaesthetized hippocampus. *J. Physiol., Lond.*, **216**, 32P.

BLISS, T. V. P. and LØMO, T. (1970). Plasticity in a monosynaptic cortical pathway. *J. Physiol., Lond.*, **207**, 61P.

BRINDLEY, G. S. (1969). Nerve net models of plausible size that perform many simple learning tasks. *Proc. R. Soc.*, B, **174**, 173–91.

DOUGLAS, R. J. (1967). The hippocampus and behaviour. *Psychol. Bull.*, **67**, 416–42.

ECCLES, J. C. (1953). *The Neurophysiological Basis of Mind*. Clarendon Press, Oxford.

ELAZAR, Z. and ADEY, W. R. (1967). Spectral analysis of low frequency components in the electrical activity of the hippocampus during learning. *Electroenceph. clin. Neurophysiol.*, **23**, 225–40.

GARDNER-MEDWIN, A. R. (1969). Modifiable synapses necessary for learning. *Nature, Lond.*, **223**, 916–19.

GLASSMAN, E. and WILSON, J. E. (1973). RNA and brain function. In: *Macromolecules and Behaviour* (ANSELL, G. B. and BRADLEY, P. B., Eds.), pp. 81–92. Macmillan, London.

GRASTYAN, E. and KARMOS, G. (1962). The influence of hippocampal lesions on simple and delayed instrumental conditioned reflexes. In: *Physiologie de l'hippocampe*, pp. 225–34. CNRS, Paris.

HEBB, D. O. (1949). *The Organisation of Behaviour*. Wiley, New York.

HYDÉN, H. (1973). In: *Macromolecules and Behaviour* (ANSELL, G. B. and BRADLEY, P. B., Eds.), pp. 3–75. Macmillan, London.

LØMO, T. (1966). Frequency potentiation of excitatory synaptic activity in the dentate area of the hippocampal formation. *Acta phsyiol. scand.*, **68**, suppl. 277, 128.

LØMO, T. (1971). Patterns of activation in a monosynaptic cortical pathway: The perforant path input to the dentate area of the hippocampal formation. *Exp. Brain Res.*, **12**, 18–45.

LORENTE DE NÓ, R. (1934). Studies on the structure of the cerebral cortex. II. Continuation of the study of the Ammonic system. *J. Psychol. Neurol., Leipzig*, **46**, 113–77.

MARR, D. (1970). A theory for cerebral neocortex. *Proc. R. Soc.*, B, **176**, 161–234.

MILNER, B. (1970). Memory and the medial temporal regions of the brain. In: *Biology of Memory* (PRIBRAM, K. H. and BROADBENT, D. E., Eds.), pp. 29–50. Academic Press, New York.

NAFSTAD, P. M. J. (1967). An electron microscope study of the termination of the perforant path fibres in the hippocampus and the fascia dentata. *Z. Zellforsch.*, **76**, 532–42.

RAISMAN, G., COWAN, W. M. and POWELL, T. P. S. (1965). The extrinsic afferent, commissural and association fibres of the hippocampus. *Brain*, **89**, 317–48.

RAMÓN Y CAJAL, S. (1911). *Histologie du système nerveux de l'homme et des vertébrés*, Vol. II. Maloine, Paris.

VINOGRADOVA, O. S., SEMYONOVA, T. P. and KONOVALOV, V. PH. (1970). Trace phenomena in single neurons of hippocampus and mammiliary bodies. In: *Biology of Memory* (PRIBRAM, K. H. and BROADBENT, D. E., Eds.), pp. 191–221. Academic Press, New York.

Conditioned evoked potential: an electrical sign of memory

G. ÁDÁM

Department of Comparative Physiology, Eötvös Loránd University, Budapest, Hungary

Our study of the electrical phenomena of information storage has its roots in a certain psychophysiological concept based on earlier experiments on visceral, interoceptive learning (Ádám, 1967). We tried to elaborate a simple model suitable for reproducible and quantitative measurements in studying the elementary electrical processes of learning and memory. A special form of conditioning proved appropriate for our purposes. This model is based on the production and recording of conditioned evoked potentials in various parts of the brain elicited by electrical stimulation of a variety of sensory nerves and delayed conditioning of afferent stimuli. These learned evoked responses were considered as electrical memory models and subjected to detailed analysis. Delayed conditioning of primary evoked deflections is thus a special variant of sensory–sensory conditioning, in which a tracing stimulus elicits a well defined electrical response. The learned deflections appear as evoked potentials which can be easily distinguished from the spontaneous electrical activity constituting the background 'noise'.

The technique of conditioned evoked potentials was first applied by Livanov and Poliakov (1945) in the form of 'assimilation' of rhythmic unconditioned stimuli. After a certain amount of training, the hypersynchronous periodic evoked activity followed the rhythm of the unconditioned stimulus. In the course of elaboration of a defensive conditioned reflex, the percentage of clearly detectable potentials evoked by the conditioned stimulus (CS) increased gradually. Both techniques, the 'assimilation of the rhythm' as well as the recording of evoked responses accompanying learned behavioural changes have been employed by many workers, the wide variety of results having been surveyed repeatedly (Morell, 1961; John, 1967; Ádám, 1967).

Our approach to conditioning evoked potentials has been substantially different from those known from the literature. We used the *delayed* association of two stimuli regarded as the CS and UCS. We considered as criterion of a learned response the fulfilment of the following two postulates: (1) if the CS evoked by itself

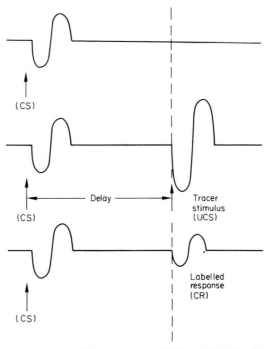

Figure 14.1. Diagram of the conditioning procedure. Curve 1, evoked potential to the conditioned stimulus (CS.) Curve 2, evoked responses to the conditioned and unconditioned stimulus (UCS). Curve 3, the application of CS alone evokes, in addition to its own potential, a second response regarded as the conditioned reaction (CR).

without unconditioned reinforcement *two* potentials—in addition to its own response, a second one corresponding to the previous UCS; (2) if the delay of this second potential (regarded as conditioned reaction) was identical to the delay of the response elicited by the former reinforcing stimulus. Thus, the parameters of the delayed conditioned evoked potential (CEP) constitute the sole and exclusive index of learning and retention (Figure 14.1). In most experiments, the response was recorded as averaged deflections, each individual curve being resolved into

256 or 512 elementary points, corresponding to a channel-width of 2 or 5 ms. In general, forty to fifty deflections were averaged, and the curve obtained was recorded photographically or plotted by an X–Y recorder. By this method, it was possible to distinguish signals from background activity (Figure 14.2).

As shown on Figure 14.2, the most conspicuous and remarkable characteristic of the learned electric response was the accurate timing of delay, that is, the fact

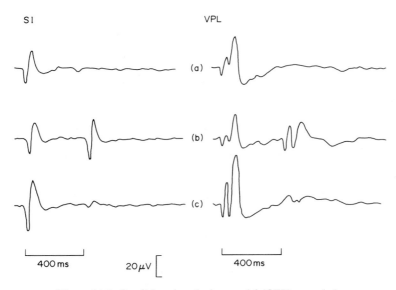

Figure 14.2. Conditioned evoked potential (CEP) recorded from the somatosensory cortical area (SI) and from the ventral postero-lateral nucleus (VPL) of the thalamus of the cat. (a), Average of 40–40 potentials to left splanchnic stimulation. (b), Association of splanchnic and sciatic stimulation with delay of 400 ms. (c), Average of forty splanchnic evoked potentials following 200 reinforcements. The CEP appears with the same delay as the previous sciatic reinforcement. Recording from the right hemisphere in the chloralosed cat. NTA 512B type computer, X–Y recorder.

that the conditioned response appeared with the same delay as the unconditioned reinforcing stimulus used for the elaboration of the CEP. This accurate timing was observed both on curves of the CEP and on the latency-histograms. Thus, it could be proved that the conditioned evoked deflection had a latency identical to the delay of the reinforcing stimulus. If, for example, the second stimulus was applied 80 ms after the first one, the conditioned response also appeared with a delay of 80 ms; if reinforcement occurred 200, 300, 400 or 500 ms after the CS, the evoked response was recorded with exactly the same delay after the CS when the latter was presented alone. This finding suggests a new interpretation of the phenomenon of delay (or delayed inhibition) described by Pavlov. Namely, in classic conditioning experiments, the process of delay ensues gradually and relatively slowly, probably as the result of the inertia of the salivary and motor efferent system. From our results, we conclude that, in the central neuronal networks, delay is a flexible and mobile process, conditioned responses appearing with the same delay as that used in applying the reinforcing stimulus, without any previous gradation (Figure 14.3).

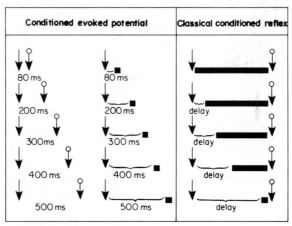

Figure 14.3. Comparison of CEP and classical conditioning. The diverse mechanism of delay schematically represented. ♀, Conditioned stimulus; ♀, unconditioned reinforcement; heavy horizontal line, conditioned response. Detailed explanation in the text.

The topography of the learned electrical response has been thoroughly studied in our laboratory. We have succeeded in demonstrating that it appears not only in the cortex and the thalamus but also in lower structures, for example in the reticular formation, both in intact and decerebrate animals (Figure 14.4). The phenomenon occurred in large areas of the cortex. In the case of unilateral stimulation, the evoked conditioned response could be recorded not only on the heterolateral but also on the homolateral cortex, on the primary projection areas of the two stimuli and also on adjacent regions of the cortex (Figure 14.5). The conclusions drawn from these observations concerning the mechanism of learning will be discussed later.

To obtain a clear picture of the mechanism of learned electric responses, attempts were made to study this phenomenon using microelectrodes at the level of small cell populations and single units. It could be demonstrated that neurones or groups of neurones which failed to respond to the first, splanchnic stimulus

Conditioned potential

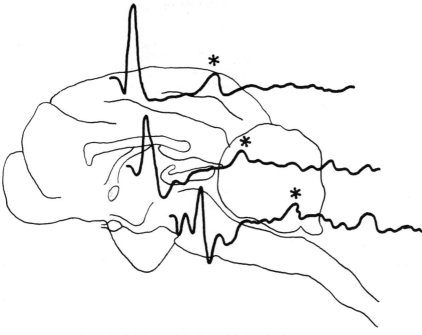

Figure 14.4. The CEP is detectable in addition to primary cortical projection areas (representing the CS and UCS) from specific nuclei of the thalamus and from the midbrain reticular formation. * CEP, delay 400 ms.

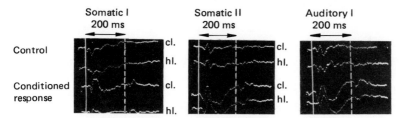

Figure 14.5. Chronic conditioned evoked potentials recorded from the somatic sensory areas I–II and from the primary auditory cortex on both hemispheres. cl, Right hemisphere, contralateral to left hind leg stimulation; hl, left hemisphere, homolateral to the peripheral stimulation. The first vertical solid line marks the administration of the auditory CS; the second, dotted line marks the time of the previous reinforcing UCS. The marked conditioned evoked response is noticeable at the site of the unconditioned potential evoked previously by the dermal stimulus. Each curve represents the average of forty potentials.

(CS), but increased or decreased their spike frequency in response to the second, sciatic stimulus (UCS), gave, after a sufficient number of reinforcements, an adequate response to the CS (Figure 14.6). By extracellular recording it was possible to establish both facilitation, that is, the appearance of a train of spikes, and inhibition, that is, the cessation of oscillation of a single unit or of groups of neurones, after appropriate conditioning.

The consolidation of this learned electric response was studied extensively in cats with chronically implanted electrodes (Figure 14.7). We have been relying on the well known theory of Hebb (1949) assuming that the storage of information begins with the formation of an unstable, short-term memory trace which is

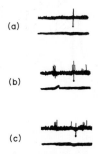

Figure 14.6. Conditioned response of a group of cortical units. Top trace, single unit activity; lower trace, artefact of sciatic stimulus. (a), Splanchnic stimulus (artefact on the top trace); (b), association of splanchnic and sciatic stimulus (notch on lower trace); (c), splanchnic stimulation following reinforcements. The unit activity of at least three cortical neurones is clearly visible. Delay 200 ms. Read figure from right to left.

followed by lasting, permanent, long-term storage. It has been shown in our experiments that, in the case of conditioned trials made after eighty reinforcements, an electroconvulsive shock (ECS) abolishes the conditioned response. There is still great controversy over the mechanism of action of ECS treatment introduced by Cerletti and Bini (1938). The most significant feature of this treatment is the total amnesia or lack of memory for the events occurring within a few minutes before shock treatment. The amnesia is lasting and indicates that this rather crude treatment affects recent memory. According to most authors, the electric shock causes oedema of the brain, leading to transient loosening and lasting disruption of synaptic connections. Others believe that ECS disrupts the functional reverberation circuits. In view of these assumptions it is easy to understand why, in our cats, the evoked potential conditioned only for one day and by a relatively small number of reinforcements was extinguished by the ECS treatment. In other cats, successive training for three or more days resulted in a lasting

Conditioned potential

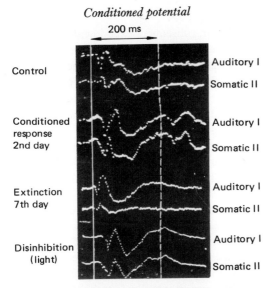

Figure 14.7. Extinction and disinhibition of the chronic CEP by additional light-stimulus. Legend as in Figure 14.5.

fixation of the electric memory trace which could no longer be extinguished by ECS (Figure 14.8).

The data from the experiments devoted to the establishment of electric memory traces within a session could be interpreted by assuming neuronal reverberating functions. It was supposed that the afferent stimuli applied with an interval of 200 to 400 ms elicited reverberational activity with a well defined time course which was finally manifested in a learned evoked response resulting from the summation

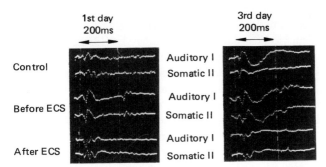

Figure 14.8. The effect of electroconvulsive shock treatment on chronic CEP. Legend as in Figure 14.5. The data of two different animals are represented, treated with ECS on the first and third day of conditioning.

of postsynaptic potentials. In subsequent experiments, an attempt was made to confirm or reject this hypothesis by a method different from that of the ECS. It has been assumed that the reversible disruption of the neuronal flux of impulses might have an effect on the learned evoked response by establishing a transient but total electric silence in the brain. A reversible isoelectric corticogram and electrothalamogram was produced by complete cessation of blood supply to the brain on one hand and by cooling on the other. According to the observation of Hirsch (1962) and others, the effect of complete ischaemia of the brain for at least one minute but no longer than four minutes may be reversible, depending on the actual temperature of the brain. Therefore, we occluded simultaneously the vertebral and carotid arteries for periods of one to four minutes.

We obtained rather unexpected results: the CEP persisted without significant diminution after the total electric silence. Moreover, in most cases the amplitude of the conditioned deflections increased (Figure 14.9). Cessation of blood supply to the brain in many cases caused some deterioration of cerebral functions, indicated by the diminution of the amplitude of the 'unconditioned' splanchnic evoked potential. Remarkably, however, the amplitude of the conditioned evoked response also increased in these cases. The CEP of the somatosensory cortex and the ventral postero-lateral nucleus of the thalamus persisted equally after the electric silence, and in the initial period after the transient ischaemia, the response was usually more marked in the thalamus than in the cortex. Cerebral electrical activity could also be successfully suspended by placing a 0°C paraffin pool on the exposed surface of the brain which reduced the temperature of the cortex at a depth of 3 to 5 mm to 25–27°C within ten to fifteen minutes. Similarly as in the cerebral 'stop-flow' experiments, previously established conditioned deflections persisted after this procedure (Figure 14.10).

The results of these experiments are not as surprising as they might have appeared initially. Although the hypothesis of self-stimulating reverberating circuits has been frequently cited as the basis of the theory of the short-term memory trace, mainly through the network diagrams of Lorente de Nó (1938) and the mathematical considerations of Rashevsky (1938), this concept seems to be much too simplified, even vulgar, in view of the intricate cerebral configuration of neurones, even though Konorski (1961) considered it as the most plausible mechanism underlying short-term learning as early as 1961. Is it conceivable that a train of impulses would reverberate if a well-defined chemical or morphological change in the structure of synapses was not leading to consolidation of the trace? Certainly it is, at least in a model experiment. However, it seems highly unlikely in view of the intricate cerebral geometry. The phenomenon has been verified only a little in physiological experiments, the best known of which are the electrophysiological studies of Verzeano and Negishi (1960). Providing that the reverberation process is a train of spikes passing along a circular neuronal path, the electrical sign studied in our conditioning experiments was certainly not the result of such a mechanism. When comparing our findings with the observations of Baldwin and Soltysik (1969) made on goats and using the classic method of delayed conditioning, we may arrive at the conclusion that the labile learned reaction is not abolished by isoelectric silence of the brain.

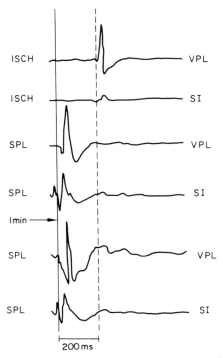

Figure 14.9. The effect of reversible cerebral isoelectrical state on previously elaborated CEP. After total cessation of the cerebral blood flow for one minute the previously elaborated CEP persists on the somatosensory cortex (SI) as well as in the thalamus (VPL). ISCH, Site of sciatic reinforcement; SPL, splanchnic stimulation. The arrow indicates the time of ligation of the carotid and vertebral arteries. Heavy vertical line, moment of administration of splanchnic stimulus; dotted vertical line, the site of sciatic reinforcement. Delay 200 ms.

A remarkable observation in these experiments was the increase in the amplitude of the learned deflection following cerebral ischaemia and sometimes following cooling. This indicates a considerable depletion of transmitters in the involved synaptic structures. It is also possible that the enhancement of protein synthesis during ischaemia observed by several investigators, and the process of microvacuolisation described recently by McGee-Russel, Brown and Brierley (1970), might be responsible for the fixation of the electrical signal. Thus, the synaptic mechanism seems to become more and more attractive as a possible explanation for some fundamental events of memory; this appears to be supported by the observation of Szentágothai (1971), according to which the complexity of synaptic surfaces increases in certain functional states in response to some hitherto unknown impact, but ultimately as the result of enhanced protein synthesis.

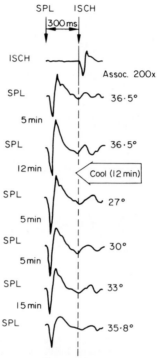

Figure 14.10. The effect of cortical cooling on CEP. The cooling of the cortical surface for twelve minutes by means of a paraffin pool of 0°C caused complete electrical 'silence'. This isoelectrical state did not affect the previously elaborated CEP. Legends as in Figure 14.9. The numbers on the right of the curves indicate the actual cortical temperature; the numbers on the left indicate the interstimulus intervals.

At this point our train of thought inevitably touches the problem of macromolecular changes, since the synaptic modifications mentioned above are based on enhancement of the rate of protein synthesis. The results of our electrophysiological observations seem to support the assumption that the various memory traces are processes borne by specific networks of neurones, the firing of which indicates the recognition of the stored information in response to the reminder stimulus. Of course, this form of memory trace postulates the involvement of a great number of cells in an intricate spatial arrangement, containing at each level an element of probability. Thus random firing of single units is very probable and must be reckoned with. In a whole system, however, the many random factors mask regularity and determination.

References

ÁDÁM, G. (1967). *Interoception and Behaviour. An Experimental Study*. Akadémiai Kiadó, Budapest.
BALDWIN, B. A. and SOLTYSIK, S. S. (1969). The effect of cerebral ischaemia or intracarotid injection of methohexitone on short-term memory in goats. *Brain Res.*, **16**, 105–20.
CERLETTI, V. and BINI, L. (1938). Electric shock treatment. *Boll. Accad. Med. Roma*, **64**, 36.
HIRSCH, H. (1962). Vulnérabilité et consommation d'oxygène du cerveau sous ischémie. In: *Actualités Neurophysiologiques* (MONNIER, A. M., Ed.), Quatrième Serie, pp. 33–53. Masson et Cie, Paris.
HEBB, D. O. (1949). *The Organization of Behaviour*, pp. 27–169. Wiley, New York.
JOHN, E. R. (1967). *Mechanisms of Memory*, p. 468. Academic Press, New York and London.
KONORSKI, J. (1961). The physiological approach to the problem of recent memory. In: *Brain Mechanism and Learning* (DELAFRESNAYE, Ed.), pp. 115–32. Blackwell, Oxford.
LIVANOV, M. N. and POLIAKOV, K. L. (1945). The electrical reactions of the cerebral cortex of a rabbit during the formation of a conditioned defense reflex by means of rhythmic stimulation. *Izv. Akad. Nauk. USSR Ser. Biol.*, **3**, 247–95.
LORENTE DE NÓ, R. (1938). Analysis of the activity of the chains of internuncial neurons. *J. Neurophysiol.*, **1**, 207–44.
MCGEE-RUSSEL, S. M., BROWN, A. W. and BRIERLEY, J. B. (1970). A combined light and electron microscope study of early anoxic-ischaemic cell change in rat brain. *Brain Res.*, **20**, 193–200.
MORELL, F. (1961). Electrophysiological contributions to the neuronal basis of learning. *Physiol. Rev.*, **41**, 443–94.
RASHEVSKY, N. (1938). *Mathematical Biophysics: Physiocomathematical Foundations of Biology*, 1st edition, University of Chicago Press, Chicago. 2nd edition, rev. ibid. (1948).
SZENTÁGOTHAI, J. (1971). Memory functions and the structural organization of the brain. In: *Biology of Memory* (ÁDÁM, G., Ed.), Akadémiai Kiadó, Budapest.
VERZEANO, M. and NEGISHI, K. (1960). Neuronal activity in cortical and thalamic networks. *J. gen. Physiol.*, 43 Suppl., **177**, 27; 33; 234.

Morphological correlates of functional activity in the nervous system

M. BERRY, T. HOLLINGWORTH, R. FLINN and E. M. ANDERSON

Department of Anatomy, Medical School, Birmingham B15 2TJ, England

Previous conferences on macromolecules and behaviour have focussed on a possible direct relationship between macromolecules and the functional status of the nervous system. This trend is expected since the classical view of the nervous system is one in which anatomical connections are thought to be permanent and immutable and where metabolic events alone are seen to be dynamic. However, recent researches have indicated that the nervous system exhibits a physiological and anatomical plasticity which is functionally determined and contingent on the integrity of the biochemistry of neurones and glia. Macromolecules undoubtedly play a role in these structural rearrangements but the extent to which learning and memory involve morphological change is unknown. This paper reviews the evidence for plasticity within the nervous system and also criticises some of the analytical techniques used.

Glial cells

Glial cells become overtly active in response to trauma, radiation and certain drugs. They also participate in neuronal metabolism, brain development, degeneration and regeneration, myelination and demyelination, the allergic response and certain electrical phenomena. The Diamond-Krech-Rozenzweig-Bennett group (1962, 1963, 1964, 1968, 1969) has found that the number of glial cells increases in the neocortex of rats exposed to 'enriched' environments while the number of neurones remains constant. The lability of glia is also demonstrated by the use of tissue culture in which glial cells and their processes are seen to be freely mobile, withdrawing processes, extending new ones and 'crawling' through the tissue and along neurones (Pomerat, 1958).

The relationships between neurones and glia at the synapse have been documented by many workers, and Galambos (1965) has suggested that synaptic activity involves glial cells directly. Drawing on information given in a paper by Koelle (1962), Galambos suggests that re-excitation of the presynaptic membrane may involve the active secretion of transmitter substance by the glial cells juxtaposed to the presynaptic terminal. Direct evidence that transmitter substance can be stored and released by glia has been given by Birks, Huxley and Katz (1960) and Birks, Katz and Miledi (1960). Their electron-microscopical studies of Schwann cells in normal and degenerating motor end-plates of the frog show that in both cases Schwann cells investing the end-plate possess small numbers of vesicles. It was suggested that the continuous release of vesicles from Schwann cells may account for the miniature end-plate potentials recorded from both normal and denervated neuromuscular junctions in the frog.

During retrograde changes in the facial nucleus of rats after section of the facial nerve there is an increase in the number of microglia about each cell body associated with complete depletion of axosomatic and axodendritic synapses (Blinzinger and Kreutzberg, 1968). It was suggested that microglia had actively denuded these chromatolytic cells of presynaptic endings and thus effectively insulated them from afferent input (Kreutzberg, 1968). Recently this work has been substantiated by Hamberger, Hansson and Sjöstrand (1970), using the scanning electron microscope. Their beautiful pictures clearly show the absence of presynaptic endings on chromatolytic hypoglossal nuclei from the rabbit. It is tempting to speculate that glial cells are normally active, in this way, in resiting synaptic contacts during learning and memory.

A new hypothesis for the genesis of the conditioned reflex includes the involvement of oligodendrocytes (Roitbach, 1970). It is proposed that 'potential synapses' establish the conditioned response by becoming functional synapses. 'Potential synapses' exist as unmyelinated collaterals terminating as presynaptic boutons on postsynaptic loci. Associated with each unmyelinated collateral is the process of an oligodendrocyte, and the whole unit is called a neurone–neuroglia module. The synapse does not work, however, because the decrement of electrotonus along the unmyelinated membrane is so great that activity reaching the synapse is too weak to release sufficient mediator for propagation. But when input converges on neurone–neuroglia modules and neurones in the focus of the unconditioned stimulation, depolarisation of the oligodendrocyte occurs. This stimulates the oligodendrocyte to form myelin about the collateral. When myelination is complete, sufficient current is conducted to the bouton, the synapse becomes functional and conditioning is achieved. In this light the results of Gyllensten and Malfors (1963) may have new significance. They found that myelination of the optic nerve was delayed in mice reared in darkness from birth.

The neuronal cell body and nucleus

It is now established that the size of the cell body and the nucleus of neurones and glia is related to function (see Rather, 1958, for review). Indeed the actual viability of neurones appears to depend on afferent input and when this is entirely lacking the cell may degenerate (Hess, 1958; Pinching and Powell, 1971). A few examples may be useful: the nuclei of neurones in an epileptic focus are smaller than in normal tissue (Westrum, White and Ward, 1964), the sizes of the nuclei of neurones in the lateral geniculate body are reduced both after rearing in darkness (Hubel and Wiesel, 1963) and by lid closure (Kupfer and Palmer, 1964) and the volume of cells in layers II–IV of the striate cortex and the diameter of their nuclei are reduced in kittens reared in darkness from birth (Gyllensten, 1959; Gyllensten, Malfors and Norrlin-Grettoe, 1965, 1967; Tsang, 1937); motor neurones in the spinal cord may increase in size after a short duration of activity (Edström, 1957; Geinsmann, Larima and Mats, 1971) but both nucleus and perikaryon become smaller after prolonged, intense activity (Geinsmann et al., 1971); increased activity in the auditory cortex of dark-reared rats produced increased nuclear size in the neurones of this area (Gyllensten, Malfors and Norrlin-Grettoe, 1966); the volume of the perikaryon of ventral horn cells is increased during myelination of the sciatic nerve of the rat and this is associated with a redistribution of RNA within the cell (Martinez and Friede, 1970). Correlated with changes in activity there occurs a change in the level of RNA and protein in the cytoplasm of the neurone (Hydén, 1943, 1960, 1964). From this point of view, the changes in RNA during regeneration may be significant since it has been shown that RNA turnover is at its highest during the sprouting growth phase of axonal regeneration (Brattgård, Edström and Hydén, 1958) although the exact stimulus for these RNA changes is little understood (Cragg, 1970).

The sizes of neurones and their nuclei differ markedly throughout the CNS and it has been shown recently that large efferent neurones, for example, ventral horn cells, Purkinje cells, pyramidal cells in the hippocampus and Betz cells in the neocortex all exhibit tetraploidy and occasionally octaploidy (Herman and Lapham, 1968, 1969). Clearly the future investigation of the metabolism of neurones with different DNA content will give some insight into the significance of macromolecules in the functioning of the nervous system.

Axons

Different functional states have a marked effect upon the structure of axons. In the retina of the cat, for example, the plexiform layers are reduced in thickness, without concomitant neurone loss in the ganglion cell layers, after rearing in darkness (Rasch, Riesen and Chow, 1959; Weiskrantz, 1958), although ganglion cell loss has been noted in the chimpanzee during dark-rearing (Chow, Riesen and Newell, 1957). The former result implies that the growth of collaterals and terminal branches of axons is influenced by ongoing intrinsic activity. Other evidence that the organisation of the terminal branching of axons is functionally determined is provided by rapid Golgi studies of degenerating dendritic spines after sensory deprivation. Colonnier (1968) has pointed out that most synaptic contacts are established on dendritic spines in the cerebral cortex, and Globus and Scheibel (1966) have shown that dendritic spines disappear (or are not impregnated) when the presynaptic bouton is lost. Thus, quantitative studies of the extent of dendritic spine loss, following fibre tract interruption, demonstrate the geometry of the fields of axodendritic contact of the fibres of the sectioned tract.

Sensory deprivation has remarkable effects on dendritic spines. In striate cortex, after visual deprivation, spines are reduced over the middle portion of the apical shafts of layer V neurones; this part of the dendrite courses through layers III and IV (Valverde, 1967, 1968; Globus and Scheibel, 1967a, b, c; Fifková, 1970a). It is precisely this area of the cortex which is supplied by the visual radiations. Although there may be differences between enucleation and dark-rearing at the levels of the retina and lateral geniculate nucleus (Gyllensten *et al.*, 1967), enucleation *vis-à-vis* lid closure appears to have an identical effect within the cortex (Fifková, 1968). However, the effects on the apical dendrites of layer V neurones traversing layer III and IV are thought to be secondary since visual projection fibres primarily engage internuncial stellate neurones located in layers IV and III, and the short axons of these cells, in turn, engage the apical dendrites of layer V neurones (Valverde and Ruiz-Marcos, 1969). But effects may be transmitted still further to the peristriate cortex receiving commissural fibres from the contralateral striate cortex primarily effected by visual deprivation (Valverde and Estéban, 1968) and to the pulvinar (Fifková and Hassler, 1969). Similar transneuronal effects are seen in the spinal cord (Illis, 1963). Thus, deafferentation may effect an anatomical change in the terminal arborisations of axons over a chain of interconnections. The terminal branches of axons engage apical spines in a precisely defined manner which can be predicted by mathematical law (Ruiz-Marcos and Valverde, 1969). Sensory deprivation in visual cortex causes simple quantitative reduction in the number of spines but does not alter their distribution. Marin-Padilla (1968) has suggested, from ontological observations, that the number of spines established over the superficial part (pial end) of apical dendrites in human neocortex is probably influenced by experience. The effect of lid closure on the number of apical dendritic spines in the visual cortex may be reversed if the eyes are opened after ten to thirty days, but beyond two months opening of the lids effects no recovery (Fifková, 1970b).

The intrinsic fine structure of the synapse may also be altered by functional change. In neuropsychiatric disorders characterised by disturbances in memory and learning, Gonatas (1967) has noted abnormal changes in presynaptic boutons in human neocortex. Deprivation of visual input and first exposure to light both effect synaptic changes throughout the visual system. Retinal receptor terminals of rats increase in width during prolonged exposure to darkness and subsequently decrease in width after exposure to daylight. Synaptic vesicles are dispersed within the large terminal profiles of dark-reared animals but are concentrated into groups in the smaller terminals of light-exposed rats (Cragg, 1969a). In the lateral geniculate body, the axon terminals of dark-reared rats become more numerous but smaller when animals are exposed to light and these effects are reversed when light-reared rats are put in darkness (Cragg, 1969b). Unilateral lid closure in the immature albino rat causes a 20 per cent reduction in synaptic density in upper neocortical layers together with a 7·5 per cent increase in the size of synaptic profiles (Fifková, 1970a). On the other hand, first exposure to light in dark-reared animals promotes the formation of new synapses of small diameter in the deeper layers, while synapses already formed in the superficial part of the cortex grow slightly larger (Cragg, 1969b). In dark-reared rats, synaptic density in the deeper cortex is reduced but remains unchanged in the superficial cortex (Cragg, 1969b). In the adult rabbit, accumulation of large numbers of vesicles around the presynaptic membrane at rod–cone–bipolar junctions occurs after twenty-four hours in darkness and more prolonged exposure produces a further decrease in the size of synaptic vesicles (de Robertis, 1958; de Robertis and Franchi, 1956). Mountford (1963) found no changes in the number of vesicles, their size or the diameter of synaptic profiles in adult albino guinea-pigs following light and dark adaption.

Szentàgothai and Rajkovits (1955) have described shrinkage in size of presynaptic terminals at the neuromuscular junction following disuse. Nerve stimulation has different effects. de Robertis (1958) investigated the effects of nerve stimulation on the morphology of the presynaptic endings of the splanchnic nerve in the adrenal medulla of the rabbit and showed that stimulation at a frequency of one hundred times per second produced an increase in the number of vesicles about the synaptic membrane while stimulation at four hundred times per second caused a reduction in the number of vesicles in the endings. Sensory stimulation during the period of spine growth differentially accelerates the maturation of synaptic spines on the dendritic tree of pyramidal cells in the rat cerebral cortex (Shapiro and Vukovich, 1970). These authors suggested that this effect might be brought about by increases in regional blood flow which causes the environment to be rich in nutrients. In this respect it is interesting that Gelfan and Tarlov (1963) and Gelfan and Rapisarda (1964) selectively destroyed internuncial neurones in the cord by transitory ischaemia thereby causing a 30 per cent reduction in synapses engaging ventral horn cells.

Sectioning of the dorsal roots in the spinal cord of adult cats stimulates collateral sprouting in the intraspinal part of the intact roots (Liu and Chambers, 1958) but functional connections do not appear to be formed (McCough, Austin and Liu, 1955). Functional connections are made, however, after corticospinal tract section in the adult cat and monkey cord, since this procedure stimulates ascending afferents to form collaterals which, in turn, make functional connections with internuncial neurones (McCough et al., 1955). Activity over these new connections may play a role in the development of the spasticity which is characteristic of an upper motor neurone lesion. Similar axon-sprouting has been seen in the superior cervical ganglion in axons which survive section of the preganglionic fibres from the roots of T 1–4. Functional connections may be formed with the postganglionic cells vacated by the degenerating terminals (Guth and Bernstein, 1961). Illis (1964) has found that after section of dorsal roots and/or transection of the cord, following an initial degenerative phase, the boutons of surviving axons undergo hypertrophy and increase their area of contact at the synapse. Similar results are obtained after section of the fibres converging on the septum, along the fimbria and medial forebrain bundle in the albino adult rat, when the synaptic sites vacated following degeneration in one tract are taken over by the terminals from fibres in the uninterrupted tract (Raisman, 1969a, b). Following complete destruction of neocortical axons by alpha and deutron irradiation, Kruger (1965) has demonstrated good 'regeneration' of axons through the lesions several days after irradiation.

Dendrites

The changes in dendritic spines after deafferentation indicate that the number of spines located on a dendrite is either a function of the level of activity converging on the dendrite or dependent on the presence of presynaptic junctions. But changes in synaptology may cause more gross effects. Many workers have noted that the volume and the thickness of neocortex and the amount of internuclear material are reduced following deafferentation (Fifková, 1967, 1970b; Fifková and Hassler, 1969; Tsang, 1937; Gyllensten et al., 1965; Krech, Rosenzweig and Bennett, 1963). By contrast, rearing in complex environments increases neocortical weight and depth but decreases neuronal density (Rosenzweig et al., 1962, 1968, 1969; Diamond et al., 1964; Bennett et al., 1964; Krech et al., 1963). These changes have been interpreted as demonstrating that dendritic branching is reduced by deafferentation and increased by the enriched experience afforded by environmental complexity. Similarly, Gyllensten et al. (1966) found that the auditory cortex was hypertrophied both in dark-reared mice and in adults kept in darkness; nuclear size and amount of internuclear material were increased. These changes were thought to indicate increased dendritic branching in the auditory areas. But, in fact, more direct evidence is available suggesting that dendritic morphology is modified by function.

Under the electron microscope, dendrites show degenerative changes following deafferentation (Grant and Westman, 1968; Le Vay, 1971). After section of the parallel fibres in the cerebellum of adult cats there occurs a diminution in dendritic branchlets of Purkinje cells (Mouren-Mathieu and Colonnier, 1969). The formation of new sprouts along Purkinje cell dendrites occurs in albino rats chronically intoxicated with sodium diphenylhydantoin (Dilantin) (Snider and Perez del Cerro, 1967). Dendrites have also been seen to regenerate across a laminar lesion in the cerebral cortex induced by alpha or deutron irradiation (Rose, Malis, Kruger and Baker, 1960; Kruger, 1965), and it is suggested that the appearance of both axons and dendrites in the irradiated area may be an expression of normal continuous growth rather than regeneration *per se*. Similarly, after lesions in the spinal cord, Bernstein and Bernstein (1971) observed normal axons and dendrites growing into a reactive area where motor and sensory neurones had suffered decrements in the density of their dendritic fields. Valverde (1968) looked at the striate cortex of enucleated mice and observed a striking change in the orientation of the dendrites of stellate cells (with ascending axons) lying in layer IV. The dendrites of these cells were quite clearly directed out of layer IV into layer III above, or layer V below, 'as if they were looking for other axons'. Normally the ramification of these dendrites is confined within layer IV where the geniculocalcarine tract actually arborises.

Unfortunately, quantitative studies of dendritic fields and the effect of function on the various parameters of the dendritic tree give conflicting results. Globus and Scheibel (1967a, b) found no quantitative difference in the dendritic fields of stellate and pyramidal cells in the striate cortex in normal and dark-reared rats other than an increased variance of all parameters in treated animals. In contrast, Coleman and Riesen (1968), also using cats, were able to show that stellate cells in layer II of the striate cortex and pyramidal cells in the posterior cingulate gyrus exhibited a reduced probability of branching although dendritic length was unaffected. Both of these measures on the stellate cells of layer V of the striate cortex were unaffected.

Valverde (1970) obtained similar results to those of Globus and Scheibel (1967a, b) when he compared entire dendritic fields of pyramids in the striate cortex of dark-reared mice with those from normal animals. But when he divided the dendritic fields into sectors he was able to show that dendritic density was reduced in an inferior sector relative to the density in the rest of the field. Thus, it appears that dendrites can reorientate their fields within an axonal array as the input over the array changes. Holloway (1966) has suggested that 'enriched' environments may allow dendrites to branch more abundantly in the cerebral cortex of rats when compared with the branching pattern of rats placed in isolation. But this latter work was, at best, a pilot study, and the results were inconclusive; too few animals were used, Golgi–Cox impregnation was very erratic and the variance between animals was large. This experiment has not been repeated to date.

Perhaps one of the most dramatic demonstrations of the effects of deafferentation on the organisation of dendrites was given by Jones and Thomas (1962). After section of the olfactory tract on one side in adult rats they noted in the ipsilateral pyriform cortex a marked reduction in the number and length of dendritic branches stemming from the pyramidal cells into layers I and II.

At this point we would like to present some of our results. Dendritic analysis is difficult and laborious but it is also grossly inaccurate. Recently we have attempted to define the inherent errors and hence the limitations of the technique (Berry, Hollingworth, Flinn and Anderson, unpublished observations).

The methods of dendritic analysis, used in the above experiments, were based on a technique first devised by Sholl (1953) who, using the Golgi-Cox stain and basing his estimates on sections 100–200 μm thick, measured the individual basal dendrites of neurones in the visual cortex of cats and corrected for three-dimensional array. The method purports to give absolute estimates of dendritic length and the positions of branching points, thus enabling dendritic density to be calculated. By this means Sholl demonstrated that dendritic density could be described in terms of an exponential decay which increased with distance from the centre of the cell body.

In 1955, Eayrs described an alternative method. Though neglecting to apply some of the finer corrections used by Sholl, he claimed the method to be sufficiently accurate for the quantitative comparison of different populations of neurones of similar generalised configuration. The outlines of selected cells, in Golgi-Cox preparations of rat cerebral cortex, were projected on paper targets made up of equidistant concentric circles each separated by a distance representing 18 μm. With the perikaryon located centrally on the target, the number of branches and dendritic terminals lying within the intervals between concentric circles and the number of intersections made by basal dendrites with each circle were counted giving results similar to those of Sholl and thus substantiating the finding that, in a three dimensional model, the density of dendritic fields decays exponentially with distance from the cell body. This technique has now become accepted as the best available for quantitative comparison of the effects of treatments on dendritic organisation although the method was never intended to give absolute results.

Since both of the quantitative methods outlined above employ the Golgi-Cox impregnation technique it is germane to recall that this procedure is empirical and not completely reliable. The mechanism of impregnation is unknown but may be associated with a particular biochemical state existing in potentially stainable neurones at the time of death. It is also questionable whether experimental procedures such as surgery, the administration of drugs or electrical stimulation modify the extent of impregnation. Impregnation of neurones may be total or partial and dendrites may be stained randomly or selectively. Until the factors regulating the uptake of this stain have been elucidated, interpretation of the results of experiments using this technique must remain guarded.

The dendritic fields of cortical neurones of layer Vb are thought to be spherical with diameters in excess of 400 μm. But section thickness of Golgi-Cox preparations used in the projection method is limited to 100–200 μm for practical reasons because, beyond this thickness, increasing opacity and the superimposition of processes from neighbouring cells precludes accurate analysis. Thus, the projected dendritic fields of neurones in sections of 100–200 μm are never complete and the dendritic losses are related to the total volume of the dendritic field under study and to the position of the cell body within the section.

Moreover, the volume into which basal dendrites grow is not a complete sphere because there is a region about the origin of the apical dendrite where basal dendrites are absent, the volume of which approximates to a cone. From an analysis of 160 fields using the target method, the apical angle of this cone has been estimated to be $105° \pm 30°$. The changes in the decay of dendritic density when correction for sectioning and projection is applied are shown in Figures 15.1 and 15.2.

If dendritic fields are spherical, it follows that volume losses due to sectioning are related to both the position of the centre of the sphere in the section and to the radius of the sphere in relation to the section thickness. It is possible to correct for this error at any vertical height within the section and at any radius by applying an appropriate correction factor. (The paper reporting the details is in preparation.)

The basic assumption of the projection method has been that the concentric circles on the Eayrs' target sample concentric spheres of the same diameter centred about the perikaryon and thus the data recorded on the target have been extrapolated to exist in three dimensions about the cell body (Figure 15.1c). However, there are two misconceptions in these arguments. Firstly, spheres are not represented beyond the section thickness because of sectioning losses (Figures 15.1a and b), and secondly, the concentric circles on the target do not represent spheres but the plan view of cylinders, the height of which is the section thickness (Figures 15.1a and b; Figures 15.2a–d). The volume of each cylinder represents the sampling volume and is made up of parts of several concentric spheres. It can be seen that the volume denominator in a density calculation for the data sampled within each concentric circle on the target should be an expression for cylindrical and not spherical volume. The height of the cylinder is the section thickness (Figures 15.2a and b).

The information losses in sections of varying thickness and the projection error are being investigated by means of a computer program involving the construction of a simplified model of a neurone and the use of the Birmingham University KDF 9 digital computer. In the model, concentric spheres, set 20 μm apart, are constructed about a central cell body. Correction is made for the error of the vertical position of the perikaryon within the section. For a given dendrite, the quantitative relationship between endings and branches is such that for N endings there are $(N-1)$ branches. Branches and endings are inserted as isolated points into the volume about the cell body according to various three-dimensional

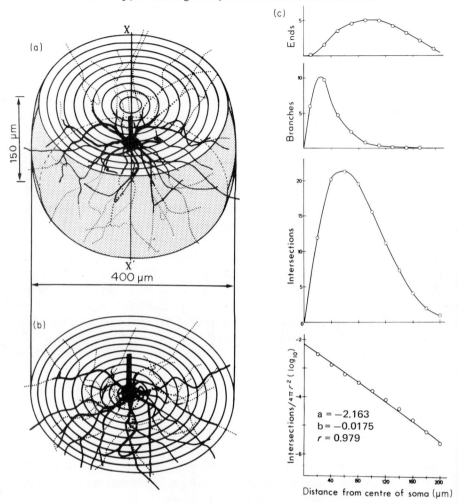

Figure 15.1. (a), Diagrammatic representation of sectioning error. A model of a neurone is placed at the centre of a sphere (400 μm in diameter) and sectioned to 150 μm in the plane of the apical dendrite. The dendrites lost from the system because of sectioning are dotted distal to the point of cutting. (b), The same cell as in (a) projected on a target; dendrites lost due to sectioning are dotted, dendrites unaffected by sectioning are black. This diagram also illustrates that the target does not sample a spherical volume but a small section of that volume. (c), The shape of plots of endings, branches and intersections at specific distances from the cell body obtained, using the Eayrs (1955) projection technique, from 160 neurones in layer Vb of the neocortex of rats. It is clear

distributions (Figure 15.3). Small slices are then removed from opposite poles and after each sectioning procedure the model is projected, through the cut faces, onto a target of the Eayrs' type, and the endings and branching points are counted and the intersections estimated from formula 1.

$$I_n = I_{(n-1)} + B_n - E_n \qquad (1)$$

where $I =$ intersections, $B =$ branches, $E =$ endings, $n =$ shell number ($I_0 =$ number of primary dendrites originating from the perikaryon). The results have shown that the best approximation to the distribution found from histological material, by the method of Eayrs (Figures 15.1 and 15.3), was given by a neurone in which both dendritic endings and branching nodes were normally distributed (Figure 15.3). The position of the means and the magnitudes of the standard deviations are now being adjusted so that, after substitution in formula 1, an exact replica of the curve of intersections against distance from the cell body can be obtained. It is then possible to compute the decrement of the dendritic density, at increasing distances from the cell body, before sectioning and before projection (Figure 15.3).

Another criticism of previous quantitative estimates is the failure to consider cell size and hence to detect the correlation which exists between the size of the perikaryon of cortical pyramids and the density of their dendritic fields. The importance of this relationship is illustrated by the results of the following experiment. The internal capsule of eight neonatal Wistar rats was sectioned at three days *post partum*, effectively isolating the cortex of one hemisphere from afferent influence except for that mediated by the corpus callosum. Eight treated and sixteen control animals were allowed to survive until thirty days *post partum*; their brains were treated by the Golgi-Cox technique and the basal dendritic fields of ten layer Vb pyramidal cells from each animal were analysed using the method of Eayrs. The results showed that dendritic density was markedly reduced (Figure 15.4), but the effect of treatment was not confined to fibres entering the cortex, for corticofugal fibres were also severed and thus an additional factor, often called the Gudden effect (Brodal, 1940), was operative, tending to cause degeneration and loss of cells. Correlation of cell size with dendritic density (Figure 15.5) presented the possibility that there was no reduction but that sampling was from a

---

from a comparison of (a), (b) and (c) that the shape of these plots can bear little resemblance to the magnitude and distribution of these parameters before section and projection have occurred. Dendritic density is usually represented as the number of dendrites/$4\pi r^2$ but with reference to part (a) of this figure it can be seen that $4\pi r^2$ is clearly the wrong denominator for this density calculation ($r =$ radii of concentric spheres; radius of each concentric sphere $=$ radius of corresponding concentric circle on the target). The plane XX' is referred to in the legend of Figure 15.2.

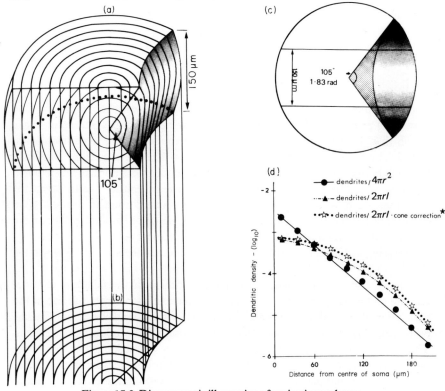

Figure 15.2. Diagrammatic illustration of projection and cone errors. (a), Hemisection of Figure 15.1 (a) along the plane XX' with the conical area about the apical dendrite removed illustrating the extent of the volume losses. (b), Cylinders are sampled by the target, the height of the cylinders being the section thickness (150 μm). (c), Sphere with the cone removed; the losses from the sphere due to sectioning to 150 μm are also shown. (d), Graphical representation of dendritic decay according to Eayrs using the $4\pi r^2$ denominator (r = radii of concentric spheres) and graphs showing the deviations from exponential linearity after correction for sectioning, cone and projection error.

★ when $r \leqslant \dfrac{l}{2\tan\theta}$ ($\simeq 60$ μm when $l = 150$ μm $\theta = 52\tfrac{1}{2}°$)

cone correction $= \pi r^2\, \theta \tan\theta$

when $r > \dfrac{l}{2\tan\theta}$

cone correction $= 2r^2\, \theta \tan\theta(\sin 2\rho + \rho)$

where $\rho = \sin^{-1}\left(\dfrac{l}{2r\tan\theta}\right)$

l = section thickness, θ = cone angle/2, r = radii of concentric cylinders.

normal population of smaller neurones. Further analysis showed that the dendritic density of the smaller cells was, in fact, reduced (Figure 15.5) and that reduction was uniform for all sizes of cell. Clearly, comparison between groups is meaningless if the size of neurones is not taken into account.

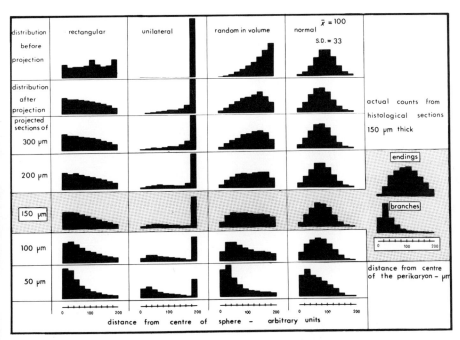

Figure 15.3. The effect of projection and sectioning on various frequency distributions. The histograms on the right are transformations of the curves for branches and endings from figure 15.1c. The distributions in the shaded area are obtained after projection of 150 μm sections (often 100 μm sections are also analysed). It can be seen that distortion of the actual distribution becomes greater as the section thickness decreases, in most cases tending towards a mirror image of the original. The projected distribution of the histological sections of 150 μm, on the right of the diagram, best approximate to the distortion of a projected normal distribution at this section thickness. The curve for branches shows marked skewness.

Cell size is also related to the number of primary dendrites arising from the perikaryon and to the total number of branches making up the dendritic field. These two parameters together with the length of dendrites determine the dendritic density. The relationship between branches and dendrites can be derived graphically from the slope of the plot of branches v. dendrites and is called the

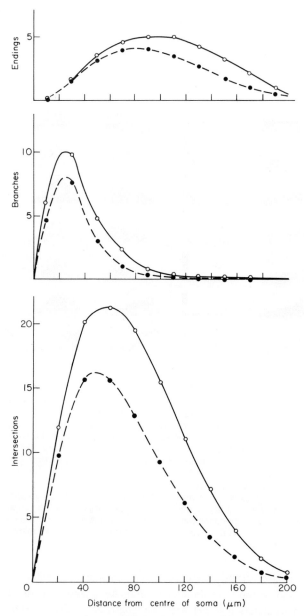

Figure 15.4. Endings, branches and intersections, at increasing distances from the cell body, as estimated by the Eayrs' (1955) technique. Note the overall reduction in the treated (--●--) group. This reduction may be real or apparent. If cell size is directly related to dendritic density then an apparent reduction may occur when small, but normal (—○—), cells are sampled in one group and normal large cells are analysed in the other group (see text and Figure 15.5).

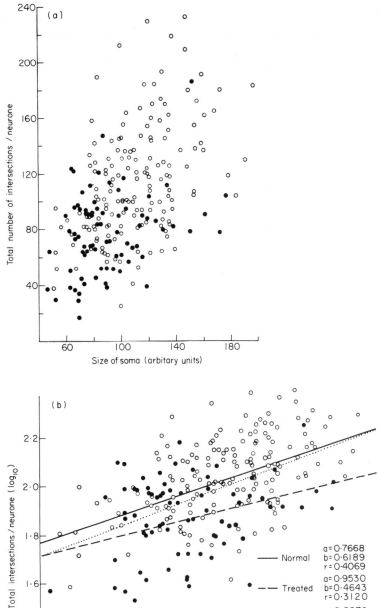

Figure 15.5. (a), Intersections against cell size (○—normal, ●—treated). (b), Intersections against cell size (logged data). All differences between normal and treated were significant ($P < 0.001$) and lines were estimated to be parallel ($P < 0.01$) (except the combined line which was calculated for the purposes of statistical testing by analysis of variance).

branching index (Figure 15.6). The branching index decreases as the number of primary dendrites increases tending to approach a factor of 2 asymptotically. This, however, is also a projection artefact and the mechanism of its production is illustrated in Figure 15.6. The quadrants labelled A are much larger than the quadrants labelled B (Figure 15.6), but dendrites will grow equally into both

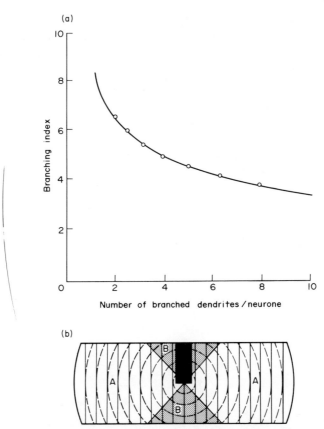

Figure 15.6. Branching index (calculated from the plot of branches v. dendrites) against number of dendrites. The observation that the branching index decreases as the number of dendrites increases is thought to be an artefact. Diagram (b), which illustrates how the branching index may vary when dendrites grow into areas A and B, may explain the production of this artefact (see text for further explanation). The dark rectangular area in the upper sector marked B is the cell body shadow (see text for full explanation). (The diagram represents a section (150 μm) through a sphere at right angles to the plane in figure 15.1. The cell body is exactly central and dendrites have equal opportunity to grow into areas A and B.)

areas. All cells may be vetted before drawing so that a reasonably uniform state of impregnation obtains for all cells sampled. If dendrites grow into the areas labelled A they appear long and many branches will be seen, but dendrites growing into areas B appear fore-shortened and few branches are seen. In assessing the state of impregnation it can be understood that cells with a small number of dendrites will only be accepted if dendrites grow into areas A, and that neurones with many dendrites will never be rejected since the numbers growing into areas A will always be sufficient for acceptance. Thus, the branching index (total branches/total dendrites per neurone) will tend to increase as the number of dendrites decreases and 'poor impregnation' may, in fact, mean inappropriate orientation of dendrites with respect to quadrants A and B, rather than a modification in the uptake of the stain. The dark region in the upper part of quadrant B (Figure 15.6) represents the shadow, formed by the cell body, within and behind which no dendrites can be seen. This will give added losses, particularly in neurones with many dendrites.

Thus, the method of Sholl and the modification of Eayrs give broad generalisations about the density of the dendritic tree which may be useful for detecting differences between groups but only if, *pari passu*, cell size is taken into account. The methods do not give any absolute information about the dendritic tree because sectioning and projection errors are too gross. Density is the product of dendritic length and branching. Absolute dendritic length may be estimated by correcting for the third dimension (although error due to section thickness is inevitable) but quantitation of dendritic branching requires a different methodology.

Conclusions

It is clear from the above account that functional activity modifies both the morphology of neurones and the synaptic geometry of their interconnections. Glial cells also appear to participate. If morphological changes are to play any part in learning and memory then the time constant of these structural rearrangements must be compatible with the consolidation time of the engram. Little attention has been directed to assessing the latency of morphological change, but Cragg (1969a) has shown that changes in retinal synapses following first exposure to light occur within three minutes while changes after placing in darkness occur after an interval of twenty-four hours (de Robertis, 1958). The factors to be considered in assessing the time constants are the site of manufacture of the proteins, lipids, etc., the distance between this site of synthesis and the site of structural change, and the speed at which metabolites can reach this site and be incorporated into new membranes, etc. The site of manufacture of proteins is within the perikaryon and involves the DNA → RNA → protein pathway. In a recent N.R.P.B. on the function of macromolecules in synaptic function (Bloom, Iversen and Schmitt,

1970), the concensus of opinion held that the macromolecules incorporated into synaptic membranes or being released with the mediator into the synaptic cleft, were produced in the cell body and travelled to the ending in the fast axonal flow stream.

Altman (1967) has suggested that internuncial microneurones are likely to be the most plastic elements, in the CNS of young animals, by virtue of their post-natal development and slow differentiation. Transport is completed sooner in a short rather than a long axon and the involvement of short-axoned internuncial neurones has been implicated in both the effects of deafferentation and theories of memory.

Changes also occur in dendrites although our results may indicate that these changes need reappraisal in the light of the errors inherent in the current methods of analysis. The recent demonstrations that dendrites and soma form, on the one hand, dendro-axonal, dendro-dendritic and dendro-somatic synapses suggests that dendritic activity need not necessarily invade the soma to be effective since axodendritic depolarisation could release mediator locally via a dendritic synapse (Ralston, 1971). Similarly, juxtaposed hyperpolarising axodendritic synapses could insulate this local activity from the soma by short-circuiting. In general, dendrites are shorter than axons (although there are obvious exceptions) and thus changes in dendritic structure could not only occur quickly but also alter markedly local connectivity which in turn would cause a re-routing of excitation with quite profound effects.

It has been pointed out that, during learning, RNA molecules with exceptional base ratios are produced and S-100 brain-specific proteins appear in the cytoplasm. Both the postsynaptic and presynaptic membranes and the synaptic vesicles contain highly specific proteins and all may exhibit structural differences which are correlated with function (Uchizono, 1965). Receptor sites can also determine the polarity of the postsynaptic membrane (in inhibitory collaterals, for example) and it is possible that specific proteins released from presynaptic vesicles may participate in attaching mediator to receptor site. The role of brain-specific mucoids in learning and memory has been discussed by Bogoch (1968).

The idea that glial cells may be active in resiting synapses or in converting potential synapses to functional ones is interesting. Professor Hydén has continually reminded us of the biochemical interrelationships between glia and neurones and has emphasised that these two cell types must be viewed as acting in concert. The theory of Roitbach (1970) concerning the conversion of potential synapses to functional synapses is of interest although it does not appear to be flexible enough to explain extinction.

The anatomy of the CNS of the young animal appears to be more susceptible to environmental manipulation than does that of the adult. This may be explained by postulating that afferent input is necessary for normal growth. Hubel and Wiesel (1963) and Wiesel and Hubel (1963) obtained neurophysiological evidence that the visual cortex of the cat was functionally quite mature at or near birth before the eyes had opened but became distorted with prolonged deprivation of visual experience. It was suggested that all connections are present at birth but become defective with disuse. However, the new electron microscope findings of Bloom and Aghajanian (cited by Akert, Gray and Bloom, 1970) indicate that afferent activity is a prerequisite for normal development. They used the EPTA method to differentiate between immature and mature synapses and found a 30–40 per cent increase of immature junctions in the cortex of dark-reared animals. It could be argued that the lack of convergence of afferent input into 'neurone-neuroglia modules' (Roitbach, 1970) prevented potential (immature) synapses from being converted into functional (mature) forms.

In this article there has been little reference to the neurophysiological evidence for changes in synaptic function during learning and memory or to the role of sleep in consolidation. These factors are obviously very pertinent to this discussion but have been omitted because of time. In conclusion it can be stated that biochemical, structural and physiological changes are correlated with changes in function and that there is experimental evidence supporting the hypothesis that biochemical events, often of a very specific nature, are involved in structural and physiological changes which may in turn be associated with storage and recall of the engram.

We greatly appreciate the stimulating interest and support given to us by Professor J. T. Eayrs and we thank Mrs S. Buckley for her excellent technical assistance.

References

AKERT, K., GRAY, E. G. and BLOOM, F. E. (1970). Synaptic ultrastructure. B. Physiological significance of specialized synaptic function. Changes in synaptic structure during development and degeneration. In: *Neurosciences Research Bulletin*, 8, No. 4, Chap. II, pp. 347–8.
ALTMAN, J. (1967). Postulated growth and differentiation of the mammalian brain, with implications for a morphological theory of memory. In: *The Neurosciences. A Study Program* (QUARTON, J. C., MELNECHUK, T. and SCHMITT, F. O., Eds.). Rockefeller University Press, New York.
BENNETT, E. L., DIAMOND, M. C., KRECH, D. and ROSENZWEIG, M. R. (1964). Chemical and anatomical plasticity of brain. *Science, N.Y.*, 146, 610–19.
BERNSTEIN, J. J. and BERNSTEIN, M. E. (1971). Axonal regeneration and formation of synapses proximal to the site of lesion following hemisection of the rat spinal cord. *Expl Neurol.*, 30, 336–51.
BIRKS, R., HUXLEY, H. E. and KATZ, B. (1960). The fine structure of the neuromuscular junction of the frog. *J. Physiol.*, 150, 134–44.

BIRKS, R., KATZ, B. and MILEDI, R. (1960). Physiological and structural changes at the amphibian myoneural junction, in the course of nerve degeneration. *J. Physiol.*, **150**, 145–68.

BLINZINGER, K. and KREUTZBERG, G. (1968). Displacement of synaptic terminals from regenerating motorneurones by microglial cells. *Z. Zellforsch. mikrosk. Anat.*, **85**, 145–57.

BLOOM, F. E., IVERSEN, L. L. and SCHMITT, F. O. (1970). Macromolecules in a synaptic function. A report on a NRP work session. *Neurosciences Research Bulletin*, **8**, No. 4.

BOGOCH, S. (1968). *The Biochemistry of Memory.* Oxford University Press, London.

BRATTGÅRD, S-O, EDSTRÖM, J. E. and HYDÉN, H. (1958). Productive capacity of the neuron in retrograde reaction. *Expl Cell Res.*, Suppl. **5**, 185–200.

BRODAL, A. (1940). Modification of Gudden method for study of cerebral localization. *Archs Neurol. Psychiat.*, Chicago, **43**, 46–58.

CHOW, K. L., RIESEN, A. H. and NEWELL, F. W. (1957). Degeneration of retinal ganglion cells in infant chimpanzees in darkness. *J. comp. Neurol.*, **107**, 27–42.

COLEMAN, P. D. and RIESEN, A. H. (1968). Environmental effects on cortical dendritic fields. I. Rearing in the dark. *J. Anat.*, **102**, 363–74.

COLONNIER, M. (1968). Synaptic patterns on different cell types on the different laminae of the cat visual cortex. An electron microscope study. *Brain Res.*, **9**, 268–87.

CRAGG, B. G. (1969a). Structural changes in naïve retinal synapses detectable within minutes of first exposure to daylight. *Brain Res.*, **15**, 79–96.

CRAGG, B. G. (1969b). The effects of vision and darkrearing on the size and the density of synapses in the lateral geniculate nucleus measured by electron microscopy. *Brain Res.*, **13**, 53–67.

CRAGG, B. G. (1970). What is the stimulus for chromatolysis? *Brain Res.*, **23**, 1–21.

DE ROBERTIS, E. (1958). Submicroscopic morphology and function of synapse. *Expl Cell Res.*, Suppl. **5**, 347–69.

DE ROBERTIS, E. and FRANCHI, C. M. (1956). Electron microscope observations on synaptic vesicles in synapses of the retinal rods and cones. *J. biophys. biochem. Cytol.*, **2**, 307–18.

DIAMOND, M. C., KRECH, D. and ROSENZWEIG, M. R. (1964). The effects of enriched environment on the histology of the rat cerebral cortex. *J. comp. Neurol.*, **123**, 111–20.

EAYRS, J. T. (1955). The cerebral cortex of normal and hypothyroid rats. *Acta anat.*, **25**, 160–83.

EDSTRÖM, J.-E. (1957). Effects of increased motor activity on the dimensions and staining properties of the neuron soma. *J. comp. Neurol.*, **107**, 295–304.

FIFKOVÁ, E. (1967). The influence of unilateral visual deprivation on optic centres. *Brain Res.*, **6**, 763–6.

FIFKOVÁ, E. (1968). Changes in the visual cortex of rats after unilateral deprivation. *Nature, Lond.*, **220**, 379–81.

FIFKOVÁ, E. (1970a). The effects of monocular deprivation on the synaptic contacts of the visual cortex. *J. Neurobiol.*, **1**, 285–94.

FIFKOVÁ, E. (1970b). The effect of unilateral deprivation on visual centers in rats. *J. comp. Neurol.*, **140**, 431–8.

FIFKOVÁ, E. and HASSLER, R. (1969). Quantitative morphological changes in visual centers in rats after unilateral deprivation. *J. comp. Neurol.*, **135**, 167–78.

GALAMBOS, R. (1965). Introductory discussion on glial function. *Progr. Brain Res.*, **15**, 267–77.

GEINSMANN, Y. Y., LARIMA, V. N. and MATS, U. N. (1971). Changes in neuron dimensions as a possible morphological correlate of their increased functional activity. *Brain Res.*, **26**, 247–57.

GELFAN, S. and RAPISARDA, A. F. (1964). Synaptic density on spinal neurons of normal dogs and dogs with experimental hind-limb rigidity. *J. comp. Neurol.*, **123**, 73–96.

GELFAN, S. and TARLOV, I. M. (1963). Altered neuron population in L7 segment of dogs with experimental hind-limb rigidity. *Am. J. Physiol.*, **205**, 606–16.

GLOBUS, A. and SCHEIBEL, A. B. (1966). Loss of dendrite spines as an index of presynaptic terminal patterns. *Nature, Lond.*, **212**, 463–5.

GLOBUS, A. and SCHEIBEL, A. B. (1967a). The effect of visual deprivation on cortical neurons. A Golgi-study. *Expl Neurol.*, **19**, 331–45.

GLOBUS, A. and SCHEIBEL, A. B. (1967b). Effects of visual deprivation on neurons of the visual cortex. *Anat. Rec.*, **157**, 248.

GLOBUS, A. and SCHEIBEL, A. B. (1967c). Synaptic loci on visual cortical neurons of the rabbit: the specific afferent radiation. *Expl Neurol.*, **18**, 116–31.

GONATAS, N. K. (1967). Axonic and synaptic lesions in neuropsychiatric disorders. *Nature, Lond.*, **214**, 352–5.

GRANT, G. and WESTMAN, J. (1968). Degenerative changes in dendrites central to axonal transection. Electron microscopical observations. *Experientia*, **24**, 169–70.

GUTH, L. and BERNSTEIN, J. J. (1961). Selectivity in the re-establishment of synapses in the superior cervical sympathetic ganglion of the cat. *Expl Neurol.*, **4**, 59–69.

GYLLENSTEN, L. (1959). Postnatal development of the visual cortex in darkness (mice). *Acta morph. neerl.-scand.*, **2**, 331–45.

GYLLENSTEN, L. and MALFORS, T. (1963). Myelinization of the optic nerve and its dependence on visual function. A quantitative investigation in mice. *J. Embryol. exp. Morph.*, **11**, 255–66.

GYLLENSTEN, L., MALFORS, T. and NORRLIN-GRETTOE, M.-L. (1965). Effect of visual deprivation in optic centres of growing and adult mice. *J. comp. Neurol.*, **124**, 149–60.

GYLLENSTEN, L., MALFORS, T. and NORRLIN-GRETTOE, M.-L. (1966). Growth alterations in the auditory cortex of visually deprived mice. *J. comp. Neurol.*, **126**, 463–70.

GYLLENSTEN, L., MALFORS, T., and NORRLIN-GRETTOE, M.-L. (1967). Visual and non-visual factors in the centripetal stimulation of postnatal growth of visual centres in mice. *J. comp. Neurol.*, **131**, 549–58.

HAMBERGER, A., HANSSON, H.-A. and SJÖSTRAND, J. (1970). Surface structure of isolated neurons. Detachment of nerve terminals during axon regeneration. *J. Cell. Biol.*, **47**, 319–31.

HERMAN, C. J. and LAPHAM, L. W. (1968). DNA content of neurons in the cat hippocampus. *Science, N.Y.*, **160**, 537.

HERMAN, C. J. and LAPHAM, L. W. (1969). Neuronal polyploidy and nuclear volume in the cat central nervous system. *Brain Res.*, **15**, 35–48.

HESS, A. (1958). Optic centres and pathways after eye removal in fetal guinea pigs. *J. comp. Neurol.* **109**, 91–116.

HOLLOWAY, JR. R. L. (1966). Dendritic branching; some preliminary results of training and complexity in rat visual cortex. *Brain Res.*, **2**, 393–6.

HUBEL, D. H. and WIESEL, T. N. (1963). Receptive fields of cells in striate cortex of very young, visually inexperienced kittens. *J. Neurophysiol.*, **26**, 994–1002.

HYDÉN, H. (1943). Protein metabolism in the nerve cell during growth and function. *Acta. physiol. scand.*, Suppl. 17, **6**, 1–136.

HYDÉN, H. (1960). The neuron. In: *The Cell* (BRACHET, J. and LURSKY, A. E., Eds.), Vol. IV, pp. 215–323. Academic Press. New York.

HYDÉN, H. (1964). RNA—a functional characteristic of the neuron and its glia. In: *Brain Function*. Vol. II. RNA and Brain Function, Memory and Learning. (BRAZIER, M. A. B., Ed.), pp. 29–68. University of California Press, Berkeley.

ILLIS, L. (1963). Changes in spinal cord synapses and a possible explanation for spinal shock. *Expl Neurol.*, **8**, 328–35.

ILLIS, L. (1964). Spinal cord synapses in the cat, the reaction of the bouton termineaux at the motorneurone synapses to experimental denervation. *Brain*, **87**, 555–72.

JONES, W. H. and THOMAS, D. B. (1962). Changes in the dendritic organisation of neurons in the cerebral cortex following deafferentation. *J. Anat.* **96**, 375–81.

KOELLE, G. B. (1962). A new general concept of the neurohumoral functions of acetylcholine and acetylcholinesterase. *J. Pharm. Pharmac.*, **14**, 65–90.

KRECH, D., ROSENZWEIG, M. R. and BENNETT, E. L. (1963). Effects of complex environments and blindness on rat brain. *Archs Neurol.*, **8**, 403–12.

KREUTZBERG, G. W. (1968). DNA metabolism in glia cells during retrograde changes. In: *Macromolecules and the Function of the Neuron* (LODIN, Z. and ROSE, S. P. R., Eds.). Excerpta Medica Foundation, Amsterdam.

KRUGER, L. (1965). Morphological alterations of the cerebral cortex and their possible role in the loss and acquisition of information. In: *The Anatomy of*

Memory. Proceedings 1st Conference on learning, remembering and forgetting. Science and Behaviour Books, Inc.

KUPFER, C. and PALMER, P. (1964). Lateral geniculate nucleus; histological and cytochemical changes following afferent denervation and visual deprivation. *Expl Neurol.*, **9**, 400–9.

LE VAY, S. (1971). On the neurons and synapses of the lateral geniculate nucleus of the monkey, and the effects of eye enucleation. *Z. Zellforsch. mikrosk. Anat.*, **113**, 396–419.

LIU, C.-N. and CHAMBERS, W. W. (1958). Intraspinal sprouting of dorsal root axons. *Archs Neurol. Psychiat., Chicago*, **79**, 46–61.

MARIN-PADILLA, M. (1968). Cortical axo-spinodendritic synapses in man. A Golgi study. *Brain Res.*, **8**, 196–200.

MARTINEZ, A. J. and FRIEDE, B. L. (1970). Changes in nerve cell bodies during the myelination of their axons. *J. comp. Neurol.*, **138**, 329–38.

MCCOUGH, G. P., AUSTIN, G. M. and LIU, C. Y. (1955). Sprouting of new terminals as a cause of spasticity. *Am. J. Physiol.*, **183**, 642–3.

MOUNTFORD, S. (1963). Effects of light and dark adaption on vesicle population of receptor-bipolar synapses. *J. Ultrastruct. Res.*, **9**, 403–18.

MOUREN-MATHIEU, A.-M. and COLONNIER, M. (1969). The molecular layer of the adult cat cerebellar cortex after lesions of the parallel fibres: An optic and electron microscope study. *Brain Res.*, **16**, 307–23.

PINCHING, A. J. and POWELL, T. P. S. (1971). Ultrastructural features of transneuronal cell degeneration in the olfactory system. *J. Cell. Sci.*, **8**, 253–87.

POMERAT, C. M. (1958). In: *Biology of Neuroglia* (WINDLE, W. F. and THOMAS, C. C., Eds.), p. 162. Springfield, Illinois.

RAISMAN, G. (1969a). A comparison of the mode of termination of the hippocampal and hypothalamic afferents to the septal nuclei as revealed by the electron microscopy of degeneration. *Expl Brain Res.*, **7**, 317–43.

RAISMAN, G. (1969b). Neuronal plasticity in the septal nuclei of the adult rat. *Brain Res.*, **14**, 25–48.

RALSTON, H. J. (1971). III. Evidence for presynaptic dendrites and a proposal for their mechanism of action. *Nature, Lond.*, **230**, 585–7.

RASCH, E., RIESEN, A. H. and CHOW, K. L. (1959). Altered structure and composition of retinal cells in dark reared cats. *J. Histochem. Cytochem.*, **7**, 321–2.

RATHER, L. J. (1958). The significance of nuclear size in physiological and pathological processes. *Ergebn. allg. Pathol. path. Anat.*, **38**, 127–99.

ROITBACH, A. I. (1970). A new hypothesis concerning the mechanism of function of the conditioned reflex. *Acta neurobiol. Exp.*, **30**, 81–94.

ROSE, J. E., MALIS, L. I., KRUGER, L. and BAKER, C. P. (1960). Effects of heavy ionizing monoenergetic particles on the cerebral cortex. II. Histological appearance of laminar lesions and growth of nerve fibres after laminar destructions. *J. comp. Neurol.*, **115**, 243–55.

ROSENZWEIG, M. R., BENNETT, E. L., DIAMOND, M. C., SU-YU, W. W., SLAGLE, R. W. and SAFFRAN, E. (1969). Influences of environmental complexity and visual stimulation on development of occipital cortex in the rat. *Brain Res.*, **14**, 427–45.

ROSENZWEIG, M. R., KRECH, D., BENNETT, E. L. and DIAMOND, M. C. (1962). Effects of environmental complexity and training on brain chemistry and anatomy: a replication and extension. *J. comp. physiol. Psychol.*, **55**, 529–37.

ROSENZWEIG, M. R., LOVE, W. and BENNETT, E. L. (1968). Effects of a few hours a day of enriched experience on brain chemistry and brain weights. *Physiol. Behav.*, **3**, 819–25.

RUIZ-MARCOS, A., and VALVERDE, F. (1969). The temporal evolution of the distribution of dendritic spines in the visual cortex of normal and dark raised mice. *Expl Brain Res.*, **8**, 284–94.

SHAPIRO, S. and VUKOVICH, K. R. (1970). Early experience effects upon cortical dendrites; a proposed model for development. *Science, N.Y.*, **167**, 292–4.

SHOLL, D. A. (1953). Dendritic organization in the neurons of the visual and motor cortices of the cat. *J. Anat.*, **87**, 387–406.

SNIDER, R. S. and PEREZ DEL CERRO, M. (1967). Drug-induced dendritic sprouts on Purkinje cells in the adult cerebellum. *Expl Neurol.*, **17**, 466–80.

SZENTÀGOTHAI, J. and RAJKOVITS, K. (1955). Die Ruchwirking der spezifischen Funktion auf die Struktur der Nervenelamente. *Acta morph. hung.*, **5**, 253–74.

TSANG, Y.-C. (1937). Visual centres in blinded rats. *J. comp. Neurol.*, **66**, 211–61.

UCHIZONO, K. (1965). Characteristics of excitatory and inhibitory synapses in the central nervous system of the cat. *Nature, Lond.*, **207**, 642–3.

VALVERDE, F. (1967). Apical dendritic spines of the visual cortex and light deprivation in the mouse. *Expl Brain Res.*, **3**, 337–52.

VALVERDE, F. (1968). Structural changes in the area striata of the mouse after enucleation. *Expl Brain Res.*, **5**, 274–92.

VALVERDE, F. (1970). The Golgi method. A tool for comparative structural analysis. In: *Contemporary Research Methods in Neuroanatomy* (NAUTER, W. J. H. and EBBESSON, S. O. E., Eds.). Elsevier, Amsterdam.

VALVERDE, F. and ESTÉBAN, M. E. (1968). Peristriate cortex of mouse: location and effects of enucleation on the number of dendritic spines. *Brain Res.*, **9**, 145–8.

VALVERDE, F. and RUIZ-MARCOS, A. (1969). Dendritic spines in the visual cortex of the mouse: Introduction to a mathematical model. *Expl Brain Res.*, **8**, 269–83.

WEISKRANTZ, L. (1958). Sensory deprivation and the cat's optic nervous system. *Nature, Lond.*, **181**, 1047–50.

WESTRUM, L. E., WHITE, L. E. and WARD, A. A. (1964). Morphology of the experimental epileptic focus. *J. Neurosurg.*, **21**, 1033–44.

WIESEL, T. N. and HUBEL, D. H. (1963). Effects of visual deprivation on morphology and physiology of cells in the cat's lateral geniculate body. *J. Neurophysiol.*, **26**, 978–93.

Learning in the lower animals

G. A. KERKUT, P. EMSON and R. J. WALKER

Department of Physiology and Biochemistry, University of Southampton, Southampton SO9 5NH, England

In 1964 a meeting was held in Cambridge to discuss the phenomenon of learning in the lower animals (Thorpe and Davenport, 1964). The accent then was mainly on the behavioural aspects of learning but since that time there has been a gradual swing towards a more neurochemical approach to the investigation of learning

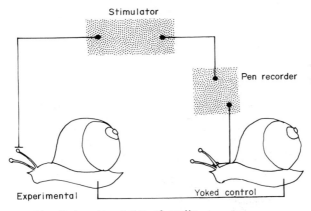

Circuit for stimulation of snails

Figure 16.1. Training circuit devised to condition snails to shock-avoidance paradigm. When the experimental animal completes the circuit it is able to associate tentacle position with shock. The yoked control animal is randomly shocked whenever the experimental animal receives a shock.

(Hydén, 1960, 1964; Flexner and Stellar, 1963; Barondes and Cohen, 1966; Deutsch, 1969; Agranoff and Klinger, 1964; Glassman, 1967, 1969; Bogoch, 1968; Lodin and Rose 1968; Peterson and Kernell, 1970; Ádám, 1970). In this symposium (1973) Dr Oliver has already discussed the study of learning in the insect *Periplaneta americana*. Today we shall describe a study on the behaviour of the

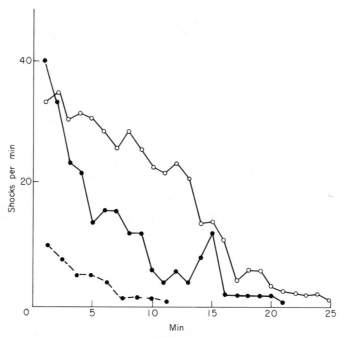

Figure 16.2. Learning curve. The response of snails to electrical stimulation. The graph shows the number of shocks received by the experimental animal (●—●) and the number of shocks received by the yoked control (○—○) and the experimental animals on retest (● - - - ●). The experimental animals learn not to extend the tentacle. The yoked control, although it receives the same number of shocks as the experimental animal, does not learn to associate shock with extension of the tentacle.

snail *Helix aspersa* and the way in which a simple yoked-control avoidance-conditioning arrangement allows us to determine which biochemical parameters to study in the nervous system associated with these behavioural changes.

An account of this work, giving full experimental details, has been published (Emson, Walker and Kerkut, 1971; Kerkut, Oliver, Rick and Walker, 1970). The experimental arrangement is shown diagrammatically in Figure 16.1. Two snails were restrained by elastic bands on a piece of wax. When the experimental snail put out its tentacle, it received a shock and retracted the tentacle. It learned in time not to put its tentacle out. The second animal, the yoked control, received a shock every time the first animal got a shock. The difference here was that the yoked control shock was independent of the position of the tentacle. The number of shocks that the animal received was recorded on a pen recorder. Thus, both animals received the same number of shocks but only the experimental snail was able to associate the shock with the position of the tentacle and to learn.

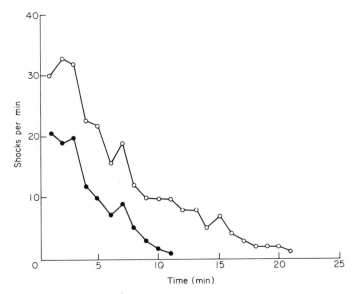

Figure 16.3. The learning curve of an animal injected with 150 μg amphetamine (●—●), compared with that of an animal injected with saline (○—○). The drugs and saline were injected one hour before training. The amphetamine-injected animal learned more quickly than did the saline-injected animal.

Figure 16.2 shows a typical learning curve of this preparation. The black circles show the curve of the experimental animal after its first testing. Initially it received about forty shocks per minute, but as time went on it received fewer and fewer shocks so that after twenty-one minutes it was receiving no shocks. If the animal was put on to retest, it initially received ten shocks per minute but by ten minutes it was receiving no shocks. When the yoked control was put on retest the animal received about thirty-eight shocks per minute and this slowly fell to zero shocks by twenty-five minutes. Thus, though the yoked control received the same number of shocks as the experimental animal, when the yoked control was put onto retest it was shown not to have learnt to retract its tentacle. Both animals had received the same number of shocks but the experimental animal had learnt and the yoked control had not.

Effect of drug injection

An experimental animal injected with saline before testing learned to retract its tentacle after about twenty-one minutes (Figure 16.3), whereas a similar animal injected with 150 µg of amphetamine one hour before testing learnt within only twelve minutes. Figure 16.4 shows a dose–response relationship between the amount of drug injected, in this case amphetamine or magnesium pemoline, and the time required for the animal to reach learning criterion. Initially, the animal

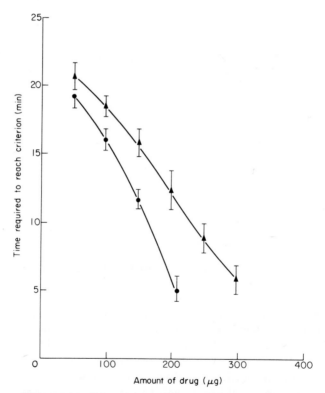

Figure 16.4. Dose–response curves for two drugs that facilitate learning. The saline-injected animal took about twenty-two minutes to learn. Amphetamine (●—●) and magnesium pemoline (▲—▲) enabled the animals to learn more rapidly. The effect depended on the dose of the drug injected.

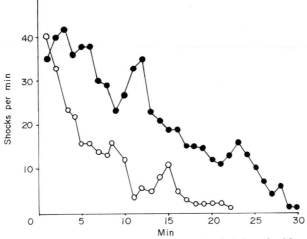

Figure 16.5. The learning curves of animals injected with either 300 μg cycloheximide (●—●) or saline (○—○) one hour before testing. The animals injected with cycloheximide took longer to learn.

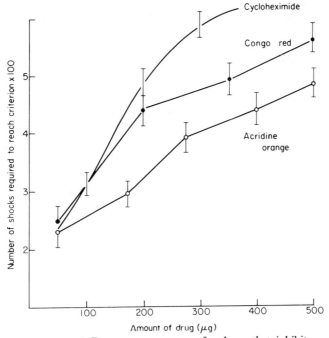

Figure 16.6. Dose–response curves for drugs that inhibit learning in the snail. The drugs shown here all increased the number of shocks required by the snail to reach learning criterion. The drugs were injected one hour before testing. Controls injected with Ringer's solution required a mean of 200 shocks to reach learning criterion.

took about twenty minutes to learn, but with the injection of increasing amounts of amphetamine the animal learned more and more quickly so that when 200 μg amphetamine was injected it learned in five minutes. Similarly, magnesium pemoline increased the speed with which the animal learned. Animals injected with 300 μg cycloheximide one hour before they were tested learned more slowly than animals injected with saline (Figure 16.5). Cycloheximide-injected animals required thirty minutes to learn whereas the saline-injected animals required twenty-two minutes. Figure 16.6 shows a dose–response relationship between the amount of drug injected and the number of shocks required for the animal to reach learning criterion. The drugs and dyes cycloheximide, congo red and acridine orange all inhibited learning and made the animals require more shocks before they could learn.

These enhancers or inhibitors of learning gave some indication of the probable biochemical stages for investigation. The amphetamines could be related to the metabolism of catecholamines in the nervous system. Magnesium pemoline could affect the nucleic acids. Cycloheximide inhibited protein synthesis and congo red and acridine orange had an effect upon the RNA polymerase and on enzymatic systems. The next stage, then, is to investigate some of the biochemical parameters that differ between the experimental and the control animal.

Incorporation of labelled uridine or labelled leucine

The differences between incorporation of labelled uridine or labelled leucine into the experimental or control animals can be studied by means of a double-labelling technique (Figure 16.7). One animal was injected with [^{14}C]uridine, the other with tritiated uridine, one being treated as the experimental animal and the other as the control. The ganglia were removed, the RNA was extracted and the tritium/carbon ratio was counted. Full details of the technique are described by Emson *et al.* (1971). Similarly, it is possible to study the incorporation of labelled leucine into proteins by a double-labelling method using ^{14}C or tritiated leucine. The results of a typical experiment can be seen in Table 16.1. The incorporation of labelled tritiated uridine into the brain RNA of experimental, yoked control and quiet control animals was such that the experimental animals had a higher incorporation (387 counts/μg RNA) than the yoked control which had received shocks but which had not learnt (343 counts) or the quiet control which had been restrained but given no shocks (295 counts). There was a greater incorporation of uridine into the RNA of the brain of experimental animals than into that of the yoked control or the quiet animals. The differences were significant at the $P = 0.01$ level.

The increased RNA production in the experimental animal was investigated using a sucrose density gradient. Figure 16.8 shows the density separation of the

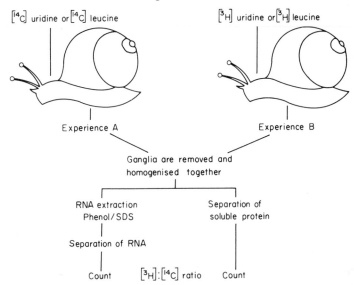

Figure 16.7. An outline of the double-labelling technique used in incorporation studies of RNA and protein during training.

RNA of experimental and control animals. The experimental animals had been injected with tritiated uridine whereas the control had been injected with [^{14}C]-uridine. The dashed line indicates the sucrose density gradient in the tubes, the continuous line the optical density of the RNA read at 280 nm and the line with circles the tritium/carbon ratio. Any values greater than 1 represent an increased incorporation into the RNA of the experimental animal. There was a considerable

Table 16.1

The incorporation of ^{3}H-labelled uridine into RNA of the snail brain in experimental, yoked control and quiet control animals.

	Counts per μg RNA	n	% increase relative to quiet control	$P^\star$
Quiet control	295 ± 10	8	0·00	
Yoked control	343 ± 9	8	14·00	0·01
Experimental	387 ± 12	8	26·40	0·01

$\star$ P is the probability of these increases not differing from a population mean of 0%. P was computed using Student's t test. Values are means plus or minus standard errors, n: the number of animals in each group.

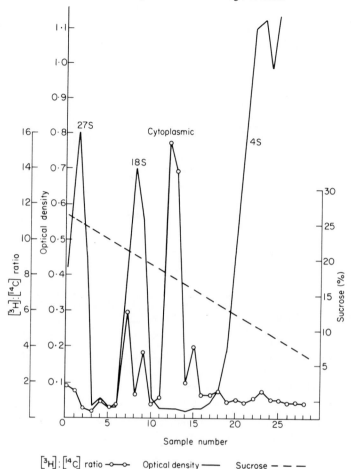

Figure 16.8. Sucrose gradient analysis of the incorporation of uridine into RNA during the training of snails. Control animals were injected with [^{14}C]uridine, experimental animals with [^{3}H]uridine. Note the peaks in the [^{3}H]:[^{14}C] ratio associated with the increased RNA synthesis.

increase in the incorporation of uridine into the 18S and the cytoplasmic fractions of the RNA of the experimental ganglia.

Autoradiography was used to identify the nerve cells with the greater incorporation of this labelled uridine. These were found in the cerebral ganglion and in the pedal and sub-oesophageal ganglia. We also used a new technique for quantifying and locating the incorporation of uridine in the brain. After incubating animals

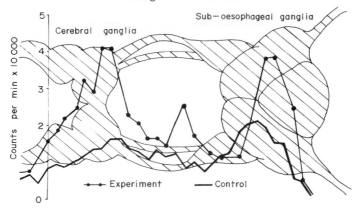

Figure 16.9. Incorporation of leucine into the snail brain. Animals were treated as control or experimental animals following the injection of labelled leucine. The brain was removed and sections were cut to determine the degree of incorporation into the different parts of the brain. The brain of the experimental animal had a higher incorporation of labelled leucine into the cerebral and sub-oesophageal ganglia than did the control animal.

with labelled uridine, they were trained or treated as controls and their brains were removed, fixed and embedded in wax. Sections were cut and the activity in each was counted. A diagrammatic representation is shown in Figure 16.9 where the lower continuous line shows the counts per minute in the sections from the control brain and the upper line with dots indicates the counts per minute of the experimental brain. Again, there was considerably greater incorporation in the experimental brain in the cerebral ganglia and in the regions of the sub-oesophageal ganglia.

Table 16.2

The incorporation of ^{3}H-labelled leucine into protein of the snail brain in experimental and yoked control animals.

	Counts per μg protein	n	% increase relative to quiet control	$P\star$
Quiet control	37·6 ± 2·0	8	0·00	
Yoked control	43·28 ± 5·0	8	11·9	0·05
Experimental	57·21 ± 4·3	8	34·33	0·01

* P is the probability of these increases not differing from a population mean of 0%. P was computed using Student's t test. Values are means plus or minus standard errors, n: the number of animals in each group.

Incorporation of tritiated leucine into the proteins of snail brain is summarised in Table 16.2. The incorporation was greater in the brain of the experimental animal (57·21 counts/μg protein) than in that of the yoked control (43·28) or the quiet control (37·6). Thus, in the experimental animal incorporation was 34 per cent greater than in the quiet control.

When the proteins from the snail brain were extracted and run on polyacrylamide gel, they appeared as several bands. Coupling this experiment with incorporation of labelled leucine we found that certain bands of the experimental

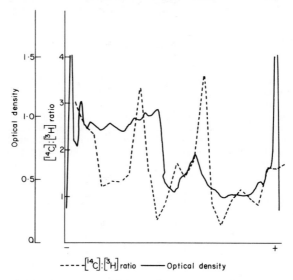

Figure 16.10. Disc gel electrophoresis analysis of leucine incorporation into proteins during the training of snails. Controls were injected with [^{3}H]leucine, experimental animals with [^{14}C]leucine. Note the peaks in the [^{14}C]:[^{3}H] ratio associated with particular protein fractions synthesised by the experimental animals.

animal protein contained more labelled leucine than corresponding bands of the control. Figure 16.10 shows such an analysis, the continuous line representing the optical density of the bands of protein and the dotted line representing the increased incorporation of [^{14}C]leucine into the brains of experimental animals. There were three distinct bands of protein that had a greater incorporation of labelled leucine in the experimental animal than into the control. This indicates that the experimental animal was synthesising some proteins at a faster rate than the control.

We studied the effect of drugs on the increase in the rate of protein synthesis in the experimental animal (Figure 16.11). In the normal experimental animal injected with saline only the rate was 36 per cent greater than in the resting animal. Animals that had been injected with congo red, actinomycin D or cycloheximide at the doses indicated in the figure showed decreased rates of learning and also a considerable decrease in the rate of protein synthesis when compared with the experimental animal. An animal injected with amphetamine, however, did not have an increased rate of protein synthesis. This suggests that the effect of congo red, actinomycin D or cycloheximide might be related to their inhibitory effects on protein synthesis.

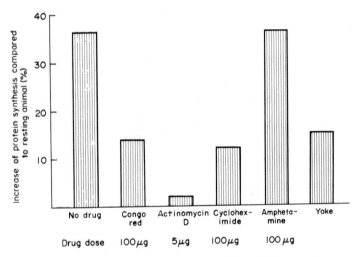

Figure 16.11. The effect of drug injection on the increased incorporation of labelled leucine into protein during training. The drugs and isotopes were injected one hour before training. The drugs that inhibit learning such as congo red, actinomycin D, and cycloheximide all prevented the increased incorporation of labelled leucine into the brain of the experimental animal. Drugs that facilitate learning such as amphetamine did not increase the degree of incorporation above that of the saline-injected experimental animal.

Cholinesterase

Although it is clear that the differences between the experimental brain and the control brain are many, the results of the labelled incorporation experiments and the effect of drugs indicates some of the enzyme systems that would be worth following up. We shall give an example of one such system now, that of the cholinesterase (ChE).

When we measured the cholinesterase activity in the brains of the resting, control and experimental animals we found that the system was quite different from

Table 16.3.

Change in activity in AChE in the brain of snail.

	AChE activity	
Resting quiet control	0·246 ± 0·023	$n = 7$
Shocked control	0·407 ± 0·027	$n = 7$
Experimental	0·592 ± 0·009	$n = 7$

AChE activity in terms of μmol ACh/100 μg protein per h.

that of the cockroach. The experimental cockroach had less ChE than the control or resting animal. In the snail the situation was the reverse. The resting level of ChE was 0·246 μmol/100 μg protein per h, that of the control animal was 0·407 and that of the experimental was 0·592 (Table 16.3). Thus, there had been an increase

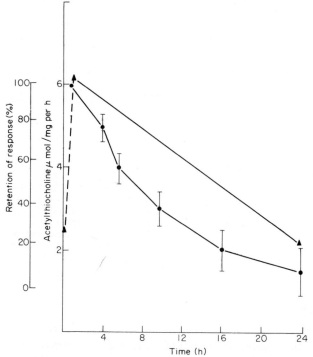

Figure 16.12. Change in ChE activity as the snail forgets. When the experimental animal learns, the ChE activity in its brain increases as shown by the line ▲——▲; as the animals forget (●——●) so the ChE activity falls back to the original level. It takes about twenty-four hours for the snail to forget.

from about 25 in the resting animal to 40 in the control and 60 in the experimental animal. This change had taken place in the twenty-five minutes of training. The ChE activity in the experimental animal diminished as the animal forgot (Figure 16.12). The animal forgot over a period of twenty-four hours during which the level of ChE slowly returned to the resting level.

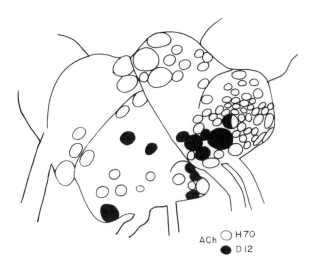

Figure 16.13. Response of neurones in the snail brain to acetylcholine (ACh). Some neurones are excited (depolarised) by ACh. These are called D cells and are shown in black. The majority of the neurones tested were hyperpolarised (H) and inhibited by ACh. H:D = 70:12.

Why should the level of ChE in the snail increase on learning yet that of the cockroach decrease? This is best answered as follows. In the cockroach acetylcholine (ACh) is entirely an excitatory transmitter. If the amount of ChE at the synapse decreases, the efficacy of the ACh as a transmitter would increase. In the snail, however, ACh is mainly an inhibitory transmitter. We have tested over a hundred different anatomically specified neurones in the snail brain to iontophoretically applied ACh. Only ten cells were excited (depolarised) by ACh. The majority of the neurones were inhibited (hyperpolarised) by the application of ACh. It is possible to produce a map of the nerve cell bodies in the snail brain indicating which neurones are H (hyperpolarised) and which neurones are D (depolarised) by ACh (Figure 16.13). The majority of neurones were H in the snail. The situation is quite different from that seen in the cockroach CNS where all the tested neurones were D to ACh (Kerkut, Pitman and Walker, 1969; Pitman and Kerkut, 1970).

A diagrammatic interpretation of what might be going on is given in Figure 16.14. The function of a synapse is to stop transmission. Normally the system would require many presynaptic action potentials before one postsynaptic action potential occurs. Thus, if it requires 20 presynaptic to 1 postsynaptic potential, the synaptic ratio could be referred to as 20:1. In the cockroach where ACh is an excitatory transmitter the decrease in the amount of ChE could reduce the synaptic ratio from 20:1 to say 5:1 or even 1:1 and thus allow excitation to be even

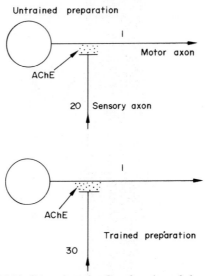

Figure 16.14. Synaptic ratio. One function of the synapse is to stop transmission. It is suggested that several presynaptic action potentials (20) are required in order to get one postsynaptic action potential. This would give a synaptic ratio of 20:1. If the AChE changes so as to become more active, this could change the synaptic ratio from 20:1 to 30:1. Since ACh is mainly inhibitory in the snail brain, the increased AChE activity would reduce the inhibitory effect and so allow excitatory pathways to become dominant.

more effective over specific pathways. Where ACh is an inhibitory transmitter, increasing the level of ChE would change the synaptic ratio from say 20:1 to 30:1 or 40:1, that is, it would reduce the inhibitory system and make the excitatory system more effective. In the experimental cockroach, not only was there a decrease in the amount of ChE but there was also a decrease in the level of GABA produced in the ganglia, GABA being the inhibitory transmitter (Oliver, Taberner, Rick and Kerkut, 1971). Thus, the experimental ganglion in the cockroach had increased excitation along some of the pathways, probably those involved in learning the leg-raising, by increasing the efficacy of the ACh (production of ChE) and by reducing the inhibitory transmitter GABA. In the snail we found an increase in the ChE which reduced the efficacy of the inhibitory transmitter ACh, thus allowing greater excitation over specific pathways.

It is clear that there are many other stages to be elucidated in the neurochemical differences between the ganglia of the experimental and control animals. The one that we have illustrated here is that involving ChE. The difference between the snail and the cockroach indicates the complexity of the system and the manner in which it is necessary to have an integrated approach. One must consider various

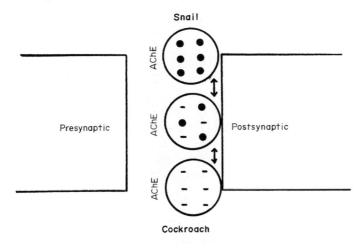

Figure 16.15. Changes in AChE at synapse. It is suggested that the enzyme AChE is able to change its activity so that it can in some cases become less active (as in the cockroach) and in other cases more active (as in the snail). Kinetic studies on the AChE indicate that the V_{max} remains the same but that the K_m changes, that is, the number of active sites is the same but the binding of the substrate has altered.

aspects of behaviour, neurochemistry, electrophysiology and neuropharmacology before one can understand the significance of the changes one observes. There are many problems still facing us. In particular how is this rapid change in the ChE activity brought about? Five possible causes are (1) a change in the rate of synthesis of ChE, (2) a change in the rate of breakdown of ChE, (3) the production of an inhibitor, that is, an anticholinesterase, (4) the production of an activator, (5) a conformational change in the enzyme which changes the activity. The differences in the properties of the ChE from the brains of experimental and control animals are at present being investigated. There is good evidence that the enzymes have the same V_{max} but different K_m values. ChE is an enzyme with an activity that can change according to the use at synapse in the CNS. Its properties change according to the functional role that ACh plays at the specific synapses (excitatory or inhibitory) (Figure 16.15). It is a link between 'macromolecules' and 'behaviour.'

It is probable that changes in substrate level and enzyme levels will also be found for the catecholamine transmitters such as dopamine and noradrenaline, and also for the glutamate and GABA systems. It is necessary, however, to locate the neurones in which these changes occur in order to understand the behavioural significance. It is likely that where a given transmitter is excitatory there will be a change in one direction and where the transmitter is inhibitory there will be a change in the opposite direction. Thus, a gross chemical analysis might fail to reveal any difference unless the transmitter is mainly excitatory, as in the case of ACh in the cockroach or mainly inhibitory as in the case of ACh in the snail. Where the transmitter is equally balanced, it is essential to carry out cellular localisation of the changes in enzymatic level before one can come to any decision as to the biochemical correlates of learning and behaviour in the CNS.

It should be stressed that this change in ChE activity is only one of many changes that take place in the CNS following stimulation. It is probable that the ChE change is a short-term change, effective over a few days until changes involving protein synthesis can be effective. Other changes that we have detected are changes in GABA synthesis, GAD activity, protein synthesis, RNA incorporation of labelled uridine. There are clearly many chapters in this story, and the present account is just one brief paragraph.

We should like to thank the Wellcome Trust for a grant to P. Emson.

References

ÁDÁM, G. (Ed.), (1970). *Brain and Memory*. Hungarian Academy of Sciences, Budapest.

AGRANOFF, B. W. and KLINGER, P. D. (1964). Puromycin effect of memory fixation in the goldfish. *Science, N.Y.*, **146**, 952–3.

BARONDES, S. H. and COHEN, H. D. (1966). Puromycin effect on successive stages of memory storage. *Science, N.Y.*, **151**, 594–5.

BOGOCH, S. (1968). *The Biochemistry of Memory*. Oxford University Press, London.

DEUTSCH, J. A. (1969). The physiological basis of memory. *A. Rev. Psychol.*, **20**, 85–104.

EMSON, P. C. and KERKUT, G. A. (1971). Acetylcholinesterase in snail brain. *Comp. Biochem. Physiol.*, **39B**, 879–89.

EMSON, P. C., WALKER, R. J. and KERKUT, G. A. (1971). Chemical changes in a molluscan ganglion associated with learning. *Comp. Biochem. Physiol.*, **40B**, 223–39.

FLEXNER, J. B. and STELLAR, E. (1963). Memory in mice as affected by intracellular puromycin. *Science, N.Y.*, **141**, 57–9.

GLASSMAN, E. (Ed.) (1967). *Molecular Approaches to Psychobiology*. Dickenson Publishing Company, Belmont, California, U.S.A.

GLASSMAN, E. (1969). The biochemistry of learning—an evaluation of the role of RNA and protein. *A. Rev. Biochem.*, **38**, 605–46.

HYDÉN, H. (1960). The Neuron. In: *The Cell* (BRACHET, J. and MIRSKY, A. E., Eds.), Vol. IV, pp. 215–323. Academic Press, New York.

HYDÉN, H. (1964). RNA a functional characteristic of the neuron and its glia. In: *RNA and Brain Function, Memory and Learning* (BRAZIER, M. A. B., Ed.), University of California Press, Los Angeles, U.S.A.

KERKUT, G. A., PITMAN, R. M. and WALKER, R. J. (1969). Iontophoretic application of acetylcholine and GABA onto insect central neurones. *Comp. Biochem. Physiol.*, **31**, 611–33.

KERKUT, G. A., OLIVER, G. W. O., RICK, J. T. and WALKER, R. J. (1970). The effects of drugs on learning in a simple preparation. *Comp. gen. Pharmac.*, **1**, 437–83.

LODIN, Z. and ROSE, S. P. R. (Eds.) (1968). *Macromolecules and the Function of the Neurone*. Excerpta Medica Foundation, Amsterdam.

OLIVER, G. W. O. (1973). Neurochemical aspects of shock-avoidance learning in cockroaches. In: *Macromolecules and Behaviour* (ANSELL, G. B. and BRADLEY, P. B., Eds.), pp. 113–31. Macmillan, London.

OLIVER, G. W. O., TABERNER, P. V., RICK, J. T. and KERKUT, G. A. (1971). Changes in GABA level, GAD and ChE activity in CNS of an insect during learning. *Comp. Biochem. Physiol.*, **38B**, 529–35.

PETERSON, R. P. and KERNELL, D. (1970). The effects of nerve stimulation on the metabolism of ribonucleic acid in a molluscan giant neurone. *J. Neurochem.*, **17**, 1075–87.

PITMAN, R. M. and KERKUT, G. A. (1970). Comparison of the actions of iontophoretically applied acetylcholine and GABA with the EPSP and IPSP in cockroach central neurones. *Comp. gen. Pharmac.*, **1**, 221–30.

THORPE, W. H. and DAVENPORT, D. (Eds.) (1964). Learning and associated phenomena in invertebrates. *Animal Behaviour Supplement*, **1**, 1–190.

ROUND TABLE DISCUSSION
Neurobiological models of learning
Chairman: S. M. Hilton
Department of Physiology, Medical School, Birmingham

Round table discussion: neurobiological models of learning

Chairman:
S. M. HILTON

Speakers:
G. Horn
H. Hydén
D. M. MacKay

P. Mandel
E. A. Turner
P. D. Wall

and

G. Ádám
B. W. Agranoff
D. A. Booth
W. E. Davies
E. Glassman

G. A. Kerkut
S. Lal
G. Raisman
S. P. R. Rose
G. Vrbová

CHAIRMAN: Those of you who have been at this meeting will have heard quite a lot about what biochemists have been trying to do over a period of years and the experiments they have been carrying out which are related to some aspects of behaviour and, hopefully, to learning. We have also heard a little from the psychologists about what is understood by learning and how it can be investigated. There has not been much in between: a little anatomy and a little physiology, and I wonder whether this might be the point where we could continue, particularly under the title we have been given today, 'Neurobiological Models of Learning'. What do we understand about the anatomy, the physiology and perhaps the pharmacology of these more elementary processes that might hopefully be thought to underlie learning? I would imagine that this would be something a biochemist would very much like to hear so that he could know there actually was a discriminating test as to whether learning of a particular task had actually taken place. Could I first ask Professor Wall if he has any concrete thoughts on this question?

P. D. WALL: I think one of the issues, if I speak only of physiology, that one has to recognise is that there has been a historical transition from looking at extremely rapid events with a duration of a millisecond to events of longer and longer duration. There has been a period of great excitement over changes of activity associated with previous behaviour which lasted for long periods of time (seconds, minutes, hours, weeks). Now we have a plethora of such changes. It is no longer the case that we know of no system to examine; we perhaps know of too many, and I think the question to ask with regard to the title of 'Neurobiological Models of Learning' is: "What long-term change would be of interest in relation to learning?"

Obviously we have to define learning. As we have heard, both physiologically and biochemically, a number of often massive changes are observed—for example, the massive change in the size of muscles following activity. Now does one want to call that learning—has a muscle learned, remembered that it was active? This is the first issue, that inactivity in some structures leads to further inactivity and to decreases of size, while activity leads to improved action and increases of size. Surely many of the biochemical, and probably many of the physiological, changes that have been observed are of that variety. By simply knowing the presence of past activity some change can be observed. This is surely a proper subject for study and a very important one, but if we are talking about learning and memory we presumably require something in addition to such a change. I am not saying that such changes should not be studied. It would be interesting enough to know why a muscle increases its size with activity or a pathway increases or decreases its excitability with activity. However, I think that, faced with the number of changes available, we should start looking round to see which might be associated with the interesting aspects of learning behaviour; and here one needs more than a simple coupling of stimulus and response.

We need to begin to ask about the other criteria for learning. In any of the simplest possible memory systems one criterion would be the means by which two sets of activity, not necessarily two stimuli, but a stimulus and a response, somehow become associated. It is not enough just to talk of a straight-through channel, input/output change. Somehow a method of investigating how two inputs are related must be found.

A second property is that the duration of the changes observed should somehow match the behavioural properties of the whole system. The changes in the parameters of stimulation needed to produce a change in behaviour can now be defined sufficiently well for us to be able to match them with particular targets within the system, to ask: "Do the time course and the other parameters suggest a matching?"

The third and last problem in an ordinary memory system is that if you wish to point to some change as being significant in terms of the memory system, you must say how this could be read. It is not enough merely to show that a change has occurred such as in staining or impedance; you must be prepared at least to guess how the nervous system could detect such a change.

Obviously we all have our favourite suggestions as to which would be the best targets for future study, but I would simply point out that if we are going to talk about 'Neurobiological Models of Learning', we are going to need to talk about the association of inputs; let us say the association of nerve impulses, not the mere presence of activity or inactivity; we are going to need to match parameters and we are going to need to be quite certain that there is a trace which can be read by the nervous system.

CHAIRMAN: We must be very grateful to Professor Wall for being brave enough to start this. I don't think he has quite answered my question, but then maybe the question is unanswerable anyway. Does anybody at the table here think that we do know enough in a particular situation for it to be regarded as an anatomical and physiological basis for the study of learning?

G. HORN: There is certainly one situation where the evidence available is very promising and where there is close parametric congruence between the item of behaviour being studied and the observed changes in the central nervous system. When an organism is presented with a novel stimulus it may respond to it, but the response usually declines as the stimulus is repeatedly delivered. There are many neurones in the central nervous system whose responsiveness to a stimulus changes in a similar way. Such cells have been described in both vertebrate and invertebrate nervous systems and careful studies (Horn and Hinde, 1970)[1] of the properties of these cells suggest that the neuronal changes adequately account for the behavioural changes. Here, then, is a behavioural response where a good start has been made in analysing its anatomical and physiological bases.

E. A. TURNER: I was interested in Professor Wall's reference to the different parameters, especially the time parameters that we are concerned with, because I think that as soon as you get to mammalian structure, and certainly to the human, you are dealing with two widely different parameters. First of all you are dealing with the long-term and almost permanent memory which we refer to as long-term memory or late recall, and secondly with a very much shorter one linked with hippocampal structures, which is associated with short-term memory or recent recall of stimuli. This fits in with the kind of experiment we have been hearing

[1] HORN, G. and HINDE, R. A. (Eds.) (1970). *Short-Term Changes in Neural Activity and Behaviour*. Cambridge University Press, Cambridge.

about in which a change takes place and persists for some hours and it really fits quite well with the timing of the functions with which we are concerned. But when we come to the trace of permanently learned behaviour, I think we need to look at a different kind of concept and I should be very surprised if it were to be accompanied by the same kind of chemical modulation.

S. LAL*: Should we not bear certain distinctions in mind? Firstly, there is the distinction between those physiological and biochemical changes that take place as a result of storing the 'image' of a situation and those that result from any ongoing stimulation and activity in the nervous system. Secondly, there is the distinction between the biochemical and organisational aspects of learning and memory. The biochemical changes associated with learning are likely to be similar in all species or at least will not differ in many ways, whereas the organisational differences in learning mechanisms are likely to be very different. Thirdly, in talking about short-term memory, or rather the temporal aspects of the process required to hold a stimulus or experience in the short-term memory, biochemists, psychologists and physiologists mean different things. To the biochemist short-term memory processes last about four hours; to the psychologist they last half-an-hour and to the physiologist tens of milliseconds. Unless we are clear about these distinctions we will not know what our arguments and disagreements are about.

CHAIRMAN: This raises a large number of general issues as well as the particular ones and I am a little disappointed that so far there seems to be very little information that would really provide us with a basis on which we could start thinking about biochemistry.

HORN: I have already given you one example of a situation that might profitably be looked at in more detail. There are others which are also specific and amenable to experimental analysis. Imprinting is one of these. The general strategy of our own work (Rose, Bateson and Horn, this volume)[1] has been to see if it is possible to identify specific brain regions which are influenced by the imprinting procedure. We have used measures of protein and RNA synthesis in the search for such regions. If our findings can consistently be related to imprinting, if the regional changes persist after we have controlled for variables that occur with, but are not necessary for, imprinting (for example, stress—see Horn, Horn, Bateson and Rose, 1971),[2] it will be worth looking at the brain regions in more detail and using anatomical, biochemical and electrophysiological techniques.

[1] ROSE, S. P. R., BATESON, P. P. G. AND HORN, G. (1973). Biochemistry and behaviour in the chick. In: *Macromolecules and Behaviour* (ANSELL, G. B. and BRADLEY, P. B., Eds.), pp. 93–104. Macmillan, London.

[2] HORN, G., HORN, A. L. D., BATESON, P. P. G. and ROSE, S. P. R. (1971). Effects of imprinting on uracil incorporation into brain RNA in the 'split-brain' chick. *Nature*, **229**, 131–2.

* Chelsea College of Science and Technology, London.

CHAIRMAN: What are the facts that have been discovered?

HORN: We have consistently found changes in protein and RNA synthesis in the forebrain roof but not in other brain regions of imprinted chicks.

CHAIRMAN: Could they be described in anatomical or physiological terms?

HORN: Ultimately, yes. You were originally asking for something to look for. I am suggesting a possible place to look for them.

P. MANDEL: I have assumed that the goal of the first question was to know if there is any model for learning which we know something about anatomically, physiologically or electrophysiologically, and psychologically, and if it is a good model for learning. This is the basic question. Then we can go to other models which are under discussion and we can hope to find more evidence about them. But first let us ask if there are any models for which we already have some anatomical, physiological, electrophysiological and behavioural evidence.

CHAIRMAN: Thank you Dr Mandel. Your scientific English is much more explicit than mine.

H. HYDÉN: I would like to make a more general comment. If we start with the phylogenetically laid down pathways in the whole of the brain, we have then to ask ourselves whether there is, in addition, a non-hereditary mechanism functioning only for a life-time, which can be used for acquisition, storage and retrieval. Retrieval of this information should be made with a high distinction, that is quite clear, and one should be able to correlate it with the function required. In the end this requires that we study gene activities of neurones in a pathway of the brain, to be able to say whether there is gross differentiation through gene depression for a considerable time, whether it stops, or another mechanism takes over. One thing is clear for advanced study, and that is that in order to have three-dimensional changes we have to look for systematic analysis of pathways of labelled or nonlabelled neurones with a mechanism of distinction.

WALL: Gabriel Horn is being rightly aggressive here in saying that he thinks there is information. I would just like to define what that information is. To take your two examples: you and your colleagues are doing this extremely interesting work on imprinting, but you should also mention that while there is a fascinating change in the behaviour of the animal, there is, at the same time, an enormous surge of anatomical development in the animal. It is not just that it points its beak at the light; its whole development changes at that stage. Here is an example of pulling of a trigger important to the whole animal's development. Imprinting in birds certainly is an extremely important and interesting thing to look at, but if you are talking about learning or relating biochemistry to behaviour, how do you propose to demonstrate a causal relationship between an increase in the amount of protein and the particular behaviour that is called imprinting rather than all this general explosion that goes on?

In your other examples of habituation, you have almost the opposite problem. It is so specific that there is no association involved. A change is demonstrated physiologically but it is not identified in detail with one pathway which is absolutely locked in with the activity so that no other pathway will influence the affected one except by overwhelming action.

GERTA VRBOVÁ*: I was really provoked by what Patrick Wall said about the muscle because, in fact, I think that the muscle is not just a tissue that can grow and become bigger with activity. It has its membrane and it has its neuromuscular junction and both are in fact extremely plastic. They are so plastic that we can actually produce changes in the chemosensitivity of the junction within a few hours. Now the reason why I am talking about it is that during conditioning or learning, whichever we call it, one assumes that a new synapse is formed on a place where there was no synapse, or that a new functional connection is formed somewhere where there wasn't one. Now a muscle accepts the innervation only when its membrane is sensitive to the transmitter; when it is desensitised, it will not accept innervation. In fact we have found that activity of the presynaptic element greatly increases the sensitivity of the junction area to the transmitter. You find a several-fold increase after an hour's stimulation and this persists for eight to ten hours. During this time, if there was another neurone, it could be imagined that sprouting would occur and a new connection would be formed.

It is extremely interesting, too, that at the neuromuscular junction the time constant of the growth of the neurone, which is really extremely fast, can be followed. A nerve fibre can grow as fast as 100 μm an hour and this rate is of an order of magnitude which is consistent with the time course of the behavioural changes that can be seen during conditioning. So I think that although the neuromuscular junction has only one input, it could be a very interesting structure to study, particularly for biochemists, because we already know a lot about it. We know what the transmitter is; we can block it selectively; we know a lot about the function of the membrane and its biochemistry and we can handle it very easily. I would greatly recommend this structure as a model of learning.

S. P. R. ROSE: It seems to me that there are several confusions about what one is really trying to do here and all of them are embraced by the fact that one is attempting to define a process called 'learning' and then trying to fit a lot of things into this, whether they fit or not. Clearly, there is a set of related processes. There are the genetically specified processes within the brain which Professor Hydén referred to. There are the maturational processes in which there is obligatory learning of something or other, like the imprinting situation. There is learning in

* Medical School, Birmingham.

the adult animal—Professor Ádám this morning produced a distinction between conscious and unconscious memory. There are questions as to whether linguistic memory is the same as visual memory and so on. If we try to lump all these together as processes we may be in danger of glossing over definitional and process differences which actually confuse the experimentation.

The one thing I think it is reasonable to say is that from what we know about the general principles of the economy of biochemistry, phylogenetically and within the individual, it is likely that if we could elucidate the biochemical sequence of events in any one of these numerous different situations, we would go some way at any rate towards finding out the mechanism which operated at several of the others as well, and we might then look for process differences which related different parts of the brain, or cellular differences which discriminated one form of situation from another.

But from the biochemical point of view, what I think we need to agree is that for the biochemist it is much easier to measure changes taking place in a system rather than something which reflects the steady state of the system, and therefore we need to look for some environmental situation (the phrase I used was 'environmental trigger' and Bernard Agranoff tells me that it was his phrase originally!) which produces some sets of defined changes in the brain and then examine the whole complex of these processes, without, I think, worrying as to whether this fitted some abstract definition of learning or not. We can then go back and see how the change itself differs as a second order of difference amongst different processes which might be defined as learning under different contexts.

MANDEL: We should talk about models which are already used; it would be useful to be told what is known about these models (what is known about their anatomy, electrophysiology and physiology, for example) and what the precise limitations of these models are. Are these models acceptable at the present time from the psychological and behavioural point of view? We should start with something we already know. Later we can try to generalise. I would like to leave this room with a model about which psychologists and behaviourists agree.

CHAIRMAN: Well, we have had one model at the neuromuscular junction proposed. Is there any other?

LAL: A model for the organisational aspects of particular memory or learning processes could be provided by looking at the techniques used in computers for labelling and indexing information, for retrieving information and storing it. Almost certainly such structural analogues would be wrong and confused but at least they could give us some reasonably definite way of thinking about the problem.

G. RAISMAN: In reference to the neuromuscular junction as a model, and the idea that learning may involve the formation of new contacts or new synapses in the central nervous system, I don't know of any evidence—unless there is some presented here—that new connections are formed during the course of learning.

W. E. DAVIES*: I would like to draw your attention to the suitability of the mammalian auditory system for studies of this nature. It is a fairly discrete system certainly at the lower levels and its sensory input can be fairly easily controlled. It has the advantage over the visual system in that its second order neurones are more easily accessible and further away from the receptor organ. The cochlear nucleus seems to be particularly amenable to study in that it receives afferent input only from the VIIIth nerve of one side.

Whilst one cannot dispute the advantages of the simplicity of the neural input of the invertebrate ganglia described by Professor Kerkut and his colleagues, it is debatable whether mechanisms functional in these situations can be extended to the more complex mammalian systems. At the other extreme, the neural input of the chick visual system during imprinting, that Professor Rose described, must be extremely complex, making it very difficult to form any functional correlates of the neurochemical changes observed.

Here, therefore, in the cochlear nucleus we have a system that is a compromise between these two extremes, having a comparatively simple sensory input while remaining a fully organised mammalian neural aggregate.

We have done some preliminary experiments with this system in an attempt to correlate changes in the protein makeup with the sensory input. To be brief, the experiments have consisted of depriving the guinea pig completely of the auditory input on one side, by fracture of one cochlea, followed by various analyses of proteins extracted from different parts of the two sides of the system after a suitable time lapse. These analyses have included disc electrophoretic analyses of the soluble proteins from the cochlear nuclei, inferior colliculi and auditory cortices of the two sides, and the measurement of the incorporation of [^{14}C]glucose into proteins of the same areas.

Preliminary results suggest that the complexity of the electrophoretic pattern of the soluble proteins is dependent on the neural input of that area. In the hemideprived animals, the more complex cochlear nucleus pattern is given by the proteins from the cochlear nucleus on the intact side. At the cortical level, where most of the neural representation is from the cochlea on the opposite side, the side contralateral to the intact side shows the more complex protein pattern. At an intermediate level, the inferior colliculi, where considerable mixing of the inputs from the two cochleae has occurred, very similar electrophoretic patterns are seen on the two sides.

Measurement of the specific radioactivity of proteins labelled with [^{14}C]-glucose from such areas gives an identical picture, namely the highest specific activity is found in the regions of greatest neural input.

* Medical School, Birmingham.

Finally, I would like to say that after the wealth of data, albeit diverse data, that has been presented at this Symposium, I am of the opinion that the most useful information will be that which can be extracted from the most simple mammalian sensory system. Furthermore, the auditory system is basically very suitable for studies of this nature. I am therefore suggesting that if one remains at the lower levels of the auditory pathway, particularly at the level of the cochlear nucleus, some very meaningful chemical correlates of information-processing will emerge.

CHAIRMAN: Thank you, Dr Davies. But can we deal with the anatomy and physiology of any other system? Is there nothing known of any invertebrate system, for instance? With this audience, there must be someone who can tell us whether we know enough to regard what goes on at any invertebrate synapse as a model of learning.

G. A. KERKUT: I think that in some ways you are asking too much, Professor Hilton. The Schrodinger equation can be solved for hydrogen and water but not for glucose and glutathione. What you are asking is for something of an equivalent complexity.

We certainly know something about the anatomy, electrophysiology, pharmacology and behaviour of some invertebrate systems, but there are still very many gaps. Even if we take the vertebrate spinal cord, what appears to be a simple 'two neurone' reflex was shown by Professor Malcolm's work[1] (1953) on the development of the reflex in the kitten to be much more complex. In the invertebrates we can find 'simple' giant axon pathways and test these but when we use more refined physiological stimulation we find the system is more complex and has additional parts interacting.

I think that over the next four years we will know something about the changes in a given group of ten anatomically specified neurones in an invertebrate ganglion during the learning process. It is likely that this will be done for the insect ganglion and also for the molluscan ganglion.

D. M. MACKAY: The conceptual gap between macromolecules and memory is a wide one, and I think we will have to develop a more refined methodological scaffolding if we are ever to fit these fragments of information into a coherent physiological theory of memory. At present, our biggest problem is to know what questions would be most profitable to ask at the physiological level. We perform experiments in which animals learn, and we find macromolecular and structural changes correlated with their learning. But like the villagers in Charles Lamb's *Essay on Roast Pig*, we find it hard to separate essential mediators of the process that interests us from incidental concomitants that throw no light on its mechanism.

[1] MALCOM, J. L. (1953). In: *The Spinal Cord* (MALCOM, J. L. and GRAY, J. A. B., Eds.), Ciba Foundation Symposium. Churchill, London.

Physiologically, we start from the notion of the modifiability of brain tissue. Some synapses, we know, are modifiable; so apparently, are some protein patterns, and doubtless other things too. But not all modifiability may be relevant to information storage. Our prior task is thus to find a way of specifying the job that has to be done by those modifications (whatever they may be) that are the basis for memory. Here, perhaps, the concepts of information engineering may have some place. An organism can be regarded in general terms as an information system in constant transition from one state to another, the relative probabilities of different transitions varying according to its current inputs and internal goal-settings. At any given time its internal structure determines a vast array (which we can picture as an n-dimensional matrix) of conditional probabilities, that if such-and-such were to happen in such-and-such circumstances, then a transition would take place to state so-and-so. The modifications that interest us can be formally defined as those that affect (for a significant period) this conditional-probability matrix or CPM. The need to distinguish these from other modifications should be a primary consideration in the design of experiments on the physiological basis of memory.

This leads naturally to the question: which modifiable parameters of a system such as the central nervous system could significantly affect its CPM? There is a temptation to assume that the only ones that matter are the synaptic couplings and the levels of excitability of nerve cells. These of course depend on many metabolic and other parameters, some of which may in turn be modifiable. I would like, however, to draw attention to one rather different parameter which seems to have been relatively neglected (MacKay and McCulloch, 1952;[1] MacKay, 1954[2]). I mean the timing, or more specifically the difference in transmission times, of correlated signals impinging on the same neurone. There is plenty of evidence, for example in the binaural auditory system, of exquisite neural sensitivity to changes in relative timing, even down to a few tens of milliseconds. Lorenté de Nó (1939)[3] reported similar evidence from the oculomotor nucleus. There is also some evidence, at least in peripheral nerve, of differential changes in fibre diameter, and hence in transmission speed, as a function of use. If, then, similar semi-permanent changes in the speed of travel of signals occurred in the central nervous system, they could have extremely powerful effects on the overall CPM. To appreciate this, think of the reduction in feasibility of a cross-country rail trip which results when British Railways speed up one of their services so that your train reaches a junction just too late to make the connection!

Here, then, may be another physiological question worth asking: what changes

---

[1] MacKay, D. M. and McCulloch, W. S. (1952). The limiting information capacity of a neuronal link. *Bull. Math. Biophys.*, **14**, 127–35; **15**, 107.

[2] MacKay, D. M. (1954). Operational aspects of some fundamental concepts of human communication. *Synthèse*, **9**, 182–98.

[3] Lorenté de Nó, R. (1939). Transmission of impulses through cranial motor nuclei. *J. Neurophysiol.*, **2**, 401–64.

in the temporal structure of neural networks accompany learning? How far can the CPM of a neural network be modified in this way? Again, are the branch-points of dendrites sensitive to the relative timing of convergent signals, and are their temporal properties similarly modifiable? What macromolecular factors determine the magnitude and the stability of such modifications (if any?) and so on.

Another point that emerges from information theory is that a system which has to develop its organisation by trial and error will do so more efficiently if its repertoire starts with relatively few degrees of freedom, and is progressively differentiated as maturation proceeds. In other words, learning in the early stages might advantageously involve more selective dissolution of connections than formation of new ones (MacKay, 1956).[1] This raises obvious questions about the sorts of changes we ought to be on the lookout for as a function of maturation, as distinct from those to be expected during learning in a mature organism.

One further point: an informational analysis can give us a useful feeling for the scale of the problem we have to tackle. It has sometimes been argued that a man (under hypnosis) can recall so many distinct items in such fine detail that his brain must store its information in some molecular code. The joker here is what the communication engineer calls redundancy (Shannon, 1948;[2] MacKay, 1969[3]). What we recall in memory, for all its variety, is highly redundant information—i.e. the elements are far from statistically independent. If we make due allowance for this, and bear in mind the complexity of the dendritic and axonal ramifications of a typical nerve cell, it is far from obvious that we need any more storage capacity than is available in the possible permutations of gross neuronal structure and connectivity. If so, there would still be plenty of questions to ask at the macromolecular level; but they would be different questions: in particular, questions about the role of macromolecules in bringing about and maintaining the long-term stability of changes in neuronal structures.

The general point I am making is that in a field such as this it isn't enough to accumulate more evidence. If we are to avoid having the evidence pile up around us in a large amorphous and unmanageable heap, we must lose no time in constructing a functional conceptual framework that sufficiently spells out the task the brain has to perform, so that ideally we know where to put the bits of evidence as they come in, and find our next questions suggested by the shapes of the gaps they leave (MacKay, 1954).[4] This will be possible only if the framework starts at a sufficiently

[1] MACKAY, D. M. (1956). Towards an information-flow model of human behaviour. *Br. J. Psychol.* **47**, 30–43.
[2] SHANNON, C. E. (1948). A mathematical theory of communication. *Bell. Syst. Tech. J.*, **27**, 279–423; 623–56.
[3] MACKAY, D. M. (1969). *Information, Mechanism and Meaning*. M.I.T. Press, Boston.
[4] MACKAY, D. M. (1954). On comparing the brain with machines. *The Adv. of Sci.*, **40**, 402–406. Also *American Scientist*, **42**, 261–8 and Ann. Report of Smithsonian Inst., 231–40.

fundamental and general level to be able itself to grow and be adapted without total destruction as fresh data come in. The development of such a framework will clearly be a long job, needing patient cooperation between many different disciplines. I have mentioned these examples to indicate how I think informational analysis may help provide some of the necessary bridge-building materials.

LAL: Is not the model of fetching and matching a template with incoming data structure an inadequate description of how we recognise and respond to previously learned situations? Surely it would be more efficient and economical to construct a 'filter' and then store either the characteristics of the filter, or the procedure for generating it? Alternatively, one could think of a set of basic descriptors which are used to construct a complex descriptor of the required complexity for the situation in hand. Then the procedure for generating the complex description is stored and information is fed back to modify or refine the basic descriptor set.

There seem to me to be at least two major defects in adopting an approach based on information theory and on conditional transitional probabilities linking inputs and outputs. Firstly, the theorems of information theory that can be applied to neurophysiological systems are of great generality and of little specific use—for example, the maximum rate at which information can be transmitted through a channel. Secondly, once one starts thinking in terms of transitional probabilities, one's interest tends to focus on formal questions about how the probability distributions connecting inputs and outputs change, or how the calculation of limiting frequencies or their realisation by a 'neural calculator' could take place.

WALL: Professor Mandel, you want to leave here with a model. Now do you mean a model or would you like a real animal really doing something because I think you have heard both here? You have had through-and-through models as a type, like the neuromuscular junction, and the cochlear nucleus. You have had a suggestion for temporal models, and many people could give you specific examples of these, and I think you have also had spectacular models like imprinting, in which we have heard that you can follow the biochemical sequence of events. Now, whether you consider these satisfactory models, I don't know. Could you specify a little more what you would like?

MANDEL: In general we have some behaviour people using neurochemical methods and some neurochemists working on behaviour. Often the neurochemist does not agree with the work done by the behaviourists and the behaviourist does not agree with the learning model used by the neurochemist. I would like to ascertain the limitations of the models about which papers have been presented at this meeting. Are behaviourists in agreement that the shuttle-box is a good model for learning experiments? Are people in agreement that the cochlear model is a good model? Are people in agreement that the imprinting model is a good model? And what do we know about these different models? It is easier to start from something about which we already know a little than to start from something about which we know nothing, and if we don't start with a precise model I think we could stay here for several days without progress.

I have heard that the approach using the shuttle-box is not correct. Let us discuss this problem. Who agrees that the shuttle-box is a learning model, how could it be improved, and what are its limitations? Afterwards the neurochemists must outline the limitations of the methods they use.

D. A. BOOTH: I am not happy with the question, "Can we please have a model of learning?" It is like asking for a model of genetics. There are many aspects to the phenomenon of learning and the mechanism of memory. A good model to work on depends on what you are looking for. If you want to be sure that you are working on memory in the strict sense (retention of skills and facts, though not necessarily anything as complex as human learning of language), you will make sure that you have a behavioural paradigm which involves behavioural change of that type, and measures which pick it out specifically. But then you may never find any biochemistry—perhaps because the neurochemical changes are so small or unspecific for memory, or even because no covalent changes are needed.

At the other extreme, if you want to be very sure you have a biochemical effect, then you will choose something which really hits the brain. Yet, if you do then get a big biochemical change, although it is reasonable to hope that it will lead to improved neurochemical understanding, what the change means behaviourally may be interesting or it may be trivial. You just have to take the risk that the neural effects relate, say, to arousal, emotion or sensory or motor processing rather than to memory, or even have no role in controlling behaviour at all.

So I think the best response here to a plea for suggestions from psychology is to point out how learning can be picked out from other behavioural phenomena. There are at least two criteria to require of any 'learning task' which we use to look for memory correlates or in which we try to disrupt memory retention (Miller, 1967 a,[1] b;[2] Booth, 1970[3]).

One is that you should be able to change the response to the situation in either direction by varying the environmental contingencies. The other one is that, over the range of perceptions, actions and knowledge within the organism's capacity, you should be able to pick an arbitrary stimulus or an arbitrary response

---

[1] MILLER, N. E. (1967a). Laws of learning relevant to its biological basis. *Proc. Am. phil. Soc.*, **111**, 315–25.

[2] MILLER, N. E. (1967b). Certain facts of learning relevant to a search for its physical basis. In: *The Neurosciences. A Study Program* (QUARTON, G. C., MELNECHUK, T. and SCHMITT, F. O., Eds.), pp. 643–52. The Rockefeller University Press, New York.

[3] BOOTH, D. A. (1970). Neurochemical changes correlated with learning and memory retention. In: *Molecular Mechanisms in Memory and Learning* (UNGAR, G., Ed.), pp. 1–57. Plenum Press, New York.

to be learnt. So what is difficult about shuttle-box performance is to know whether the biochemistry is specifically related to response to onset of the warning light—whether, for example, antibiotics suppress movement to a light of a colour that does not predict shock in a markedly smaller proportion than they suppress movement to light of another colour which is predictive. Or, the important point for the memory problem about biochemical correlates of the disappearance of an overt reaction, such as holding a leg raised or keeping on withdrawing a tentacle, is to know what would happen (as was queried this morning) if you tried to work it the other way. This is applying the bi-directional criterion and the shuttle-box example applies the arbitrariness criterion.

Now this is just offering a couple of criteria, not necessarily sufficient and only crudely stated. But I don't see why biochemists wanting to work on memory should not be able to apply these criteria to the design of experiments or in the evaluation of existing data for its relevance to memory biochemistry.

G. ÁDÁM: I refer to the question of Professor Mandel. The experiments described yesterday and today in the different lectures delivered in this room dealt predominantly with several avoidance conditioning techniques: jumping tests, shuttle-boxes, etc. In my opinion for all kinds of biochemical analyses and molecular purposes the approach training would be more effective. The avoidance situation always implicates in some form the element of stress that Professor Mandel mentioned yesterday. Thus, I suggest that you change your techniques and choose some kind of approach situation, for example, operant conditioning, classical alimentary conditioning, etc.

Speaking generally about models of learning, we can outline two categories of such plastic phenomena. The first category can be characterised by the arrival of a single flow of impulses to the central nervous system. Imprinting in the early ontogenesis is an example of this type of learning. The psychologists call it sensory, or perceptual learning. The negative side of this 'one channel' learning is habituation, proposed by Dr Horn as a suitable model. The other category of models consists of associative phenomena. In this case two sets of inputs are acting simultaneously on central nervous structures, as for instance in classical Pavlovian conditioning and in operant conditioning. This type of learning is characterised obviously by the contiguity of the two channels of impulses arriving at the central neurones at the same time. The negative mirror of this type of learning is extinction, discrimination, or delay response. Each research worker: biochemist, physiologist, pharmacologist, or psychologist should choose his preferred adequate model from the rich variety of the above outlined learning phenomena according to the concrete and actual task of his investigation.

CHAIRMAN: Can I ask why we have to use operant conditioning, because this introduces such complications into any learning situation?

BOOTH: What is difficult about operant training?

CHAIRMAN: It is too easy, I think.

BOOTH: Too easy to run. But if you start putting the bi-directionality tests and the arbitrary experimental and control stimuli, to give the results a real chance of relating to memory, it will not be quite so offhand.

In fact truly classically conditioned reactions may not be easier to observe than acquired instrumental behaviour, for example in invertebrates. Also there is little reason to believe that the learned components of involuntary reactions have to be different in neurology or neurochemistry from those of intentional acts, although of course the use of the memory must be different.

One experimental option is to ignore or even prevent the animal's reactions or actions at the actual time of learning. Elicit changes in the brain with different sorts of sensory inputs and merely presume from other observations that the animal is learning. Rensch and co-workers (1968)[1] have presented different visual patterns to restrained goldfish and found indications of anatomically differentiated biochemical effects by autoradiography. Similarly, in the imprinting work, I did not see any behavioural measure of what was going on during the period over which the biochemistry was examined. Here, too, the stimulus should be varied—for example, between flashing object and flashing general illumination, as mentioned this morning. On-off causes massive retinal activity, unlike continuous light. Differences between the degrees of imprinting after the two sorts of flashing could be compared with differences in their immediate biochemical effects. A consistent correlation in such an experiment would be far better evidence that the biochemical changes related to instruction of behaviour, rather than being merely a consequence of a particularly demanding sort of sensory processing.

B. W. AGRANOFF: I would like to respond to several of the questions, including one of the Chairman. In regard to the shuttle-box, we have run the same test letting the animals go into the light instead of the dark and have obtained identical results, and of course we have run the usual sorts of activity control experiments such as a Gellerman schedule in which the light and shock were dissociated.

I would like to agree, however, that shuttle-boxes in general have certain disadvantages. Activity phenomena cannot be ruled out as easily as they can in discrimination tests. Why then do we prefer the shuttle-box over discrimination and why do we use avoidance instead of some positive reward system? The answer is that the shuttle-box is highly convenient. We can teach an animal an avoidance task much more rapidly than positive reward learning, and with the shuttle-box significant difference can be obtained more easily than in a discrimination task,

---

[1] RENSCH, B., RAHMANN, H. and SKRZIPEK, K. H. (1968). Autoradiographische Untersuchungen über visuelle 'Engramm'-Bildung bei Fischen (II). *Pflügers Arch. ges. Physiol.*, **304**, 242–51.

particularly with partial learning. I think many of you know that the protein inhibitors block much more effectively with labile, if you will, fresh memory than they do in overtrained animals. In our shuttle-box we have a 'go no-go' situation. It is easy to get very large behavioural changes quickly. On the other hand, if I were to work on the field of memory transfer, I think I would use a discrimination task because of the possibility that some nonspecific activator is responsible for the effect. Unless stimulus specificity is shown, a brain-active peptide cannot be distinguished from any other hormone.

In regard to memory models, I must first confess that I am basically an empiricist. What we need, and I think I may be paraphrasing Professor MacKay, is constraints. When we know the imposed limitations, both from the standpoint of biological fact and from what we know about intimate details of neuronal physiology, we can begin to consider models. I tried to communicate yesterday some differences, which we are fortunate enough to see by means of antimetabolites, between short-term and long-term memory. We are now learning from studying axonal flow how long it takes for a message to get from the nucleus to the presynaptic terminals.

This has been a meeting on macromolecules and behaviour and I presume that we came here to learn the 'state of the art'. Those who have come to reassure themselves that nothing momentous is going on in the field of macromolecules and behaviour may leave reassured that the time is not yet ripe for them to enter this area. We can only wonder at the frequency with which they require the reassurance. To critics and enthusiasts alike, I extend my sympathies. It is very difficult to work in interdisciplinary areas with different languages and different methods of quantitation. I know this because I come from an interdisciplinary institute where we deal with this issue every day. The problem for the researcher is how to avoid a phenomenon called cross-sterilisation.

E. GLASSMAN: I have a number of remarks, the first of which concerns Professor Ádám's suggestion that appetitive tasks are less stressful than conditioned avoidance tasks where electric shocks are used. I would also agree intuitively that shocks are stressful, but there is little evidence that an animal learning an appetitive test is not under the same sorts of crucial stresses as an animal that is shocked. After all, in an appetitive task a mouse is placed under a state of partial starvation, or partial thirst, for several days, and then is required to perform in an apparatus in order to eat and drink. It certainly is not clear that the specific stresses associated with learning are less evident here than in an apparatus where the animal is shocked.

Now fortunately, Bowman (1970)[1] has used an appetitive task in which he used

[1] BOWMAN, R. E. and KOTTLER, P. D. (1970). Regional brain RNA metabolism as a function of different experiences. In: *Biochemistry of Brain and Behaviour* (BOWMAN, R. E. and DATTA, S. P., Eds.), pp. 301–26. Plenum Press, New York.

water as a reward in a maze; he has been able to cut down the time of training by using reversal training; and he has shown chemical responses similar to the sorts of data that we presented. That is, he does get increased incorporation into RNA in areas that we do. It is very hard to say that the changes are in the same cells, because we do not know exactly which cells are involved. But the appetitive test also yielded data consistent with those I reported the other day. The question of which type of task is more stressful is not relevant since the results do come out with some consistency.

One thing I would like to emphasise, but which we seem to be ignoring in this discussion, is that the architecture of the brain is, as we know, very complex. If a chemical response is observed in the cortex, in the cerebellum or in the limbic system, there is a tendency to conclude that the underlying stimuli and mechanism of response are the same in all three parts of the brain. The same assumptions are made when investigators compare changes in mammals with fish or with invertebrates. I doubt that these assumptions are correct. The variety of biochemical changes in a cell are limited, but the significance of the response can vary widely. In other words, the assumption seems to be that similar chemical changes have the same causes and effects in a wide variety of cells. This may be correct, but it seems equally possible that, because the cells are so different and the function of the various areas of the nervous system are so different, similar chemical changes may have different causes and effects. This is probably where the specificity of the chemical correlates of behaviour lies. That is, the electrical activity of the neurones in the nervous system does not, of itself, produce the chemical changes that we are reporting, and these changes occur in specific cells in response to specific stimuli.

For example, we know that during a learning experience massive firing takes place all over the brain, and yet people do not report chemical changes all over the brain. Rose, Bateson and Horn (1973)[1] report very specific localisation in the forebrain of the chick with imprinting. We report in the mouse localised responses in limbic system components and other structures in that region of the brain. We do not see changes in the cortex and we do not see changes in the cerebellum, and it seems unlikely that these are nonspecific changes. They are very specific to the training test. In a number of our experiments we did put an animal through classical conditioning in the yoke side of the jump-box, that is light and buzzer followed by shock for periods of up to half an hour, and these by themselves were not sufficient to cause the kind of increases that we see when the animal goes through instrumental conditioning. This may indicate a difference between the effects of classical conditioning and instrumental conditioning. Why that is true, I don't know.

Let me change the topic now and come to the question concerning simpler

---

[1] ROSE, S. P. R., BATESON, P. P. G. and HORN, G. (1973). Biochemistry and behaviour in the chick. In: *Macromolecules and Behaviour* (ANSELL, G. B. and BRADLEY, P. B., Eds.), pp. 93–104. Macmillan, London.

models of learning. To me the simplest model of learning would be two isolated nerve cells with a synapse between them. If you can change the efficiency of transmission across the synapse by conditioning, and thus produce a change in the behaviour of that synapse with respect to synaptic transmission, then you would have the simplest preparation possible, and it is hoped, an opportunity to examine the cells for macromolecular changes or any other changes responsible for these changes. This is why many molecular biologists going into neurobiology are studying nerve cells in tissue culture; they hope to be able to produce functional synapses in tissue culture that they can then manipulate and study.

I think that anything more complex than that is going to be so confusing as to be impossible to analyse.

WALL: What is wrong with the neuromuscular junction? Why bother with the central nervous system?

GLASSMAN: If you can produce changes in the synapse at the neuromuscular junction then I agree that perhaps this is a preparation that should be looked at also.

My final comment is directed to the statement that the chemical changes are nonspecific and therefore trivial. I do not quite know what nonspecific means, and I don't understand why they are trivial. I should think that we should look in awe at the fact that input into the brain can cause these kinds of macromolecular changes, whether they occur as a result of training in the jump-box, tickling a snail's tentacle, shocking a cockroach leg, or injecting amphetamine. I should think we would be very excited to discover that the brain has this capacity, and we should be full of curiosity as to the role of this phenomenon in different parts of the brain. I would not call such chemical responses trivial at all, and indeed, they may be very important for the function of the brain. I think that rather than focusing on such changes as correlates of learning and memory, we really should be focusing on the role of macromolecules in brain function, hoping that they are going to be important, that they are going to have a more significant role than just keeping cells healthy and able to respond, and that they do play an important part in nerve cell response and interact with each other to control behaviour.

HORN: I have one or two things to say that are relevant to several of the comments that have been made so far. The first relates to work on the neuromuscular junction to which Dr Vrbová referred. I am sure she would agree that it is absurd to extrapolate from an observed change at the neuromuscular junction to changes in the central nervous system that are presumed to occur during the acquisition of a new behavioural response. Studies of neuromuscular junctions will certainly tell us something about the fundamental properties of synapses and membranes; but it is possible that modifiable synapses in the central nervous system have properties different from those possessed by neuromuscular junctions. We do not know, so we need to find out.

The second thing relates to the issues that Professor McKay raised. Problems about the neural basis of learning are surely susceptible to experimental analysis. This analysis has not been going on for a long time, so that it is unreasonable to argue that the experimental approach has failed, that we should give up this approach and turn to model making. Men have been making models of cerebral function since the time of Aristotle, but experimental studies have been going on for only a decade or so.

The last thing I want to say relates to the issue that Pat Wall raised about the "surges in anatomical development" that may be taking place at the time learning occurs. He is saying, in an emphatic way, that when an animal is exposed to a learning situation, large numbers of different changes may be taking place not all of which are necessary for learning. This is surely correct (see, for example, Bateson, 1970),[1] but it is not insuperably difficult to devise controls through which it will be possible to distinguish between changes which are necessary for the learning process from those which are not.

HYDÉN: I would like to make a more general comment. In the phylogenetically laid down pathways of the brain, there is a lot of information stored which is used for integrated brain function before birth and after. Some of this is not used for complex reflexes and action until a trigger situation releases the function. A question then is whether the same mechanisms are used for both genetically programmed activity and for storage of new information in the brain during only one life-cycle, or if another mechanism takes over. One way to attack this problem from one angle is to study gene activities of brain cells in different brain areas. To get a real insight into these problems we have to know both the molecular changes of the brain cells and also get a grasp of the dynamics of the hierarchically organised system which is the brain.

Why have we discussed macromolecules and learning during these two days? Primarily there are properties which are inherent in these molecules and which make them so interesting from our point of view. There is also the localisation of the macromolecules within the brain structure to consider.

One should not forget that the brain is a three-dimensional hierarchic system of an enormous complexity. So when we are discussing macromolecules and behaviour, an understanding requires that we know where, in which brain areas, certain types of macromolecular changes occur in specific structures in neurones and glia and in a certain time sequence. This is such a complex problem that we have to look for a new analytic tool to deal with the phenomenon. One way to

[1] BATESON, P. P. G. (1970). Are they really products of learning? In: *Short-Term Changes in Neural Activity and Behaviour* (HORN, G. and HINDE, R. A., Eds.), Cambridge University Press.

phrase it is to ask how a thermodynamically open system creates order, decreases entropy and stores new information by means of an information-carrying system in restricted structures. A guess is that a theory of dynamic hierarchic order would be needed to get a picture of what goes on during memory formation.

Now there are certain intrinsic properties of macromolecules which make them so interesting from a behavioural point of view, especially since macromolecules in brain cells do respond at establishment of new behaviour.

The properties I have in mind are hysteresis cycles due to metastable conformations. They are time-independent but dependent upon previous experience and render the molecules a higher state of information. Hysteresis phenomena require only a small investment in free energy and can be seen in macromolecules as a result of pH changes, as Katchalsky and Oplatka (1966)[1] have shown. This property could make macromolecules particularly suited as identification molecules in synaptic or nerve cell membranes and why not in glia?

MACKAY: I must try to clear up a couple of misunderstandings of what I was saying. The last thing I am suggesting is "let's turn to model making because we have not got data". It is exactly the opposite. The danger as I see it is that unless we have a conceptual framework, not a predictive model, but a functional conceptual framework that can suggest good questions to us, we may find ourselves knee-deep in data we don't know what to make of. What is needed is some kind of skeleton outline of the overall function of the system such that, when you look at it, it suggests an experiment—an experiment whose results then will, if you have started on the right principles, suggest a refinement or extension of the framework, which in turn will suggest another question, and so on.

This is very different from model making in the sense of hooking up computers to behave like idealised nervous systems, a pastime for which I have never been able to work up any enthusiasm. No, the question is: how do you set about having your experimental curiosity stirred in a profitable way, and how can you avoid confusing the issue in your interpretation of your results?

Let me give you an example. Take the question of changes in the central nervous system, not now at a simple monosynaptic level, but the widely-distributed changes that might accompany learning in an enriched environment, versus those in an impoverished one. It may seem natural to expect many more neural 'connections' to be formed in the enriched environment, and to look for correspondingly increased macromolecular changes for that reason. If you look at the brain just as an information network with a modifiable conditional probability matrix (CPM), however, it becomes clear that the sorts of change in CPM that correspond to getting to know one environment rather than another might well require as many defacilitations as facilitations of connections. In order to change what the animal

---

[1] KATCHALSKY, A. and OPLATKA, A. (1966). Hysteresis and macromolecular memory. *Neurosci. Res. Progr. Bull.* Suppl. 4, 71–93.

is likely to do in a given circumstance, such a system may need to have as many couplings increased in some areas as decreased in other areas, so in this case a gross chemical assay of the macromolecular contents of a cubic centimetre of brain tissue might tell us nothing. Now that is an example of what I mean. You need to have an appropriate formal conceptualisation of what is likely to be going on in order to see which experiments have a good chance of yielding an informative result, and which possible suspects are eliminated by the outcome. That is the function of what I was describing as the conceptual framework.

I fear that my mention of transition probability matrices has led Dr Lal off on a quite spurious associative track. I agree with him that "fetching and matching a template" would be a misleading model, and I have argued for many years in favour of 'generative' models of perception and recall (MacKay, 1951;[1] MacKay, 1952[2]). I also agree (and have often insisted!) that the quantitative theorems (as distinct from the qualitative concepts) of communication engineering are of limited use in biology. But to characterise learning in terms of changes in transition probabilities does nothing *per se* to drive us to the pointless task of calculating limiting frequencies (in a nonstationary situation!). It is simply a more neutral and less question-begging way of formalising our problem, which keeps open, or even suggests, options that might be ignored if we adopted the more specific concepts of information storage and retrieval in digital computer technology, or library technology, or what have you. It helps to keep in mind, for example, the old pre-computer analogy of remembering, in terms of the way the desert rain finds its way down the old dry river bed whenever there is a storm. That's a useful corrective to a preoccupation with digital retrieval models—though again it's only one of a great range of possible catalytic images.

So I would say, don't let us spend too much effort in making models; let us do experiments. But let us at least take care that we are as well prepared as we can be to envisage and profit from the range of alternative implications that our experimental results might have. Only experiment can answer the question 'What?'. But only an adequate conceptual model can deal with the question 'So what?'.

CHAIRMAN: Mr Turner, would you like to make a short summary statement of your reaction to the discussion?

TURNER: I have been experiencing a little interdisciplinary difficulty with language, but I have been following the drift.

We have been concerned here with the bricks and mortar of the structure of the nervous system and, of course, I get concerned with the architectural plan and I

---

[1] MACKAY, D. M. (1951). Mindlike behaviour in artefacts. *Br. J. Phil. Sci.*, II, 105–21; In: *The Modeling of Mind* (SAYRE, K. R. and CROSSON, F. J., Eds.), pp. 225–41. University of Notre Dame Press, 1963.

[2] MACKAY, D. M. (1952). Mentality in machines. *Proc. Aristot. Soc.* Suppl. XXVI, 61–86; In: *Brain and Mind* (SMYTHIES, J. R., Ed.), pp. 163–200. Routledge and Kegan Paul, London, 1965.

think that the models that have been spoken of have been models of the connections at cellular level. It seems to me that the most useful way in which the different behavioural and biochemical approaches to this problem could be correlated would be on the question of this time-scale, because we do know a little bit about the time-scale used in the nervous system at different anatomical structures and in different behavioural situations. If we then find a biochemical model which works in the same time-scale and find that it correlates with the anatomical structure, we can begin to narrow the problem to one that is comprehensible to us. Viewing it as I do with regard to the function of the nervous system as a whole, I think that this seems to be the most useful way to approach the dilemma over the kind of model that is needed.

The limbic system, for example, can act in itself on different time-scales, and that is only one system that is supposed to be related with emotional states. For example, the short time-scale deals with the emotion at the time, the longer time-scale deals with the mood which overruns in time from the specific stimulus for a limited time; and then temperament is the more organically distributed function of this single system. So we are looking at different time-scales all over the nervous system, and it seems to me that examination of this temporal problem would prevent us from getting too muddled about the experimental situation.

MANDEL: Everything which concerns the central nervous system is extremely complex and wonderful. Now, the questions are why and how does the central nervous system work? To learn why and how, as Dr MacKay has told us, we need experiments. And to do experiments we have to choose an experimental design. To get a useful answer we need a good question and a good question shouldn't be too complex. For instance, in molecular biology there are people who have been working only on ribosomal proteins for several years. Knowledge of ribosomal proteins cannot give an answer about the whole mechanism because the information is not all in the proteins, nor all in the messenger. It has therefore been necessary to cut the whole complex question up into parts in order to get a valid answer. Of course we should take into account the main characteristics of the functional activity of the nervous system—the time-scale, the circuits, the organisation, the integration and so on.

Going back to my question about the use of the shuttle-box, I feel that some people here are quite happy with the shuttle-box and the criticism of the shuttle-box which exists is not strong enough to stop its being used. So we can hope that future studies on the shuttle-box will take into account the limitations which we have talked of at this Symposium—emotion, the need for discrimination, and so on.

It would be interesting to discuss in the same way other experimental projects —such as the imprinting system, the cockroach system and the snail system— about which we already have some data. But we cannot do this today. What we can do is to avoid what the picture shows.

Round table discussion: neurobiological models of learning

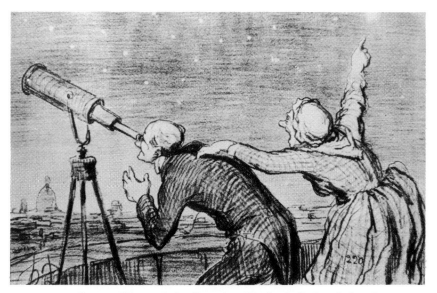

From a lithograph by Daumier. Charivari, Paris, 1858.

General summing-up: G. A. Kerkut

I think that if we had been lucky enough to have had in our audience over the past two days, Sherrington, Pavlov and Ramón y Cajal, they would have been very happy to hear of the developments that have taken place and impressed by the steps that we have taken since their time.

Ramón y Cajal would have been especially thrilled by the way that the electron microscope has shown us new details and the manner in which the synaptic endings change on denervation. Sherrington and Pavlov would have been delighted at the changes shown in the conditioned responses that Professor Ádám described in his lecture. They would all have been pleased with Professor Hydén's beautiful dissections and his and Professor Mandel's studies showing the importance of using tracers for localisation of functional changes. The use of radioactive tracers has given us the powerful tool of making a statistical survey of the activity of parts of the nervous system, and this together with electrical analysis gives the most powerful methods for studying the functions of the central nervous system. I am sure that Sherrington, Pavlov and Ramón y Cajal would have been very optimistic about the future development of their subject. Having seen what has happened over the past thirty years, one would ask what the next stage forward could be?

It would be a mistake if everyone tried to work on exactly the same experiment. It is most important that we study different preparations and use different methods of study. But what is even more important, and it has been well demonstrated at this meeting, is that as biochemists, physiologists, anatomists, pharmacologists and psychologists we should realise that we have common ground and common problems. If we can work on related preparations and discuss the results of our experiments with each other, I am sure that we will make much more rapid progress. It is by such arguments, and, as Professor Agranoff said, heated agreement and not cross-sterilisation, that the subject will develop more rapidly. It is a greater mistake to expect that the answers will appear instantly. But a greater mistake is to think that disciplines such as biochemistry, physiology, anatomy, pharmacology and psychology are in themselves of importance. What is important is the living system itself. The solution to its problems will come from a combined attack or in a word—biochemicopharmacophysiolanatopsycholoneurochemistry.

I should like to end first of all by thanking our visitors from abroad. They have given us very freely of their knowledge and experience. I would also like to thank the organisers for the excellent way in which they organised the lectures and the commissiariat. I should also like to thank the audience for sitting so patiently through these two days of lectures and discussions, and listening so attentively.

Concluding remarks: H. Hydén

Finally, I would like to say a few words of thanks. We in this field can all be pleased that we are in a boiling period with many crucial experiments still waiting and, we hope, some reward for the labour. But then at which level are these brain problems not pertinent! Think of the man who said that my wife worries about my bad memory but I am perturbed about what she remembers.

In your beautiful Barber collection at the museum here, there is a wonderful Rembrandt painting full of darkness and of light. We could be very pleased if we had added one single ray in some corner of the brain picture during these days, at least by posing questions and being together.

I would also like on behalf of the visitors to thank most sincerely for the exciting experience of the Symposium and, personally, for these fourteen days; let us once more thank the organisers, Professor Bradley, Dr Ansell and all their collaborators.

Author index

Ádám, G.	205, 274	Lal, S.	264, 267, 272
Agranoff, B. W.	143, 275	Lømo, T.	see Bliss
Anderson, E. M.	see Berry		
		Mandel, P.	163, 265, 267, 272, 282
Bateson, P. P. G.	see Rose		
Berry, M.	217	McKay, D. M.	269, 280
Bliss, T. V. P.	193		
Booth, D. A.	105, 273, 275	Oliver, G. W. O.	113
Davies, W. E.	268	Pilcher, C. W. T.	see Booth
Di Carlo, R.	see Mandel		
		Raisman, G.	183, 267
Emson, P.	see Kerkut	Randrianarosa, H.	see Mandel
		Rick, J. T.	133
Flinn, R.	see Berry	Rose, S. P. R.	93, 266
Gardner-Medwin, A. R.	see Bliss	Simler, S.	see Mandel
Glassman, E.	81, 276, 278		
		Turner, E. A.	263, 281
Hilton, S. M.	261, 263, 264, 265, 267, 269, 274, 275, 281		
		Ungar, G.	151
Hollingworth, T.	see Berry		
Horn, G.	263, 264, 265, 278, see Rose	Vrbová, G.	266
Hydén, H.	3, 27, 51, 265, 279, 287	Walker, R. J.	see Kerkut
		Wall, P. D.	262, 265, 272, 278
Kerkut, G. A.	241, 269, 285	Wilson, J. E.	see Glassman

Subject index

A

Acetoxycycloheximide
  effect on long-term memory, 173
  effect on protein synthesis, 173
  (see also Glutarimide derivatives)
Acetylcholine
  as excitatory transmitter in cockroach, 253
  as inhibitory transmitter in snail, 253
Acetylcholinesterase, activity in cockroach after learning, 120
ACh (see Acetylcholine)
AChE (see Acetylcholinesterase)
Acquisition
  of conditioned response in goldfish, 145
  of learning
    and protein synthesis, 134
    and RNA synthesis, 134
    anticholinergics, 126
    anticholinesterases, 123
    atropine, 126
    edrophonium, 125
    gallamine, 126
    hemicholinium, 126
    in cockroach, 114
    neostigmine, 125
    physostigmine, 123
Acridine orange, effect on avoidance conditioning in snails, 246
Actinomycin D
  and decreased protein synthesis in snail, 251
  and memory, 109
  as RNA-synthesis blocker, 143
Adenine, incorporation into RNA, 62
Adenosine triphosphatase
  activity in Deiters' nucleus nerve cells and glia, 34
  in nerve cell and glial membranes, 35
  ouabain, 37

Age and RNA in nerve cells, 62, 63
Amino acid
  incorporation in glia, 41
  incorporation in nerve cell, 41
γ-Aminobutyric acid and protein changes, 113
Amino-isobutyric acid
  concentration by glia, 39
  concentration by nerve cell, 39
Ammonium sulphate used in measurement of RNA polymerase activity, 167
Amnesia
  antibiotic-induced, 147
  due to puromycin, 173
  induced by electroconvulsive shock, 210
Amphetamine
  avoidance conditioning in snails, 244
  protein synthesis in snail, 251
  RNA metabolism, 168
Anisomycin (see Glutarimide derivatives)
Antibiotics
  and production of amnesia, 147
  and retrograde amnesic effects, 108
Anticholinergics and acquisition of learning in cockroach, 126
Anticholinesterases and acquisition of learning in cockroach, 123
Antiserum
  against nerve and glial cells of Deiters' nucleus, 11
  against S-100 protein, 9, 19
Apical spines, interconnections with axons, 220
Aplysia neurones, RNA synthesis after stimulation, 70
Arabinosyl cytosine as DNA-synthesis blocker, 143
Astrocytes, 33
  role in reinnervation of deafferented neuronal sites, 190

ATPase (see Adenosine triphosphatase)
Atropine and acquisition of learning in cockroach, 126
Audiogenic seizures and RNA metabolism, 170
Audiogenic stimulation, [³H]uridine incorporation in mice during, 171
Auditory system as neurobiological model of learning, 268
Autoradiography
　of changes in RNA in brain, 86
　of labelled uridine in nerve cells of snail, 248
Avoidance conditioning
　of snail, 242
　　effect of
　　　acridine orange on, 246
　　　amphetamine on, 244
　　　congo red on, 246
　　　cycloheximidine on, 246
　　　magnesium pemoline on, 244
　　　inhibition of, 246
　　techniques as learning models—stress elements, 274
　　using shuttle-box, 275
AXM (see Acetoxycycloheximide)
Axodendritic synapses in septal neuropil, 185
Axon
　interconnections by apical spines, 220
　regeneration and functional determination, 220
　regeneration and RNA turnover, 219
　regeneration in peripheral nervous system, 183
Axon-sprouting, 222
Axosomatic synapses in septal neuropil, 189

B

Barracuda, RNA in motor neurones of, 64
Base ratio changes in RNA during learning, 71
Behaviour changes in relationship to RNA synthesis, 163
Biogenic amines in learning, 6
Blood–brain barrier in chick, 94
Brain
　conditioned evoked potentials in, after ischaemia, 212
　extracts from dark-avoidance rats, 155
　extracts from dark-avoidance rats, injected into mice, 155
　function, role of RNA in, 81
　ischaemia, reversibility and temperature, 212

Brain—*continued*
　protein changes during learning, 3–26
　protein identification mechanisms in, 23
　RNA changes during learning, 85
　RNA extracts from trained rats, 155
　RNA extracts from trained rats, gel-filtration of, 155
　RNA extracts from trained rats, thin-layer chromatography of, 155
　RNA polymerase activity of, 167
　scotophobin extracts from trained rats, 157
　uridine, incorporation of orotic acid into, 136
Branching index of dendrites, projection artefact due to staining, 232

C

Calcium
　and S-100 protein, 9
　effect on S-100 protein of, 9
　in hippocampus, 17, 19
Central nervous system
　coding of, molecular mechanisms in, 151
　function of, neurone involvement in, 219
　of mammals, collateral sprouting of axons in, 184
　plasticity of, 183, 217
CEP (see Conditioned evoked potential)
Cerebellum, Purkinje cells in, 64
ChE (see Cholinesterase)
Chemical correlates of behaviour, specificity of, 277
Chemical transmission of vagus, effect on heart of, 154
Chick
　biochemistry and behaviour of, 93
　blood–brain barrier in, 94
Cholinesterase
　activity and retention of memory, 120
　activity in cockroach during learning, 252
　activity of snails during learning, 251
　changes in cockroach ganglia during learning, 117
CNS (see Central nervous system)
Cochlear nucleus, protein changes with sensory input, 268
Cockroach
　ACh as excitatory transmitter in, 253
　AChE activity after learning in, 120
　acquisition of learning by, 114
　　anticholinergics, 126
　　atropine, 126
　　edrophonium, 125
　　gallamine, 126

Subject Index

Cockroach—*continued*
  acquisition of learning by—*continued*
    hemicholinium, 126
    hexamethonium, 126
    neostigmine, 125
    physostigmine, 123
  ChE activity during learning by, 114
  learning, effect of anticholinesterases on, 123
  pseudocholinesterase activity and training in, 119
  shock-avoidance and extinction in, 135
  shock-avoidance learning by, 114
Collateral sprouting
  of axons in peripheral nervous system, 184
  in mammalian CNS, 184
Computer program, estimation of dendritic fields by, 225
Conditional-probability matrix
  facilitations and defacilitations of connections in, 280
  of neural network, 270
Conditioned avoidance (see Avoidance conditioning)
Conditioned evoked potential
  as electrical sign of learning, 205
  in brain after ischaemia, 212
Conditioned reflex, genesis of, and oligodendrocyte involvement, 218
Conditioned response
  acquisition of, in goldfish, 145
  effect of orotic acid on extinction of, 135
Conditioned stimulus, 153, 159
  and evoked potential, 206
  in goldfish training, 144
Conditioning
  and tetanic stimulation in dentate area, 196
  myelin formulation during, 218
Congo red
  and avoidance conditioning in snails, 246
  and decreased protein synthesis in snail, 251
Consolidation of short-term memory, 153
CPM (see Conditional-probability matrix)
CS (see Conditioned stimulus)
Cycloheximide
  and decreased protein synthesis in snail, 251
  effect on
    avoidance conditioning in snails, 246
    handedness in rats, 106
    long-term memory, 6, 173
      retention mechanism, 106
    negative reinforcement in rats, 108
    protein synthesis, 6
    RNA synthesis, 6

Cycloheximide—*continued*
  -induced retrograde amnesia, 107
  (see also Glutarimide derivatives)
Cytidine, incorporation into RNA, 62
Cytochrome oxidase activity in glia and nerve cells, 34
  after stimulation, 42
Cytosine in RNA of nerve cells and glia, 57

D

Dark-avoidance in rats, bioassay of brain extracts, 155
Deafferentation and dendritic branching, 222
Defacilitation of connections in conditional-probability matrix, 280
Deiters' nucleus
  antibody, 14
  glial antiserum, 14
  nerve and glial cell antigenicity of, 11
Delayed association of conditioned and unconditioned stimuli, 206
Delayed inhibition and conditioned response, 208
Dendrites
  and reorientation of fields due to change in input, 223
  arising from the perikaryon, 225, 229
  branching, deafferentation and experience, 222
  density after internal capsule sectioning, 227
  field
    determination of, by computer program, 225
    in internal capsule, 227
  impregnation of, with Golgi-Cox stain, 224
  spines of, effect of sensory deprivation on, 220
Dentate area, stimulation of, 195
DNA
  coding for new RNA species during learning, 164
  synthesis, block by arabinosyl cytosine, 143
Double isotope-labelling technique
  and incorporation of labelled compounds in snail, 246
  and shock-avoidance, 84

E

ECS (see Electroconvulsive shock)
Edrophonium and acquisition of learning in cockroach, 125

Subject Index

Electric shock as unconditioned stimulus, 145
Electroconvulsive shock
   and disruption of memory to conditioned response, 145
   block of retention by, 108
   extinction of short-term memory by, 210
   production of amnesia by, 210
Electron microscopy of synaptic knobs, 11
Electrophoresis
   discontinuous, isolation of S-100 and 14-3-2 proteins by, 13
   in analysis of [^{3}H]leucine incorporation, 250
   microdisc, 15
Engram, 5, 106, 164
Environmental situation producing changes in brain, 267
Enzyme activity in nerve cell and glia during sleep and wakefulness, 43
EPSP (see Excitatory postsynaptic potential)
Evoked potential, 196
Excitatory postsynaptic potential of dentate area, 195
Extinction
   loss of acquired response, 133
   of conditioned response, effect of orotic acid on, 135
   of shock-avoidance in cockroach, 135
   of short-term memory by electroconvulsive shock, 210
   RNA synthesis during, 135
   studies with yoked controls, 134

F

Facilitation
   of connections in conditional-probability matrix, 280
   of learning in snail
      effect of amphetamine on, 244
      effect of magnesium pemoline on, 244
Filaments in nerve cell, 57
Fimbria
   destruction of fibres of, 185
   lesions of, 189
Flaxedil (see Gallamine triethiodide)
Fluorescence of S-100 antiserum, 21
Forebrain, RNA polymerase levels in, 101

G

GABA (see γ-Aminobutyric acid)
Gallamine triethiodide, effect on acquisition of learning in cockroach, 126
Gamma globulin and S-100 antiserum, 21
Ganglia of cockroach, ChE levels of, after training, 117
Gangliosides in nerve cells and glia, 37
Gel filtration of RNA extracts of trained rat brain, 155
Glia
   and relationship with nerve cells, 27–49
   as potassium regulator, 34
   ATPase activity of, 35
   biochemical differences from nerve cells of, 33–42
   changes in RNA in, during Parkinson's disease, 67
   changes in, with vestibular stimulation, 42
   concentration of amino-isobutyric acid by, 39
   cytochrome oxidase activity of, after stimulation, 42
   cytosine in RNA of, 57
   early studies on, 27–29
   enzyme activity in, during sleep and wakefulness, 43
   function of, 47
      at synapse, 218
   gangliosides in, 37
   incorporation of amino acid into, 41
   isolation of, by micro and macro-procedures, 29–33
   manual separation of, 11
   oxygen consumption of, 33
   RNA in, 37
      content of, in Huntington's chorea, 45
      content of, in Parkinson's disease, 45
      polymerase activity in, 167
Globus pallidus, RNA base ratios in, 45
[^{14}C]Glucose, uptake of, by proteins in auditory system, 268
Glutamate, effect on oxygen uptake by nerve and glia, 34
Glutarimide derivatives as protein-synthesis blockers, 144, 147
Glycoproteins in nerve cell membranes, 53
Goldfish
   conditioned response, acquisition of, 145
   effect of conditioned stimulus on, 144
   effect of puromycin and acetocyclo-heximide
      on long-term memory in, 172
      on protein synthesis in, 173
   shock-avoidance by, in shuttle box, 144
   unconditioned stimulus of electric shock to, 145
Golgi-Cox stain, impregnation of dendrites by, 224

H

Handedness
  in rats, with cycloheximide, 106
  reversal of, in rats, 7
    RNA changes during, 70
Heart, action of the vagus on, 154
Helix aspersa (see Snail)
Hemicholinium and acquisition of learning in cockroach, 126
Hexamethonium and acquisition of learning in cockroach, 126
Hippocampus, 8, 195
  CA3 region of, 13–18
  calcium content of, 17
  calcium in, 19
  potassium in, 19
  14-3-2 protein in, and training, 22
  protein synthesis in, and training, 9
  role of, in long-term memory, 4
  sodium in, 19
  synaptic plasticity of, 193
Huntington's chorea, RNA content of nerve cell and glia during, 45
Hybridisation experiments to detect new RNA species, 165
Hysteresis cycles as a result of pH changes, 280

I

Imipramine hydrochloride, effect on RNA content of nerve cells, 67
Imprinting
  and perceptual learning, 274
  and protein and RNA synthesis, 264
  in chicks, 94
Information processing in nervous system, 151
Inhibition of avoidance-conditioning in snails, 245
Internal capsule, analysis of basal dendritic fields in, 227
Ischaemia
  conditioned evoked potentials of brain after, 212
  enhanced protein synthesis after, 213

K

α-Ketoglutarate, oxidation of, by glia and nerve cells, 34
Kidney, RNA of, in trained and untrained mice, 85

L

Learning
  and synaptic facilitation, 153
  changes in brain protein during, 3–26
  changes in S-100 protein during, 172
  in cockroach
    and ChE activity, 252
    and ChE levels, 117
    effect of anticholinergics on, 126
    effect of anticholinesterases on, 123
  in lower animals, 241
  in snail and ChE activity, 251
  models of, 261
  neural code, 153
  neuronal RNA changes during, 70
  protein synthesis during, 8–23
  RNA involvement with, 164
  RNA polymerase activity during, 167
  stress association, 276
Lesions of nerve pathways of septal nucleus, 185
[^{14}C]Leucine, incorporation into snail during training, 246
[^{3}H]Leucine
  incorporation into
    glial protein, 39
    nerve cell protein, 39
    protein during reversal of handedness, 8
    snail during training, 246
    injection into lateral ventricles of rat, 13
Limbic system
  action on different time-scales, 282
  and memory formation, 4
Liver
  RNA of, in trained and untrained mice, 85
  RNA polymerase activity of, 167
[^{3}H]Lysine, incorporation into protein during imprinting in chicks, 95

M

Magnesium pemoline, effect on avoidance-conditioning in snail, 244
Mammals, localisation of memory in, 4
Medial forebrain bundle, destruction of, 185
  effect on septal nucleus, 185
Memory
  and conditioned evoked potentials, 205
  association of stimuli with, 262
  disruption of
    by electroconvulsive shock, 145
    by puromycin, 145
  effect of actinomycin D on, 109

Memory—*continued*
  formation
    and the limbic system, 4
    temperature dependence, 146
    long-term, 82, 106, 143, 263
      effect of
        cycloheximide on, 6, 173
        protein synthesis inhibitors on, 146
        puromycin on, 6, 172
      fixation of electric memory trace, 210
      involvement of hippocampus in, 4
    neural code and, 153
    neurones and, 153
    retention
      and ChE activity, 120
      in cockroach, 116
    RNA involvement in, 164
    short-term, 82, 143, 263
      consolidation of, 153
      extinction by electroconvulsive shock, 210
Messenger RNA, coding of proteins by, 164
Metathoracic ganglion of cockroach, ChE reduction in, during training, 118
Methylene blue, staining of nerve cells by, after isolation, 11
Mice
  injection with 'dark-avoidance' brain extracts, 155
  submitted to audiogenic stimulation, 170
Midbrain, RNA polymerase levels in, 101
Modifiable neurones, 153
Modifiable synapses and protein patterns, 270
Motor neurones of Barracuda, RNA in, 64
Mouse, shock-avoidance training and brain RNA levels, 83
Muscle changes in size following activity, 262
Myelin formation during conditioning, 218

N

Negative reinforcement and cycloheximide in rats, 108
Neostigmine, effect on acquisition of learning in cockroach, 125
Nerve cell
  amino-isobutyric acid concentration by, 39
  and relationship with glia, 27–49
  ATPase activity in, 35
  biochemical difference from glia of, 33–42
  changes with vestibular stimulation, 42
  cytochrome oxidase activity of, after stimulation, 42

Nerve-cell—*continued*
  cytosine in RNA of, 57
  enzyme activity of, during sleep and wakefulness, 43
  filaments in, 37–60
  gangliosides in, 37
  incorporation of amino acid into, 41
  in functioning of CNS, 219
  in tissue culture, a learning model, 278
  orthograde degeneration of, 183
  oxygen consumption of, 33
  reverberation of, and establishment of electric memory, 211
  ribosomal RNA content of, 53
  RNA in, 37
    base composition and synthesis of, 57
    changes in
      during Huntington's chorea, 45
      during Parkinson's disease, 45, 67
    content of, after sensory stimulation, 65
    effect of
      imipramine hydrochloride on, 67
      psychotomimetics on, 67
      tranylcypromine on, 67
    variations with age, 57, 62
  polymerase activity in, 167
  synaptic knobs, 11
Nerve cell membrane
  and glycoproteins, 57
  ATPase in, 35
Neural code, 151
Neuromuscular junction
  as neurobiological model of learning, 266, 278
  synapse formation at, during learning, 266
Neuronal perikarya, manual isolation and staining of, 11
Neurone (see Nerve cell)
Novel stimulus, change in response with time to, 263
Nucleus hypoglossus, 44
Nucleus reticularis giganto-cellularis, 44
Nucleus reticularis pontis oralis, 44
Nucleus trigeminus mesencephalicus, 44

O

Oligodendrocytes, 33
  involvement in genesis of conditioned reflex of, 218
Operant conditioning, 274
Orotic acid
  incorporation into brain uridine, 136
  increase of extinction of conditioned response, 135
Orthograde degeneration of nerve cells, 183

Subject Index

Ouabain, effect on ATPase activity of, 37
Oxygen consumption of nerve cell and glia, 33
Oxygen tension, effect of decrease of, on RNA content, 44

P

Parkinson's disease
  RNA changes in nerve cells and glia, 67
  RNA content of nerve cells and glia in, 45
Parnate (see Tranylcypromine)
Perceptual learning, 274
Perikaryon, dendrites arising from 225, 229
Peripheral nervous system
  collateral sprouting of axons in, 184
  regeneration of nerve cells in, 183
Periplaneta americana (see Cockroach)
Physostigmine, effect of, on acquisition of learning in cockroach, 123
Plasticity
  in CNS, 217
  of adult rat, 183
  in hippocampus, 193
Polysomes in nerve cell, ribosomal content of, 53
Population spike of evoked potential in dentate area, 196
Potassium in hippocampus, 19
Potentiation of spike amplitude after stimulation, 199
Presynaptic terminal, disuse and stimulation of, 221
Protein
  changes and GABA, 113
  changes in auditory system with sensory input, 268
  coding by messenger RNA, 164
  in learning and memory, 6
  [³H]leucine, incorporation of into snail, 250
  [³H]lysine, incorporation of during imprinting in chicks, 95
  of auditory system, uptake of [¹⁴C]glucose into, 268
  14-3-2 protein
    electrophoresis of, 15
    in hippocampus during training, 22
    isolation of, 13
  S-100 protein, 6, 73
    and calcium, 18
    antibodies to, 21
    changes in, during learning, 172
    conformational changes in, during learning, 18
    effect of calcium on, 9

Protein—*continued*
  S-100 protein—*continued*
    electrophoresis of, 15
    isolation of, 13
    localisation of
      in the brain, 9
      in nerve cells and glia, 37
  synthesis
    and acquisition of new response, 134
    and learning, 6–23, 82
    block by
      glutarimide derivatives, 144, 147
      puromycin, 144, 147
    during imprinting, anatomical effects on, 265
    during reversal of handedness in rats, 8
    effect of
      imprinting on, 264
      puromycin on, 6
      puromycin and acetoxycycloheximide on, 173
    enhancement of, during ischaemia, 213
    environmentally determined, 171
    inhibitors and long-term memory, 146
    in hippocampus during training, 9–23
    in snail, effect of
      actinomycin D on, 251
      amphetamine on, 251
      congo red on, 251
      cycloheximide on, 251
Pseudocholinesterase activity in cockroach during training, 119
Psychotomimetics, effect of, on RNA content of nerve cell, 67
Purkinje cells
  in cerebellum, 64
  RNA content of, after sensory stimulation, 63
Puromycin
  amnesic effect in goldfish, 173
  as protein synthesis blocker, 144, 147
  disruption of memory of conditioned response by, 145
  effect of
    on long-term memory, 172
    on protein synthesis and long-term memory, 6
    on RNA synthesis and long-term memory, 6
Pyramidal nerve cells and S-100 protein, 9

R

Rat
  brain extracts from, 155
  dark-avoidance experiments with, 155
  handedness experiments in, 7, 70, 106

Rat—*continued*
    injection of [^{3}H]leucine into lateral ventricles of, 13
    plasticity of CNS of, 183
    reversal of handedness in, 7
        RNA changes during, 70
    scotophobin extracts from brain of, 157
Reinforcement, removal of, and extinction, 134
Reinnervation
    of septal nucleus after deafferentation, 189
    role of astrocytes in, 190
Retention
    block by electroconvulsive shock, 108
    effects of cycloheximide on, 106
    of memory
        and ChE activity, 120
        in cockroach, 116
Reticular formation, 8
Retrograde amnesia
    after cycloheximide, 107
    antibiotic-induced, 108, 148
Reverberation of nerve cells, establishment of electric memory by, 211
Reversal training, increased incorporation of label into RNA during, 277
RNA
    and brain function, 81
    and changes in behaviour and function, 51–73
    and information storage, 51
    and learning, 82
    and shock-avoidance, 83
    base composition of, in nerve cells, 61
    changes in
        base ratios of, on learning, 71
        brain
            autoradiography of, 86
            during learning, 85
            during behavioural experiments, 6
        kidney, during learning, 85
        liver, during learning, 85
    content of
        nerve cell and glia in Huntington's chorea, 45
        nerve cell and glia in Parkinson's disease, 45
        nerve cell, effect of tranylcypromine on, 67
        Purkinje cells after increased sensory activity, 63
    density gradient fractionation of, 69
    extract from trained-rat brain, 155
    incorporation of
        adenine into, 62

RNA—*continued*
    incorporation of—*continued*
        ^{14}C and ^{3}H into, during shock-avoidance, 84
        cytidine into, 62
        [^{3}H]uracil into, during imprinting in chick, 97
        [^{3}H]uridine into, in snail, 246
        increased labelling of, during reversal training, 277
    in motor neurones
        of Barracuda, 64
        effect of age on, 63
    in nerve cells, 53–63
        and glia, 37
        after sensory stimulation, 65
        base composition and synthesis of, 57–63
        changes in, during learning, 70
        effect of imipramine hydrochloride on, 67
        effect of psychotomimetics on, 67
    involvement in memory and learning, 164
    labelled, sedimentation of by sucrose gradient, 87
    metabolism
        effect of amphetamine on, 168
        effect of audiogenic seizures on, 170
    ribosomal, 70
        in nerve cells, 53
    separation on sucrose density gradient, 169
    species, detection by hybridisation experiments, 165
    synthesis
        block of, by actinomycin D, 143
        effect of cycloheximide on, 6
        effect of imprinting on, 264
        in *Aplysia* neurones after stimulation, 70
        in brain during shock-avoidance, 84
        in mouse brain during extinction, 135
        in relation to behavioural changes, 163
        puromycin effects on, 6
    turnover during axonal regeneration, 219
    variation in nerve cells with age, 57, 62
RNA polymerase
    activity
        during learning, 167
        in liver, nerve cells and glia, 167
        in imprinted chicks, 100
        measurement using ammonium sulphate, 167
    level in
        forebrain base, 101
        forebrain roof, 101
        midbrain, 101

S

Scotophobin
  from trained-rat brain extracts, 155
  isolation and purification of, 155
Sensory deprivation and dendritic spines, 220
Septal neuropil, axosomatic and axodendritic synapses in, 185, 189
Septal nucleus
  deafferentation and new synaptic connections, 184
  effect of destruction of
    fimbrial fibres on, 185
    medial forebrain bundle fibres on, 185
  reinnervation of, after deafferentation, 189
Shock-avoidance
  ^{14}C and ^{3}H uptake during, 84
  in cockroach, and extinction, 135
  in mice, incorporation of radioactive precursors into RNA, 84
  learning in cockroach, 114
  training in goldfish, 144
Shuttle-box
  as neurobiological model of learning, 273
  avoidance conditioning by, 275
  goldfish training with shock-avoidance in, 144
  limitations of, as a learning model, 282
Silver impregnation of nerve cells and glia after isolation, 11
Sleep, enzyme activity in nerve cells and glia during, 43
Snail
  ACh as inhibitory transmitter in, 253
  autoradiography of labelled uridine in, 248
  avoidance conditioning and effect of
    acridine orange in, 246
    amphetamine in, 244
    congo red in, 246
    cycloheximide in, 246
    magnesium pemoline in, 244
  behaviour of, in avoidance conditioning tests, 242
  ChE activity in, during learning, 251
  double-labelling techniques in, 246
  electrophoresis of [^{3}H]leucine in, 250
  incorporation of
    [^{14}C]leucine into ganglia during training, 246
    [^{3}H]leucine into ganglia during training, 246
    [^{14}C]uridine into ganglia during training, 246

Snail—*continued*
  incorporation of—*continued*
    [^{3}H]uridine into ganglia during training, 246
  inhibition of avoidance conditioning in, 246
  protein synthesis in, 250
    effect of
      actinomycin D on, 251
      amphetamine on, 251
      congo red on, 251
      cycloheximide on, 251
Sodium in hippocampus, 19
Specificity of chemical correlates of behaviour, 277
Split-brain chick, imprinting and incorporation of [^{3}H]uracil in, 102
Stimulation
  effect on presynaptic terminals of, 221
  of dentate area, 195
  vestibular, changes in nerve cell and glia during, 42
Stress associated with learning, 276
Striate cortex, dendritic spine reduction in, after visual deprivation, 220
Succinate oxidation in nerve cells and glia, 34
Succinoxidase
  in glia, 44
  in nerve cell, 44
Sucrose density gradient
  for cerebral RNA fractions, 169
  sedimentation of ^{14}C- and ^{3}H-labelled RNA, 87
Synapse
  alterations of by functional changes, 220
  axosomatic and axodendritic, 189
  excitatory, 5
  facilitation of, and learning, 153
  function of glia, 218
  inhibitory, 5
  knobs
    electron microscopy of, 11
    on isolated nerve cells, 11
  plasticity of, in hippocampus, 193
  plasticity of collateral sprouting in mammalian CNS, 184

T

Temperature dependence
  of memory formation, 146
  of reversibility of brain ischaemia, 212
Thalamus, 8
Thin-layer chromatography, purification of RNA extracts from trained-rat brain, by, 155

Time-scale, importance of, in learning models, 282
Time-sequence analysis, protein changes during learning, 6
Tofranil (see Imipramine hydrochloride)
Training
  and effect on protein synthesis in hippocampus, 9
  and 14-3-2 protein in hippocampus, 22
Transmission times of signals impinging on neurones, 270
Transprinting in processing of acquired information, 159
Tranylcypromine, effect on RNA content of nerve cells, 67
Tricyanoaminopropene, effect on RNA content of nerve cells and glia, 47
Tritium, determination of, 17

U

UMP (see Uridine monophosphate)
Unconditioned stimulus, 153, 159
  intermittent electric shock in goldfish training, 145
  with conditioned stimulus, evoked potential, 206
[^{3}H]Uracil, incorporation into
  RNA during imprinting of chicks, 97
  split-brain chicks, 102
Uridine, brain, incorporation of orotic acid into, 136
[^{14}C]Uridine, incorporation into
  RNA during shock-avoidance, 84
  snail ganglia during training, 246

[^{3}H]Uridine, incorporation into
  mice during audiogenic stimulation, 171
  RNA during acquisition and extinction, 134
  RNA during shock-avoidance, 84
  snail ganglia during training, 246
Uridine monophosphate, incorporation of label into during shock-avoidance, 84
US (see Unconditioned stimulus)

V

Vagus, chemical transmission in, effect on heart of, 154
Vestibular nucleus, 42
Vestibular stimulation, changes in neurone and glia during, 42
Visual system as neurobiological model of learning, 264

W

Wakefulness, enzyme activity in nerve cells and glia during, 43

Y

Yoked control
  in cockroaches during shock-avoidance testing, 115
  study of extinction with, 134
Yoked mice
  in shock-avoidance experiment, RNA content of brain of, 84
  incorporation of uridine in, 72